Progress in Pain Research and Management
Volume 12

Assessment and Treatment of Cancer Pain

Mission Statement of IASP Press

The International Association for the Study of Pain (IASP) is a nonprofit, interdisciplinary organization devoted to understanding the mechanisms of pain and improving the care of patients with pain through research, education, and communication. The organization includes scientists and health care professionals dedicated to these goals. The IASP sponsors scientific meetings and publishes newsletters, technical bulletins, the journal *Pain*, and books.

The goal of IASP Press is to provide the IASP membership with timely, high-quality, low-cost publications relevant to the problem of pain. These publications are also intended to appeal to a wider audience of scientists and clinicians interested in the problem of pain.

Previous volumes in the series
Progress in Pain Research and Management

Pharmacological Approaches to the Treatment of Chronic Pain: New Concepts and Critical Issues, edited by Howard L. Fields and John C. Liebeskind

Proceedings of the 7th World Congress on Pain,
edited by Gerald F. Gebhart, Donna L. Hammond, and Troels S. Jensen

Touch, Temperature, and Pain in Health and Disease: Mechanisms and Assessments, edited by Jörgen Boivie, Per Hansson, and Ulf Lindblom

Temporomandibular Disorders and Related Pain Conditions,
edited by Barry J. Sessle, Patricia S. Bryant, and Raymond A. Dionne

Visceral Pain, edited by Gerald F. Gebhart

Reflex Sympathetic Dystrophy: A Reappraisal,
edited by Wilfrid Jänig and Michael Stanton-Hicks

Pain Treatment Centers at a Crossroads: A Practical and Conceptual Reappraisal, edited by Mitchell J.M. Cohen and James N. Campbell

Proceedings of the 8th World Congress on Pain, edited by Troels S. Jensen, Judith A. Turner, and Zsuzsanna Wiesenfeld-Hallin

Molecular Neurobiology of Pain, edited by David Borsook

Sickle Cell Pain, edited by Samir K. Ballas

Progress in Pain Research and Management
Volume 12

Assessment and Treatment of Cancer Pain

Editors

Richard Payne, MD

Department of Neuro-Oncology
University of Texas M. D. Anderson Cancer Center
Houston, Texas, USA

Richard B. Patt, MD

Department of Anesthesiology
University of Texas M. D. Anderson Cancer Center
Houston, Texas, USA

C. Stratton Hill, Jr., MD

Department of Neuro-Oncology
University of Texas M. D. Anderson Cancer Center
Houston, Texas, USA

IASP PRESS • SEATTLE

Library of Congress Cataloging-in-Publication Data

Assessment and treatment of cancer pain / editors, Richard Payne, Richard B. Patt,
  C. Stratton Hill, Jr.
     p. cm. — (Progress in pain research and management ; v. 12)
     "A satellite meeting of the 8th World Congress on Pain in August 1996."—Pref.
     Includes bibliographical references and index.
     ISBN 0-931092-21-3
     1. Cancer pain—Congresses.   I. Payne, Richard, M.D. II. Patt, Richard B.
III. Hill, C. Stratton, 1928–   .   IV. Series.
     [DNLM: 1. Neoplasms—therapy congresses. 2. Pain—prevention & control
congresses. WI PR677BL v. 12 1998 / QZ 266 A8458 1998]
     RC262.A84 1998
     616.99'4—dc21
     DNLM/DLC
     for Library of Congress   98-12346

Published by:

IASP Press
International Association for the Study of Pain
909 NE 43rd St., Suite 306
Seattle, WA 98105 USA
Fax: 206-547-1703

Printed in the United States of America

Contents

List of Contributing Authors   vii

Preface   ix

Part I Cancer Pain: A Global Perspective

1. Palliative Care in Latin America
   I. Status of Palliative Care Initiatives
   Roberto Wenk   3

   II.The Impact of the Illegal Drug Market and Parallel Distribution
   Systems on the Availability of Opioids for Pain Relief in Colombia
   Liliana De Lima   11

2. Cancer Pain Clinical Practice Guidelines for Clinicians and Patients:
   Rationale, Barriers to Implementation, and Future Directions
   Richard Payne and Judith A. Paice   17

Part II Cancer Pain Assessment: Research and Clinical Issues

3. Culture and Pain Assessment in Hispanic Patients
   Guadalupe Palos   35

4. Pain Management among Elderly Persons
   Bruce A. Ferrell   53

5. Radiological Imaging in the Cancer Patient with Back Pain
   Norman E. Leeds and Ashok J. Kumar   67

6. Medical Decision Making: Application to Pain Assessment
   and Treatment
   Scott B. Cantor   91

7. Psychological Interventions for Pain: Potential Mechanisms
   C. Richard Chapman   109

Part III Impact of Pain on Survival: What Do We Know?

8. Pain Kills: Animal Models and Neuro-Immunological Links
   Gayle Giboney Page and Shamgar Ben-Eliyahu   135

9. The Pain–Mortality Link: Unraveling the Mysteries
   Peter S. Staats   145

Part IV Clinical Assessment and Management of Cancer Pain

10. Neuropathic Pain: Mechanisms and Clinical Assessment
Robert R. Allen   159

11. Key Issues in Anesthetic Techniques in Cancer Pain
Michael J. Cousins   175

12. Methodological Issues in the Design of Clinical Trials
Perry G. Fine   189

13. The Current Status of Anesthetic Approaches to Cancer Pain
Management
Richard B. Patt   195

14. Neurosurgical Considerations and Options for Cancer-Related Pain
Ehud Arbit   213

15. Intrathecal Opioid Therapy and Implantable Devices
Sannichie Quaicoe, Russell McLaughlin, and Samuel Hassenbusch   223

16. Mechanisms of Bone Metastasis
*Randy N. Rosier, David G. Hicks, Lisa A. Teot, J. Edward Puzas,
and Regis J. O'Keefe*   257

17. Management of Metastatic Bone Pain
Richard Payne and Nora Janjan   269

18. Opioid Pharmacology: Tolerance, Receptor Modulation,
and New Analgesics
Charles E. Inturrisi   275

19. Nonopioid Analgesics for Cancer Pain: Update on Clinical
Pharmacology
Richard Payne   289

20. Alternative Routes for Administering Analgesics at Home
Porter Storey   309

Index   321

Contributing Authors

Robert R. Allen, MD *Department of Neuro-Oncology, The University of Texas M. D. Anderson Cancer Center, Houston, Texas, USA*

Ehud Arbit, MD *Department of Neurosurgical Oncology, Nalitt Cancer Institute, Staten Island University Hospital, Staten Island, New York, USA*

Shamgar Ben-Eliyahu, PhD *Department of Psychology, Tel Aviv University, Tel Aviv, Israel*

Scott B. Cantor, PhD *Ambulatory and Supportive Care Oncology Research Program, Section of General Internal Medicine, Department of Medical Specialties, The University of Texas M. D. Anderson Cancer Center, Houston, Texas, USA*

C. Richard Chapman, PhD *Departments of Anesthesiology, Psychiatry, and Behavioral Sciences, University of Washington School of Medicine, Seattle, Washington, USA*

Michael J. Cousins, MD *Department of Anaesthesia and Pain Management, University of Sydney, Royal North Shore Hospital, St. Leonard's, New South Wales, Australia*

Liliana De Lima, MS *Non-communicable Diseases Program, Pan American Health Organization, Washington, DC, USA*

Bruce A. Ferrell, MD *Departments of Medicine and Geriatrics, School of Medicine, University of California at Los Angeles, and Sepulveda VA Geriatric Research Education and Clinical Center, Sepulveda VA Medical Center, Sepulveda, Calfornia, USA*

Perry G. Fine, MD *Department of Anesthesiology and Pain Management Center, University of Utah, Salt Lake City, Utah, USA*

Samuel Hassenbusch, MD, PhD *Department of Neurosurgery, The University of Texas M. D. Anderson Cancer Center, Houston, Texas, USA*

David G. Hicks, MD *Departments of Orthopaedics and Pathology, The University of Rochester, Rochester, New York, USA*

C. Stratton Hill, Jr., MD *Department of Neuro-Oncology, The University of Texas M.D. Anderson Cancer Center, Houston, Texas, USA*

Charles E. Inturrisi, PhD *Department of Pharmacology, Cornell University Medical College, New York, New York, USA*

Nora Janjan, MD *Department of Radiation Oncology, The University of Texas M. D. Anderson Cancer Center, Houston, Texas, USA*

Ashok J. Kumar, MD *Department of Radiology, The University of Texas M. D. Anderson Cancer Center, Houston, Texas, USA*

Norman E. Leeds, MD *Department of Radiology, The University of Texas M. D. Anderson Cancer Center, Houston, Texas, USA*

Russell McLaughlin, MD *Department of Anesthesiology, The University of Texas M. D. Anderson Cancer Center, Houston, Texas, USA*

Regis J. O'Keefe, MD *Department of Orthopaedics, The University of Rochester, Rochester, New York, USA*

Gayle Giboney Page, RN, DNSc *College of Nursing, The Ohio State University, Columbus, Ohio, USA*

Judith A. Paice, PhD, RN *Department of Neurosurgery, Rush Neuroscience Institute, Rush Medical Center, and College of Nursing, Rush University, Chicago, Illinois, USA*

Guadalupe Palos, DrPH(c), LMSW, RN *Department of Neuro-Oncology, Pain Research Group, The University of Texas M. D. Anderson Cancer Center, Houston, Texas, USA*

Richard B. Patt, MD *Departments of Anesthesiology and Neuro-Oncology, and Anesthesia Pain Services, The University of Texas M. D. Anderson Cancer Center, and the Cancer, Pain and Wellness Institute International, Houston, Texas, USA*

Richard Payne, MD *Pain and Symptom Management Section, Department of Neuro-Oncology, The University of Texas M. D. Anderson Cancer Center, Houston, Texas, USA*

J. Edward Puzas, PhD *Department of Orthopaedics, The University of Rochester, Rochester, New York, USA*

Sannichie Quaicoe, MD *Department of Anesthesiology, The University of Texas M. D. Anderson Cancer Center, Houston, Texas, USA*

Randy N. Rosier, MD, PhD *Department of Orthopaedics, The University of Rochester, Rochester, New York, USA*

Peter S. Staats, MD *Division of Pain Medicine, Departments of Anesthesiology and Critical Care Medicine and Oncology, The Johns Hopkins University School of Medicine, Baltimore, Maryland, USA*

Porter Storey, MD *The Hospice at the Texas Medical Center, Houston, Texas, USA*

Lisa A. Teot, MD *Departments of Orthopaedics and Pathology, The University of Rochester, Rochester, New York, USA*

Roberto Wenk, MD *Programa Argentino de Medicina Paliativa–FEMEBA, Unidad de Cuidados Paliativos Hospital de E. Tornu, Buenos Aires; and Centro de Cuidados Paliativos Lalcec, San Nicolás; Argentina*

Preface

The problem of cancer pain is an enormous one throughout the world. Despite the difficulty of successfully managing this common and important problem in oncology, cancer pain treatment provides an opportunity for immense professional satisfaction because the relief of pain provides immediate benefit to patients and their families and complements cancer therapy. With this goal in mind, a satellite meeting of the 8th World Congress on Pain in August 1996 was organized in Houston, Texas, on the topic of "How to Assess and Treat Pain in Cancer Patients." This symposium provided a timely opportunity to assemble leading clinical scholars and to exploit their knowledge to advance the field.

We have selected for this book the most important topics discussed at the meeting, with an emphasis on new knowledge that has been accumulated on the assessment and treatment of cancer pain. We have emphasized areas that are normally ignored by books on cancer pain, choosing to cover such topics as strategies to implement clinical practice guidelines into practice, critical analysis and review of the current state of knowledge regarding the impact of pain treatment on survival, the interdisciplinary management of neuropathic and metastatic bone pain, neuroradiographic assessment of common cancer pain syndromes, and the science of medical decision making and pharmaco-economic analysis as related to pain and palliative care.

A variety of treatments are discussed, both noninvasive and invasive. Thorough assessment is a prerequisite to tailoring treatment for a specific patient. Anesthetic and neurosurgical treatment options are discussed from the point of view of correct patient selection. We particularly focused on the opportunities for improved interdisciplinary assessment and treatment of cancer pain. Traditional topics such as analgesic, anesthetic, and neurosurgical management of cancer pain are included, but with an emphasis on newer aspects of the clinical pharmacology of analgesic therapies, the evaluation of the timing of specific anesthetic and neurosurgical interventions, and the use of analgesic agents in the home environment in terminally ill patients.

Since most cancer patients experiencing pain will not be treated by pain specialists, it is important that all physicians, especially oncologists, become familiar with the modern use of pain-relieving drugs, especially opioids. Several chapters address this issue, including alternative routes of administering analgesics in homebound and home hospice patients. This monograph will complement rather than duplicate other books on cancer pain and will extend the base of practical knowledge for clinicians to improve their ability to successfully treat patients who have this devastating complication of cancer, enabling them to make a real difference in the quality of their patients' lives.

The completion of this monograph required the efforts of many persons. We thank the International Association for the Study of Pain for the opportunity to publish it. We thank the administrative and secretarial staffs in the Section of Pain and Symptom Management at The University of Texas M. D. Anderson Cancer Center. And we recognize the specific efforts of Pamela Jones, Program Coordinator for the Section of Pain and Symptom Management, without whose organizational skills and professionalism this book would not have been possible.

The editors wish to acknowledge Janssen Pharmaceutica, Knoll Pharmaceutical, and the Purdue Frederick Company for the unrestricted grants that provided the major support for the 1996 meeting in Houston and for this publication. We also thank the following companies for their unrestricted support: Abbott Laboratories, Anesta Corporation, Hoffman-LaRoche, Inc., Medtronic, Inc., and Roxane Laboratories, Inc.

RICHARD PAYNE, MD
RICHARD B. PATT, MD
C. STRATTON HILL, MD

Part I

Cancer Pain:
A Global Perspective

Assessment and Treatment of Cancer Pain,
Progress in Pain Research and Management,
Vol. 12, edited by R. Payne, R.B. Patt, and
C.S. Hill, IASP Press, Seattle, © 1998.

1

Palliative Care in Latin America

I. Status of Palliative Care Initiatives

Roberto Wenk

Programa Argentino de Medicina Paliativa–FEMEBA,
Unidad de Cuidados Paliativos Hospital de E. Tornu, Buenos Aires;
and Centro de Cuidados Paliativos Lalcec, San Nicolás; Argentina

Treatment of pain in cancer patients and palliative care (PC) have been priority issues for the WHO Cancer Control Program since 1984. The WHO Palliative Care Program for Latin America (based in Edmonton, Alberta, Canada) has responsibility for promoting the concepts of cancer pain control and palliative care in this region (Bruera 1992).

Since then, several PC programs have been developed in Latin America under the leadership of physicians from diverse specialties that use different administrative methods. The success of these programs reflects the high personal motivation and considerable time and resources that these leaders have devoted to developing operative models adapted to their distinctive situations (Bruera 1992; Wenk 1993b).

All Latin American groups face the same difficulties; they lack resources, professional education programs on symptom control, inexpensive analgesics, and an official health policy oriented to changing this situation. However, each group is solving its problems according to its own possibilities, and is adapting operational models to the local conditions. It was hard to understand and to accept that our socioeconomic and cultural situation differs from that of Europe and North America and that health care models appropriate for those regions are of questionable value in Latin America. We needed to design operative models whose organization and functioning could be adapted "in situ." This report on palliative care in Latin America describes and analyzes the following issues:

- common problems
- progress made in the past eight years

- the status of palliative care in Argentina: the Argentine Program (Medical Federation of Buenos Aires, FEMEBA)
- the effectiveness of a proposed health care model.

COMMON PROBLEMS IN LATIN AMERICA

This section reviews common problems that interfere with the interdependent factors that the WHO has identified as necessary to develop of a palliative care program (Stjernsward et al. 1992): education, national policy, and drug availability.

Education. Health care professionals are often unaware of the accepted methods for controlling pain and other cancer-related symptoms: most have not received proper instruction on the principles of symptom's control, either during medical school, residency, or continuing medical education programs. Neither have they been trained in communication skills; consequently, most patients do not understand their diagnosis and prognosis, which complicates their management and care.

Drug availability. In some countries, commercial or pharmaceutical preparations of morphine are widely available. In others, distribution of opioids is limited to large centers and city hospitals. In selected countries, the medical use of opioids is handicapped by legislation and bureaucratic requirements (requiring triplicate prescription pads and limits for the duration of therapies) (De Lima et al., unpublished data). A common factor to all Latin America is that opioids are still too expensive.

National policy. Most countries still lack official efforts to develop effective nationwide palliative care programs. The reasons include social and economic realities, bureaucracy and passivity in the official health systems, and lack of motivation at various organizational levels. All these deficiencies are dramatically amplified by poverty, a pervasive problem characterized by the lack of adequate living conditions (comfortable home, good nutrition) and inadequate health coverage.

PROGRESS REPORTED DURING THE PAST EIGHT YEARS

Every two years since 1990, the WHO has sponsored a meeting of its Palliative Care Program members in Latin America (Table I). During these congresses, members discuss issues and explore problems and possible solutions. WHO monitors the results of these programs and their success in producing changes.

Table I

Latin American palliative care congresses

Congress	Year	Place	Teams	Reports
1st	1990	San Nicolás, Argentina	10	—
2nd	1992	Cali, Colombia	20	—
3rd	1994	Florianópolis, Brazil	32	Declaración de Florianópolis
4th	1996	Santo Domingo, Dominican Republic	86	(Stjernsward et al. 1995) Reporte de Santo Domingo (De Lima et al., unpublished)

The reports of the 1996 Congress at Santo Domingo (De Lima et al., unpublished data) describe changes made since the issues were first presented at San Nicolás in 1990, and since the report of the 1994 congress in Florianópolis (Stjernsward et al. 1995). The most important changes are:

Progress in education. The number of health professionals interested in PC issues is increasing (Table I), as is their mutual cooperation. Many multidisciplinary seminars and courses are being organized, and some countries have modified some of the syllabuses for specific health care careers. Some groups produce and distribute supportive literature in Spanish.

Increase in the use of opioids. More opioids are available in different concentrations and pharmaceutical forms. In some countries, national laboratories prepare inexpensive preparations of immediate-release opioids; some others import opioid analgesics (Table II). In most countries local pharmacists prepare simple opioid solutions.

Progress in national policies. Chile, Colombia, and Mexico have developed national programs regarding palliative care. In other countries health authorities are increasingly interested in PC and the hope is that new programs will soon develop (De Lima et al., unpublished data).

The most significant changes have occurred in countries with PC programs that are not affected by political or social situations. These changes demonstrate the impact of professionals motivated to take action in the area of palliative care (Bruera 1992).

Table II

Consumption of morphine in Latin American countries (in kilograms)

Year	Global	Argentina	Chile	Colombia	Mexico
1990	7206	17	1	12	5
1991	8673	22	3	9	1
1992	10109	14	1	22	1
1993	12861	20	6	18	n.d.
1994	14042	40	10	26	15

Source: Joranson and Smokowski 1996.

STATUS OF PALLIATIVE CARE IN ARGENTINA:
THE ARGENTINE PROGRAM (FEMEBA)

In Argentina, palliative care activity began in 1984–1985 and it is in the hands of a highly motivated group of health care professionals. They follow the WHO guidelines and work in many cities at various health care facilities, both private and public (Wenk 1993a).

The patients treated by these groups receive adequate care, but has this focal activity been able to generate major changes in pain management for Argentine patients? A study conducted at a PC center in 1987 (Wenk et al. 1991) found that most patients (69%) reported "severe" or "unbearable" pain when first seen by the team. They had experienced pain for long periods (median 90 days) despite the administration of analgesics. Previous inadequate pain therapies shared common features: they were mostly parenteral, almost exclusively used mild analgesics, and did not include adjuvants or coanalgesics.

A second study conducted in 1992 at three PC centers in major cities (Wenk 1993c) revealed that patients were in severe pain when first seen by the doctor, and had been prescribed the same type of inadequate analgesic treatment. In addition, nausea, vomiting, and constipation remained untreated.

The third and latest study, conducted in 1995, extended over 120 days and included 306 calls to a hot line (Wenk and Pussetto 1995). It showed that 75% of patients undergoing oncologic treatment received ineffective symptomatic therapy (pain and other symptoms were not controlled). The remaining 25% were receiving treatment without symptomatic care.

These three studies show that various initiatives over approximately 11 years have failed to generate important changes in the management of pain in advanced cancer patients in Argentina. Which factors stand in the way of change? A priority list follows.

- Education of health care professionals is scattered and incomplete. Seminars, lectures, and courses offered by unofficial groups are available in some cities, but they lack quality control.
- Although oral opioids are available, commercial preparations are expensive. The monthly cost of treatment with 180 mg/day morphine is US$580 for slow-release preparations, $378 for immediate-release preparations, $45 for magistral preparations, and $19 when prepared by a volunteer pharmacist. Although some health care plans partially cover these costs, they are still excessive when compared with the average monthly income of workers ($400).
- Argentina lacks a health care policy addressing palliative care, which poses major obstacles to the implementation of a program. Other

obstacles to care for patients with advanced cancer include (Wenk and Marti 1996):

- Most health insurance systems do not recognize PC as a medical practice that can be invoiced, and thus professionals are unable to charge fees.
- Most PC professionals are volunteers or are underpaid, which leads to a lack of interest in PC as a part-time activity.
- Only a few health insurance systems pay for chronic treatments or domiciliary continuous care.

PC cannot be implemented in an environment with the above characteristics. No health professional can be expected to devote time, effort, and concern to an activity that is not even minimally compensated, nor can the population in such an environment demand adequate care as long as it is not duly recognized by the health authorities.

FEMEBA (a nongovernmental organization) is now supporting the Argentine program at the national level. Plans to implement PC include a continuing education program, changes in the health care policy, and the development of jobs in this field.

The continuing education program began in 1994 and consists of a PC hot line; printing and distribution of literature on PC directed to professionals, patients, and their families; courses offered to PC professionals (at clinics and hospitals, using case studies); and a clinical training program at a university hospital in Buenos Aires. Its main goal is to train family physicians.

The changes proposed in the health care policy include coverage of chronic illnesses, setting limits to curative treatment of advanced cancer patients, and recognition of PC as a medical practice, with monthly fees for continuing domiciliary care (regardless of the number of home visits). The creation of new jobs will start in 1997–98 to compensate physicians who have completed their PC training program and are managing cancer patients in their place of residence.

It is hoped that the above-mentioned unofficial medical initiative will increase the number of PC facilities and drastically improve the quality of palliative care for Argentine patients. It is also expected that it may favorably influence a future official policy.

RESULTS OBTAINED WITH A VOLUNTEER, HOME CARE PROGRAM

An example of the "on site" development of PC follows. This model of health care operates only within one level of the health care system: that of motivated professionals who assist patients. This "site" development is time consuming, but it is responsible for both the medical and teaching activities in many cities in Argentina (Wenk 1987, 1993a).

The CCP (Centro de Cuidados Paliativos) team is based in San Nicolás, a city of 170,000 inhabitants. It is a nonprofit program that does not interfere but rather interfaces with the existing health institutions. Its goals are to provide care for poor patients, to train lay volunteers as the primary liaison between physicians and patients, and to provide home care and secure its continuity.

The team is staffed by three anesthesiologists, a psychologist, a priest, a nurse, and six volunteers. Only the nurse is compensated. The costs of drugs and equipment and the nurse's salary are financed by philanthropic sources and by the city authorities.

The volunteers represent the first line in patient care. Their background is nonmedical, but over a six-month period they receive training in terminal care (Table III). The main activity of the volunteers is to monitor the condition of patients and their responses to therapy. This activity completes the "information loop" during the time between weekly medical consultations. Volunteers are the first line controlling the well-being of patients at home, and also provide support to the family through telephone contacts. Table IV summarizes the duties of volunteers. Three groups of two volunteers each visit the patients at their homes and are responsible for their telephone

Table III
Volunteer training program

Home care
Patient and family needs
Communication with the patient and the family
Monitoring of:
    Analgesia
    Nutrition
    Cognitive status
    Bowel movements
    Mouth care
    Skin care
    Sleep pattern
Prophylaxis and management of:
    Constipation
    Decubitus ulcers
    Oral Problems
    Pruritus
    Nausea and vomiting

Table IV
Duties of volunteers

Patient care

Patient and family support (at CCP offices)	Thursdays, 5–9 P.M.
Patient control at home	Scheduled (Mondays and Saturdays) on request
Telephone assistance	7 days, 24 hours

Other activities

Prescriptions, drugstore   Thursdays, 5–9 P.M.
Preparation of morphine solutions
Daily recording form reception
Data collection, computer data entry
Secretarial activities (mailing, library)
Volunteer recruiting and training

follow-up and support: two groups work while the third is on leave, on alternate three-month periods.

The volunteers are supervised by the team physicians, who are the second line in patient care, and are called when the clinical condition of a patient exceeds predetermined limits. This system reduces the demand on physicians, and consequently allows more effective attention to a greater number of patients.

Table V lists the results obtained through the team approach, which are acceptable. We strongly believe that this model may facilitate the introduction and growth of PC in developing countries, and also shows that limited resources by no means represent an absolute barrier for the development of a health care program in PC.

Table V
Results obtained through the Centro de Cuidados Paliativos (CCP) approach

Assistance activity
In 1994, 260 patients died of cancer in San Nicolás (24 % of all deaths). CCP treated 93 cancer patients (36 % of patients who died of cancer). Of these, 48 died at their homes (51% of the patients treated by CCP).

Teaching activities
Annual training program for volunteers
Translation, printing, and distribution of articles and monographs on palliative care
Increase in the number of doctors using oral morphine in San Nicolás (1 in 1982; 15 in 1995)

REFERENCES

Bruera E. Palliative care programs in Latin America. Palliat Med 1992; 6:182–184.

De Lima I, Bruera E, Stjernsward J, et al. Opioid Availability in Latin America: The Santo Domingo Report. Progress since The Declaration of Florianópolis. [Working draft and personal communication.]

Joranson DE, Smokowsky PR. Opioid Consumption Trends in Latin America [monograph]. Division of Policy Studies, University of Wisconsin Pain Research Group, WHO Collaborating Center, Madison, Wisconsin, 1996.

Stjernsward J, Koroltchouk V, Teoh N. National policies for cancer pain relief and palliative care. Palliat Med 1992, 6:293–298.

Stjernsward J, Bruera E, Joranson D, et al. Opioid availability in Latin America. The Declaration of Florianópolis. J Pain Symptom Manage 1995; 10:3:233–236.

Wenk R. Programa piloto de atención continua para el control del dolor y otros sintomas anpacientes con cancer. Rev Arg Anest 1987, 45(4): 267–273.

Wenk R. Argentina: status of cancer pain and palliative care. J Pain Symptom Manage 1993a; 8:385–387.

Wenk R. Cancer pain management problems in developing countries. In: Patt R (Ed). Cancer Pain. Philadelphia: J.B. Lippincott Co., 1993b, p 501.

Wenk R. Los Cuidados Paliativos en la República Argentina: la necesidad de centros de asistencia y entrenamiento. Rev Arg Anest 1993c, 51(2): 107–111.

Wenk R, Marti G. Palliative care in Argentina: deep changes are necessary for its effective implementation. Palliat Med 1996, 10:263–264.

Wenk R, Pussetto J. Resultados de la actividad de una hot-line de cuidados paliativos. IV Congress of the European Association for Palliative Care, Barcelona, Spain, 1995.

Wenk R, Diaz C, Echeverria M, et al. Argentina's WHO Cancer Pain Relief Program: a patient care model. J Pain Symptom Manage 1991; 6:40–43.

Correspondence to: Roberto Wenk, MD, Belgrano 585, 2900 San Nicolás, Argentina. Tel/Fax: 54-461-23680; email: wenk@intercom.com.ar.

II. The Impact of the Illegal Drug Market and Parallel Distribution Systems on the Availability of Opioids for Pain Relief in Colombia

Liliana De Lima

Non-communicable Diseases Program, Pan American Health Organization, Washington, DC, USA

MAGNITUDE OF THE PROBLEM

Cancer incidence in Colombia increased by 11% during the past five years, and cancer mortality jumped from the fifth cause of death in 1973 to third in 1994, accounting for 13% of all deaths after violence (20%) and cardiovascular diseases (30%). The prevalence rate of acquired immuno-deficiency syndrome (AIDS), which can involve tumors and pain, is also increasing (Pan American Health Organization 1995). As in other developing countries, most patients are diagnosed in advanced stages of their disease, when they do not respond to curative treatments. In Colombia, the resources to prevent, diagnose, and treat these diseases are in short supply. The funds for health allocated in the country in 1994 accounted for only 2.5% of the gross domestic product (GDP), 0.5% less than the mean for all developing countries and far below the 4% of the GDP allocated in developed countries (Fedesarrollo 1995).

THE SINGLE CONVENTION ON NARCOTIC DRUGS

Colombia is a member of the 1961 Single Convention on Narcotic Drugs (United Nations 1961), the multilateral treaty that regulates the use of controlled substances, including opioids. The Single Convention establishes rules concerning their importation, manufacture, distribution, storage, handling, and use. One of the objectives of the Single Convention is to ensure the availability of opioids for medical and scientific purposes, while minimizing the possibility of abuse and diversion to parallel markets.

THE DRUG DISTRIBUTION SYSTEM

The Single Convention requires governments to set up national drug control agencies to perform functions similar to those given to the International Narcotics Control Board (INCB) (United Nations 1961). The entity responsible for this control in Colombia is the Fondo Nacional de Estupefacientes (FNE, national narcotics office). This office is in charge of importing the medication with previous authorization from the INCB, and distributing it to the departamentos (states). The departamentos are under the control of the Fondos Regionales de Estupefacientes (FRE, regional narcotics offices), which are in turn responsible for distributing the opioid analgesics to the authorized institutions or pharmacies, which provide them to patients. In many rural areas this acquisition process can take three to five months, and physicians are forced to prescribe less potent, over-the-counter analgesics. The government offices are overloaded with work, are usually inefficient, and lack the resources to guarantee an effective distribution of medications.

OPIOID AVAILABILITY

In many countries, including Colombia, drugs are not always available to most of the population due to factors such as insufficient funding for health services, lack of health care delivery infrastructure, inadequate facilities for storage and distribution, and restrictive legislation and regulations that impede the access of patients to adequate pain relief (Joranson et al. 1996).

Colombia has a List of Essential Drugs (Ministerio de Salud 1992), as recommended by the World Health Organization (WHO 1988). The list is aimed at establishing medications that are essential for most of the population, and thus should always be available and accessible throughout the national territory. In 1992, the health ministry included codeine and morphine in its List of Essential Drugs in recognition of their importance and benefit. Unfortunately, the inclusion of these drugs has not had a significant effect on the availability of the medications, specially in the regional areas.

In the past seven years, several palliative care and pain relief programs, both public and private, have developed in Colombia. Among significant actions: the government adopted a National Palliative Care and Cancer Pain Relief Program through the National Cancer Institute (Ministerio de Salud 1993); several universities modified their curricula at the graduate and undergraduate levels to include pain assessment and treatment; publications were translated and distributed to health professionals; several symposia and international workshops were organized; and a local chapter of the International Association for the Study of Pain (IASP) and a National Association for Pain and Palliative Care were established (De Lima 1993; Moyano 1996). These actions and programs increased the demand for the use of opioids, for which the government was unprepared.

NATIONAL ESTIMATE OF OPIOID SUPPLY

The national estimate of the opioid supply is inadequate to satisfy the needs of the population. Supply patterns of potent opioids are inconsistent, with periods of availability of different opioids in several presentations, and other periods when not a single ampoule of morphine could be found (Joranson et al. 1996). The method used to determine the national estimate is based solely on past consumption data, which does not reflect unmet needs of the population or increases in the cancer and AIDS mortality and morbidity rates. An important factor in this supply pattern is the lack of financial resources. Even though the FNE may know that the opioid supply is diminishing, and that a new provision is needed, the FNE depends upon the ministries of Health and Treasury to allocate the necessary resources. It is not always easy to convince the government officials in these bureaucracies (often a different one for each new request) of the public health benefits of opioid use.

DRUGS AND LEGISLATION

In Colombia, more than in any other country in the world, the availability of opioids for medical purposes is also affected by the fear of diversion and the influence of the illegal drug market on national legislation. An analysis of the Colombian law (Ministerio de Salud 1986), performed to identify the legal and regulatory barriers that impede the access of patients to adequate palliative care and pain treatment, revealed a misuse of terms and definitions concerning opioid use, the failure to acknowledge in the law the benefits of adequate pain treatment, the lack of legal responsibility and accountability for the parties involved in each process, and the establishment of time limits for opioid prescription (Joranson and DeLima 1994). Although many of these laws were enacted before opioids were identified as essential analgesics, the negative effectexerted by parallel markets and illegal drugs continues in the minds of the regulators, legislators, health professionals, and the general public.

The war on drugs in Colombia has extended over 25 years, but has intensified in the past 10, to the extent that the country is now identified as the biggest exporter and producer of illegal drugs in the Western

Hemisphere. In this war Colombia has enacted and passed legislative reforms intended to impede the use of illegal drugs and the abuse or diversion of legal ones into illicit channels. Such legislation has affected the availability of opioids for pain patients and interfered with the capacity to receive analgesics in a regular and consistent manner. In fact, a joint report by the United Nations International Drug Control Programme (UNDCP) and the World Health Organization states that insufficient opioid availability may be a factor that facilitates the emergence of parallel markets (UNDCP-WHO 1993). According to the report, patients who are incapable of finding adequate analgesics in the legal distribution system, or who cannot afford expensive pain relievers, are willing to buy analgesics in the illegal market to obtain relief.

Much of the fear felt by the general public, patients, health care professionals, and regulators comes from the actions taken by international and national drug control authorities to fight the emergence of illegal plantations of poppy flowers grown to extract heroin. Their war is against the drugs in general, not their abuse or misuse, and thus restricts medical access to those who need them to alleviate suffering. This perception is worsened by the presence of narcoguerrillas who control specific regions and give the opium an illegal connotation in the public mind.

Unavailability of opioids for medical use does not necessarily guarantee prevention of abuse, and overly restrictive approaches may block access to opioid medications for most of the population. The WHO Expert Committee has acknowledged the need to explore the extent to which restrictive programs inhibit the prescribing of opioids to patients who need them (Angarola 1990). Health care workers may be reluctant to prescribe, stock, or dispense opioids if they feel the governing authority may suspend or revoke their professional licenses if they provide a large quantities of opioids to a patient, even though the medical need for such drugs can be proven.

CONCLUSION

The lack of availability of opioids in Colombia is a complex problem that cannot be justified or explained with the same reasons used in other countries. The illegal drug market has forced the country to constantly try to demonstrate to the world its commitment to fight the war against drugs. This situation has placed the Colombian legislators and regulators in a restricted position, where they fear that facilitating the access of opioids for medical and scientific use may be interpreted as a softening position toward the misuse and abuse of drugs.

Regardless of the increases in physician education, and the support and interest from the National Cancer Institute and the FNE, physicians are still reluctant to prescribe opioids and patients are still reluctant to use them, because they are associated with addiction. The war on drugs has unwillingly turned the pain patients into its victims, and in trying to decrease abuse, legislators and administrators have taken actions that have reduced the availability of opioid analgesics to the population.

Ensuring the supply of opioids requires effective assessment and monitoring systems, and prevention of drug diversion into illicit channels requires a special infrastructure, neither of which the country has. The availability of opioids needs to be improved through legislative and administrative measures designed to achieve a better balance between the control of opioids and their supply for medical purposes, easier access to improved health care services, and the education of health professionals regarding the rational use of opioids.

REFERENCES

Angarola RT. National and international regulation of opioid drugs: purpose, structures, benefits and risks. J Pain Symptom Manage 1990; 5:1:7–11.
De Lima L. Colombia: status of cancer pain and palliative care. J Pain Symptom Manage 1993; 8:6:404–406.
Fedesarrollo. Fondos para la Salud en Colombia siguen siendo insuficientes. El Tiempo 1995; May 27:p C4.
Joranson DE. New international efforts to ensure availability of opioids for medical purposes. J Pain Symptom Manage 1996; 12:2:85–86.
Joranson DE, De Lima L. Analisis Preliminar de la Legislación Colombiana en Relación a los Principios Internacionales de Disponibilidad de Opioides [Monografía]. Madison, Wisconsin: University of Wisconsin Pain and Policy Studies Group, Comprehensive Cancer Care Center, WHO Collaborative Center, 1994.
Joranson DE, Smokoski PR, De Lima L. Tendencias en el Consumo de Opioides en Sur America [Monografía]. Madison, Wisconsin: University of Wisconsin Pain and Policy Studies Group, Comprehensive Cancer Care Center, WHO Collaborative Center, 1996.
Ministerio de Salud. Ley 30 de 1986: Estatuto Nacional de Estupefacientes del Ministerio de Salud de Colombia. Congreso Nacional de la República, 1986.
Ministerio de Salud. Listado de Medicamentos Esenciales, Resolución 7328 del Ministerio de Salud de Colombia (Sept. 6, 1992). Bogotá: Imprenta Nacional, 1992.
Ministerio de Salud. Programa Nacional de Alivio de Dolor y Cuidados Paliativos. Resolución 013 del Instituto Nacional de Cancerología. Bogotá: Ministerio de Salud, 1993.
Moyano J. Status of cancer pain and palliative care. J Pain Symptom Manage 1996. 12:2:104–105.
Organización Panamericana de la Salud. Estadísticas de Salud en las Americas: Mortalidad, Estimaciones y Proyecciones Demográficas (Publicación Científica No. 556). Washington DC: OPS, 1995.
Pan American Health Organization. Health statistics from the Americas. PAHO Scientific Publication no. 556. Washington, DC: Pan American Health Organization, 1995.
UNDCP-WHO (United Nations International Drug Control Programme and World Health Organization). Joint UNDCP-WHO Technical Consultation Meeting on Parallel Distribution

Systems for Narcotic Drugs and Psychotropic Substances at the National Level [report]. Vienna: United Nations, 1993.

United Nations. Single Convention on Narcotic Drugs, as amended by the 1972 Protocol 93, Vienna: United Nations, 1961.

World Health Organization. The Use of Essential Drugs. Technical Report Series 770. Geneva: World Health Organization, 1988.

Correspondence to: Liliana De Lima, MS, 803 Heathcliff Ct., Houston, TX 77024, USA, Tel: 713-465-3498; Fax: 713-465-5215.

Assessment and Treatment of Cancer Pain,
Progress in Pain Research and Management,
Vol. 12, edited by R. Payne, R.B. Patt, and
C.S. Hill, IASP Press, Seattle, © 1998.

2

Cancer Pain Clinical Practice Guidelines for Clinicians and Patients: Rationale, Barriers to Implementation, and Future Directions

Richard Payne[a] and Judith A. Paice[b]

[a]Pain and Symptom Management Section, Department of Neuro-Oncology, The University of Texas M. D. Anderson Cancer Center, Houston, Texas; and [b]Department of Neurosurgery, Rush Neuroscience Institute, Rush Medical Center, and College of Nursing, Rush University, Chicago, Illinois; USA

RATIONALE FOR DEVELOPMENT OF GUIDELINES

Pain caused by a neoplasm or as a complication of cancer therapy occurs commonly (Payne et al. 1996). Many epidemiological surveys have concluded that approximately 25% of patients with localized disease report pain and that the prevalence of pain can be as high as 90% in patients with advanced cancer (Jacox et al. 1994a). Although recent studies have reported that adequate pain control can be achieved in as many as 88% of patients with cancer-related pain (Zech et al. 1995), in reality many patients have inadequate pain management (Cleeland et al. 1994). For example, a recent study used the Brief Pain Inventory to assess 1308 ambulatory cancer patients and compared their reported pain intensity to the potency of analgesics prescribed to calculate a pain management index. Results showed that 46% were undermanaged by this standard (Cleeland et al. 1994).

Because such data reveal major variations in clinical management of cancer pain, this condition meets criteria for guideline development delineated by the Institute of Medicine (1990) (Table I). More than two million copies of the Clinical Practice Guidelines for clinicians and patients have been disseminated by the Agency for Health Care Policy and Research (AHCPR), which confirms the demand for this information. However, it is

Table I

Institute of Medicine criteria for the development of clinical practice guidelines

---

Primary Criteria

1. Potential to improve individual patient outcome
2. Potential to affect a large patient population
3. Potential to reduce unit or aggregate costs
4. Potential to reduce unexplained variations in medical practice

Secondary Criteria

1. Potential to address social and ethical implications for the disease
2. Potential to advance medical knowledge of the condition
3. Potential to affect policy decisions
4. Potential to enhance the national capacity for assessment of the disorder
5. Potential to be readily conducted

Source: Institute of Medicine Committee 1990.

unclear how effectively the guidelines have been put into practice, so this chapter will present strategies for effective implementation.

THE PROCESS OF GUIDELINE DEVELOPMENT

The process of clinical practice guideline development as suggested by the IOM and the AHCPR has multiple components (Table II). The process is intended to facilitate the creation of a credible document, based on the most rigorous examination of the available scientific evidence, that also meets the needs for the flexibility required in typical clinical settings (Institute of Medicine Committee 1990). The core of the development process is an exhaustive literature review of the available scientific evidence by experts in the field and an explicit grading of the quality of the studies and the overall

Table II

Steps in the development of clinical practice guidelines
by the U.S. Agency for Health Care Policy and Research

---

1. Define the clinical condition
2. Assemble multidisciplinary committee
3. Define goals and principles of the guideline
4. Conduct literature review
5. Evaluate the evidence
6. Conduct peer review of guideline drafts
7. Prepare final draft of document
8. Conduct internal review by AHCPR and other relevant government agencies
9. Publish guidelines
10. Disseminate guidelines
11. Revise guidelines

Source: Institute of Medicine Committee 1990.

scientific evidence for specific recommendations. The committee chairpersons select the committee members, who are appointed by the AHCPR following a thorough review of credentials. Criteria include absence of academic or financial conflicts of interest that might impugn the integrity of the process and the ultimate credibility of the clinical practice guidelines.

Ideally, the panel or committee of experts represents a multidisciplinary perspective that is national in scope and free from many of the suspected professional and economic biases identified in guidelines developed by single-discipline professional societies. This approach is a great strength of the AHCPR clinical practice guideline process. From one perspective, clinicians who are active in the field have an inevitable bias and at least an apparent "conflict of interest" in the interpretation of the literature and creation of the recommendations, given that their practice patterns and even income may be directly affected by specific recommendations. Viewed from this perspective, the "least biased" expert might be someone with a background in biostatistics and health services outcomes research who is not involved in direct patient care for the clinical condition being evaluated. The more traditional perspective posits that only those who work in the specific field and have some contact with the nuances of patient care in the clinical condition under study can accurately interpret the literature. The traditional perspective also assumes that objective systems for grading the weight of the scientific evidence make explicit the rationale for specific guideline recommendations. The expert panel that wrote the cancer pain clinical practice guidelines was composed exclusively of health care professionals representing many disciplines (e.g., neuro-oncology, anesthesiology, oncology, nursing, psychology) and patients who worked in the field of cancer pain management or were directly affected by the disorder (Appendix I). Recently, the AHCPR has conducted workshops to elaborate on these and other issues associated with the methodological aspects of clinical practice guidelines development (Schriger 1994).

The creation of evidence-based guidelines is dependent on some criteria for grading the strength of the scientific data that provided the foundation for a specific recommendation. The types of evidence that constituted the basis for the guidelines in cancer pain management (and for acute pain) are listed in Table III. The panel evaluated approximately 9000 references and used about 600 core references to develop the final recommendations. Each recommendation was given a letter grade from A to D, as defined by Table III, to indicate the strength and consistency of the scientific evidence supporting the advice.

For example, the chapter on pharmacological management of cancer pain includes the following recommendation: "Medications for persistent

Table III
Types and ratings of scientific evidence used to create
the AHCPR cancer pain clinical practice guidelines

Types of evidence

I.   Meta-analysis of multiple well-designed controlled studies

II. At least one well-designed experimental study

III. Well-designed quasi-experimental studies such as nonrandomized controlled, single-group pre-post, cohort, time series, or matched case controlled studies

IV. Well-designed nonexperimental studies, such as comparative and correlational descriptive and case studies

V.   Case reports and clinical examples

Rating of strength and consistency of evidence

A.   There is evidence from type I or consistent findings from multiple studies of types II, III, or IV.

B.   There is evidence of types II, II, or IV, and findings are generally consistent.

C.   There is evidence of types II, III, or IV, but findings are inconsistent.

D.   There is little or no systematic empirical evidence.

Source: Jacox et al. 1994a.

cancer-related pain should be administered on an around-the-clock basis with additional 'as needed' doses, because regularly scheduled dosing maintains a constant level of drug in the body and helps to prevent a recurrence of pain (A)" (Jacox et al. 1994b). This recommendation is supported by the strongest possible scientific evidence, based on randomized controlled clinical trials and meta-analysis, and the user of the guidelines can be confident that clinical practice based on this recommendation will likely produce a satisfactory outcome.

However, in that same chapter on pharmacological management, the following recommendation also appears: "The oral route is the preferred route of analgesic administration because it is the most convenient and cost-effective method of administration. When patients cannot take medications orally, rectal and transdermal routes of administration should be considered because they are also relatively noninvasive (panel consensus)." Although this guideline recommendation is consistent with common clinical practice and is supported by substantial anecdotal and experimental evidence that oral administration of analgesics, particularly opioid analgesics, is safe and effective, the evidence is lacking in sufficient weight and consistency to justify an "A" grade for this specific statement. In fact, it might be argued that transdermal and transmucosal routes of administration—which were much less common when the cancer pain guidelines were released in 1994—

may be more desirable in some patients as "first-line" therapies (e.g., in a patient with known intolerance to morphine or hydromorphone).

The reader thus has a clear statement of the strength and consistency of the evidence to guide individual clinical decision making; such clarity adds to the effectiveness, ease of use, credibility, and flexibility of the document. It should also be apparent that guideline recommendations based on panel consensus only, and with relatively weak evidence (e.g., grade "B" or lower), are targets for reevaluation in future revisions and signal research opportunities.

Peer-review of guideline drafts are important to determine clarity and credibility of the recommendations and the document's ease of use. For the cancer pain guidelines, 186 health care providers and consumers served as peer reviewers. An additional 16 persons served as site testers for various phases of document development. Following revisions based on multiple sources of feedback, and review of the final document by relevant governmental agencies such as the National Cancer Institute, the Food and Drug Administration, and the AHCPR, the guidelines were released and disseminated. The initial dissemination involved widespread media publicity via television, radio, and print media and the publication of articles in professional journals. Importantly, the media campaign targeted specific ethnic groups, and the clinician and patient versions of the guidelines have been translated into Spanish, French, Italian, and Chinese for use in the United States and in other countries.

The endorsement of key advocacy groups was obtained from the American Cancer Society, the National Cancer Institute, the American Association of Retired Persons, the American Pain Society, the Oncology Nursing Society, the American Nursing Association, and many other important professional associations. These organizations also played important roles in the dissemination of the completed guidelines. The pharmaceutical industry had no role in the development of the clinical practice guidelines (although the Pharmaceutical Manufacturer's Association reviewed the final draft), but and individual companies have printed and provided copies of the guidelines at no cost to patients and health care providers.

CONTENT OF CLINICAL PRACTICE GUIDELINES

A detailed explanation of the contents of the clinical practice guidelines is beyond the scope of this chapter. Perhaps the best summary of the contents is embodied in the following ABCDE mnemonic:

A: *A*sk about pain regularly. *A*ssess pain systematically.

B: *B*elieve the patient and family in their reports of pain and what relieves it.

C: Choose pain control options appropriate for the patient, family, and setting.
D: Deliver interventions in a timely, logical, and coordinated fashion.
E: Empower patients and their families. Enable them to control their course to the greatest extent possible.

Cardinal principles emphasized in the cancer pain clinical practice guideline are to assess pain appropriately and to make rational treatment decisions based on assessments that are individualized to the needs and particular circumstances of the patients and their families. The flow chart outlining the basic issues in cancer pain assessment (Fig. 1) and the pyramid illustrating the hierarchy of pain management strategies (Fig. 2) also serve as useful summaries. Details concerning the assessment and treatment of cancer pain are covered elsewhere in this book.

BARRIERS TO IMPLEMENTATION
OF CLINICAL PRACTICE GUIDELINES

There are no data regarding the extent to which the cancer pain guidelines have been implemented into clinical practice. Many potential barriers could hinder their widespread adoption. An example is the recommendation that clinicians spend additional time talking to patients and families to evaluate pain and its effect on the family. Third-party payors may inadequately reimburse for such additional time, or may not reimburse it at all. The guidelines generally call for more aggressive and increased use of controlled substances, such as opioids and psychostimulants, which may inhibit widespread adoption into practice by clinicians who have not overcome unfounded fears of iatrogenic addiction to these substances. Although the assessment strategies call for the use of simple tools such as 0–10 self-report scales, the major determinant of adequate pain relief ultimately depends on the patient's subjective report; subjective outcomes have not traditionally been tracked in large-scale epidemiological and outcome studies. The lack of more "objective" outcomes that confirm the usefulness of the guidelines may limit their acceptance. Finally, the guidelines indicate that pharmacotherapy, specifically the aggressive use of multiple potent psychoactive substances with potential additive toxicities, is the mainstay of treatment for many, if not most cancer patients with pain. If clinicians do not use appropriate skills in administering these pharmacotherapies, patients may suffer severe side effects and a worsened quality of life, which will not enhance the adoption of the guidelines.

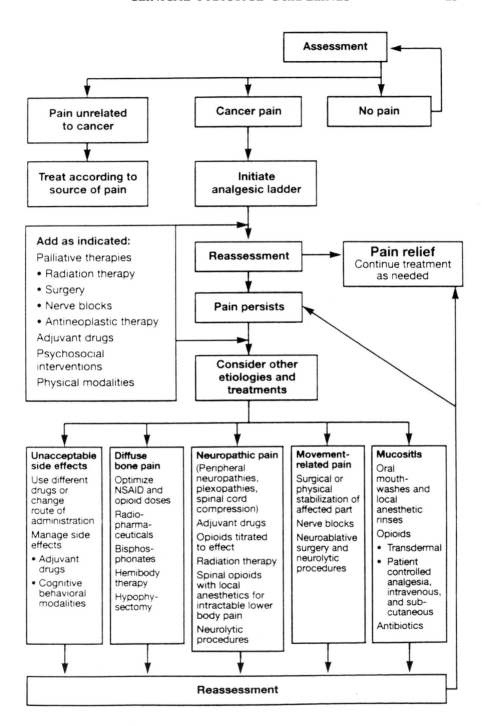

Fig. 1. Continuing pain management in patients with cancer (Jacox et al. 1994b).

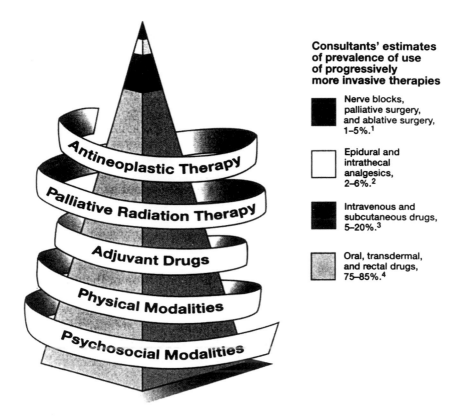

Consultants' estimates of prevalence of use of progressively more invasive therapies

- Nerve blocks, palliative surgery, and ablative surgery, 1–5%.[1]
- Epidural and intrathecal analgesics, 2–6%.[2]
- Intravenous and subcutaneous drugs, 5–20%.[3]
- Oral, transdermal, and rectal drugs, 75–85%.[4]

[1] Hiraga, Mizuguchi, and Takeda, 1991; Portenoy, 1993; Ventafridda, Caraceni, and Gamba, 1990.
[2] Hiraga, Mizuguchi, and Takeda, 1991; Ventafridda, Caraceni, and Gamba, 1990.
[3] Keller, 1984; Paice, 1993; Portenoy, 1993.
[4] Goisis, Gorini, Ratti, et al., 1989; Hiraga, Mizuguchi, and Takeda, 1991; Scug, Zech, and Dörr, 1990; Takeda, 1986; Ventafridda, Caraceni, and Gamba, 1990; Walker, Hoskin, Hanks, et al., 1988.

Note: The pyramid depicts a hierarchy of pain management strategies from least invasive (at the base) to most invasive (at the apex). Therapies depicted on the ribbon may benefit many patients who are receiving concurrent treatments at any level of invasiveness. Estimates presented in the sidebar are based on published data and consultants' estimates for various clinical populations in industrialized nations but may not reflect all settings and do not necessarily reflect what is optimal.

Fig. 2. Pain management strategies: a hierarchy (Jacox et al. 1994b).

However, several factors could counterbalance these potential barriers to more widespread adoption of the guidelines. Perhaps most important is the increased consumer demand for better pain relief, which will arise from a greater public understanding of the possibilities for improved treatment. Furthermore, the endorsement of the guidelines by many important and credible patient advocacy groups and professional societies such as the American Cancer Society and the American Pain Society should facilitate better public understanding of the need for improved pain management and hence more widespread adoption of the guidelines. Institutional pride and commitment to quality of care and pain management, will, of necessity, involve adoption of many of the guideline principles (American Pain Society Quality of Care Committee, 1995; Ferrell et al. 1996). Successful adoption by clinician "role models" will also lead to more widespread adaptation. Finally, recent innovative strategies to implement analgesic practice protocols and collaborative care pathways will have the effect of "institutionalizing" good pain management practices.

The recognition of the importance of educated patient "consumers" was a major factor in the development of the patient version of the guidelines, which is described below.

CANCER PAIN MANAGEMENT PATIENT GUIDE

Patient-related barriers to adequate pain management are largely related to fear and misinformation. Fears of addiction and tolerance and misinformation regarding side effects to analgesics cause patient reluctance to report and treat their pain. In one study of patient-related barriers, greater levels of concern about addiction, side effects to pain medications, and "complaining" about pain were associated with higher pain intensity scores (Ward et al. 1993). Therefore, education regarding the importance of reporting and treating pain might overcome these barriers and provide improved pain relief. Education directed toward family members might also improve pain relief. In a study conducted by the Minnesota Cancer Pain Initiative, family members who were not concerned about addiction and who believed that cancer pain relief was possible reported less pain experienced by their loved one with cancer (Elliot et al. 1996). Professional organizations recognize the need for patient education to provide optimal pain relief. The American Pain Society Quality of Care Committee recommended that patients be promised responsive analgesic care and be urged to communicate their pain to health care professionals (American Pain Society Quality of Care Committee 1995). Encouraging patients to report and quantify their pain is best conducted through educational efforts. The Oncology Nursing Society published a position paper on cancer pain that strongly advocated the importance of education for families and their caregivers (Spross et al. 1990). The AHCPR *Management of Cancer Pain* clinical practice guidelines also recognized the importance of patient education in ABCDE mnemonic discussed above, in which the "E" symbolizes the need to empower patients families to enable them to control pain to the fullest extent possible.

Development of patient guide

Recognizing that empowerment can best be achieved by education, the AHCPR included patient guides with most of the clinical practice guidelines released to date. The *Managing Cancer Pain Patient Guide* that accompanies the *Management of Cancer Pain* clinical practice guideline is a 21-page pamphlet for patients and their caregivers that was developed after extensive literature review (Table IV). Many educational materials are quite lengthy, written at a sophisticated level, or specific to a particular population (e.g., children or adolescents). *Managing Cancer Pain Patient Guide* provides introductory information to a broad population of patients with cancer and their caregivers. The information is purposefully brief so that ill, fatigued patients can easily read and comprehend the material. Patients who master this material and wish additional information might then seek other sources.

After considering the essential components, the committee developed a draft of the guide. Because myths are so pervasive, concerns and facts about cancer treatment were included in the introductory material. Other information covered why pain should be treated, the causes of cancer pain, and

Table IV
Patient education materials

Booklets
Cancer Pain Can Be Relieved
Children's Cancer Pain Can Be Relieved
Jeff Asks About Cancer Pain
   Wisconsin Cancer Pain Initiative
   3675 Medical Sciences Center
   University of Wisconsin Medical School
   1300 University Avenue
   Madison, WI 53706, USA

Get Relief From Cancer Pain (NIH Publication No. 94-3735)
Questions and Answers About Pain Control: A Guide for People with Cancer
   and Their Families
   Available from the American Cancer Society and the National Cancer Institute.
   Copies can be obtained by calling 1-800-4-CANCER or 1-800-ACS-2345

Books
Cowles J. *Pain Relief: How to Say No to Acute, Chronic & Cancer Pain!* New York:
   Mastermedia Ltd., 1993. Call 800-334-8232 to order.
Long SS, Patt RB. *You Don't Have to Suffer.* New York: Oxford Press, 1994.
Stacy CB, Kaplan AS, Williams G. *The Fight Against Pain.* New York: Consumer
   Reports Books, 1993. To order write: Consumer Reports Books, 101 Truman Ave.,
   Yonkers, NY 10703, USA.
Wall PD, Jones M. *Defeating Pain. The War Against a Silent Epidemic.* New York:
   Plenum Press, 1991.

treatment methods. Strategies for managing side effects and nondrug interventions were also incorporated. The guide offered a space for questions, a format for developing a treatment plan, and a pain diary for documenting pain intensity and response to treatment. The draft was then critiqued by a panel of experts, including physicians, nurses, psychologists, educators, and patients. Additions, deletions, and other revisions were incorporated into subsequent drafts, which were pilot-tested in a variety of settings throughout the United States: inpatient units at a large university hospital, university hospital outpatient clinics, a hospice serving an urban and suburban population, an inpatient and outpatient community hospital in a rural setting, and a national cancer survivors' support group. An evaluation tool that accompanied the patient guide requested demographic data and patients' perceptions regarding the utility of the tool and the ease of its use.

Sixty-nine patients completed the evaluation, with slightly more women represented (65%) than men. The average age of the sample was 53 years (± 14.7) and average years of education was 13.5 (± 2.99). The average time since cancer diagnosis was more than two years (mean 28.62 months; range 1–240 months; SD ± 44.99). Breast cancer (25%), lymphoma (15%), and lung cancer (15%) were the most common diagnoses represented. Most patients (nearly 87%) felt the guide would help them talk more openly about their pain with a doctor or nurse. Almost all of the participants (94%) also reported that the guide helped them better understand the different ways in which cancer pain could be relieved and as a result they felt more comfortable taking pain medication (nearly 93%). Most felt the information in the guide was clear and easy to read (96%), and 76% found the guide to be an appropriate length. Qualitative comments offered to data collectors were then used to develop final drafts of the guide.

Dissemination and implementation of patient guide

Since release of the patient guide in 1994 (in both English and Spanish versions), large-scale dissemination efforts have been conducted by the AHCPR and organizations such as the National Cancer Institute, the American Cancer Society, and the cancer pain initiatives in many states. Local efforts include making guides available in hospital and clinic waiting rooms and on posters displayed in areas where patients and family members congregate. To encourage use of the American Pain Society Standards for Cancer Patients, which emphasize the promise of attentive analgesic care to individual patients, many institutions now provide copies of the guide to patients and their families on admission to hospital or visits to the outpatient clinics (Bookbinder et al. 1996). Thus, dissemination efforts not only educate

Table V
Dissemination strategies for patient care guidelines

- Include in hospital and nursing home admission packets for patients and families.
- Include in orientation information to outpatient clinics and physician offices.
- Include in orientation materials and staff meetings of all health care providers (e.g., nurses, clergy, clerical staff, physicians, pharmacists).
- Distribute in retail and hospital pharmacies at the time of physician dispensing.
- Distribute to churches and other community organizations.

---

individual patients, but also assist institutions in meeting quality assurance standards.

Other dissemination strategies (Table V) include making all health care professionals, including physicians, nurses, pharmacists, psychologists, occupational and physical therapists, pastoral care personnel, volunteers, and others, aware of the guide and its contents. This effort ensures that patients and their family members receive consistent information from all persons who provide care to those with cancer. For example, distribution during new employee orientation, with the expectation that all persons with cancer be given this information, reinforces the importance of the material. Retail pharmacists who serve patients with cancer can be asked to display and distribute patient guides. Nursing homes, hospices, and support groups are logical settings for dissemination to patients with cancer and their caregivers.

Public awareness of cancer pain is key to solving the problem. For this reason, outreach efforts into the community are essential. Providing copies of the guide to church groups and other lay organizations assists in dissemination. Patient guides can also be distributed at health fairs and other screening activities. Radio and television stations are mandated to provide public service messages, and many program directors actively seek this information. Brief announcements regarding the availability of the patient guide, with appropriate telephone numbers, can fill this need.

Dissemination alone is not sufficient; implementation is essential and can be accomplished through various means. For example, patient education efforts, specifying use of the patient guide, should be incorporated into clinical pathways. Specific personnel responsible for distributing the tool and educating patients must be identified and held accountable for these tasks. In most settings, nurses are key, due to their exposure to patients, their own educational preparation, which emphasizes patient education, and their ability to synthesize complex information into lay terminology. Different personnel may be more appropriate, however, in other settings.

METHODS TO OVERCOME BARRIERS

Several barriers hinder use of the patient guide, but most are easily reconciled. Although availability of the patient guide has been an occasional barrier, this document is part of the public domain, so copies can be generated without fear of copyright violation. Copies of the patient guide can be obtained 24 hours a day, seven days a week by using the AHCPR Instant FAX (301-594-2800 using a fax machine with a telephone headset). The patient guides are also available on-line by visiting the AHCPR's Home Page at URL http://www.ahcpr.gov (click on "Consumer Health").

Given that many persons with cancer are elderly, patients or their caregivers may be visually impaired. The AHCPR has produced an audiotape narrating the publication *Pain Control After Surgery: A Patient's Guide*. Similar tapes can be made to supplement the cancer pain guide, which would allow patients to listen to small pieces of information at a time or to replay sections.

Cancer patients are often too fatigued, ill, or distressed to retain much information. Family members or other caregivers should be included during educational efforts to provide reinforcement of the material. Additionally, family members may harbor fears of their own regarding addiction, tolerance, or side effects, and these can be addressed during educational efforts.

To overcome barriers related to comprehension, adult learning principles should be considered when teaching patients and their caregivers. Individualize the content of educational efforts to meet the educational, cognitive, and cultural background of patients and their caregivers. Deliver the material in a relaxed, quiet setting, ask patients and caregivers to summarize the material, and encourage questions. These and other barriers to the dissemination and implementation of the *Managing Cancer Pain Patient Guide* can be overcome through coordinated efforts incorporating all health care professionals, adopting novel marketing techniques to reach patients and lay persons, identifying those accountable for making guides available, and employing effective teaching principles.

SUMMARY AND FUTURE DIRECTIONS
FOR CLINICAL PRACTICE GUIDELINES

The AHCPR clinical practice guidelines for cancer pain management are evidence-based and have been widely disseminated to clinicians and patients. Although immediate widespread adoption will lead to improved pain management, there are opportunities to revise the document (now almost four years old) and to implement creative and innovative strategies to ensure more widespread use of these important principles of pain assessment and treatment.

Refinement of the methodological approaches to guideline development, and rigorous examination of the effect of clinical practice guidelines on the quality and cost of care are important areas for future growth. The AHCPR has conducted and published workshops on clinical practice guidelines focused on topics such as methodological perspectives (McCormick et al. 1994); quality improvement (Schoenbaum et al. 1995), and cost analysis (Grady and Weiss 1995). These are critical areas for which clinical practice guidelines in general, and the cancer pain guidelines specifically, must focus when revised in the future. Recently, the quality of the evaluation of the efficacy of cancer pain therapies as required by the World Health Organization (WHO) three-step ladder approach has been called into question (Jadad et al. 1995). The WHO three-step ladder approach is a foundation for the pharmacological principles of cancer pain management elucidated in the AHCPR clinical practice guidelines. The criticisms expressed by Jadad and others apply equally to the evaluation of AHCPR guideline principles, and emphasize the need for prospective and controlled evaluation of specific guideline recommendations with clear statement of outcomes being studied. Finally, as noted above, the American Pain Society has published an important study evaluating the quality of pain management in several practice settings, which uses many of the principles emphasized in the AHCPR cancer pain guidelines (APS Quality of Care Committee 1995).

REFERENCES

American Pain Society Quality of Care Committee. Quality improvement guidelines for the treatment of acute pain and cancer pain. JAMA 1995; 274:1874–1880.

Bookbinder M, Coyle N, Kiss M, et al. Implementing national standards for cancer pain management: program model and evaluation. J Pain Symptom Manage 1996; 12:334–347.

Cleeland CS, Gonin R, Hatfield AK, et al. Pain and its treatment in outpatients with metastatic cancer. N Engl J Med 1994; 330:592–596.

Elliott BA, Elliott TE, Murray DM, et al. Patients and family members: the role of knowledge and attitudes in cancer pain. J Pain Symptom Manage 1996; 12:209–220.

Ferrell B, Dean G, Grant M, Coluzzi P. An institutional commitment to pain management. J Clin Oncol 1995; 13:2158–2165.

Goisis A, Gorini M, Ratti R, Luliri P. Application of a WHO protocol on medical therapy for oncologic pain in an internal medicine hospital. Tumori 1989; 75:470–472.

Grady ML, Weis KA (Eds). Conference Proceeding: Cost Analysis Methodology for Clinical Practice Guidelines, AHCPR Publication no. 95-0001. Rockville, MD: U.S. Department of Health and Human Services, Public Health Service, Agency for Health Care Policy and Research, 1995.

Hiraga K, Mizuguchi T, Takeda F. The incidence of cancer pain and improvement of pain management in Japan. Postgrad Med 1991; 67(Suppl.):S14–25.

Institute of Medicine Committee. Clinical Practice Guidelines: Directions for a New Program. Washington: National Academy Press, 1990.

Jacox A, Carr DB, Payne R. New clinical practice guidelines for the management of cancer pain. N Engl J Med 1994a; 330:169–173.

Jacox A, Carr DB, Payne R, et al. Management of Cancer Pain. Clinical Practice Guideline no. 9, AHCPR Publication no. 94-0592. Rockville, MD: U.S. Department of Health and Human Services, Public Health Service, Agency for Health Care Policy and Research, 1994b.

Jadad AR, Browman GP. The WHO analgesic ladder for cancer pain management (stepping up the quality of its evaluation). JAMA 1995; 274:1870–1873.

Keller M. A retrospective review of patients receiving continuous morphine infusion. PRN Forum 1984; 3:5–6.

McCormick KA, Moore SR, Siegel RA (Eds). Clinical Practice Guideline Development: Methodology Perspectives. AHCPR Publication no. 95-0009. Rockville, MD: U.S. Department of Health and Human Services, Public Health Service, Agency for Health Care Policy and Research, 1994

Paice J. Personal communication. May 5, 1993.

Payne R, Weinstein SM, Hill CS. Assessment and management of pain. In: Levin VA (Ed). Cancer in the Nervous System. New York: Churchill Livingstone, 1996, pp 448.

Portenoy RK, Southern MA, Gupta SK, et al. Transdermal fentanyl for cancer pain. Repeated dose pharmacokinetics. Anesthesiology 1993; 78:36–43.

Schoenbaum SC, Sundwall DN, et al. Using clinical practice guidelines to evaluate quality of care. Vol. 1 and 2. AHCPR Publication no. 95-0046. Rockville, MD: U.S. Department of Health and Human Services, Public Health Service, Agency for Health Care Policy and Research, 1995.

Schriger DL. Training panels in methodology. In: McCormick KA, Moore SR, Siegel RA (Eds). Clinical Practice Guideline Development: Methodology Perspectives. AHCPR Publication no. 95-0009. Rockville, MD: U.S. Department of Health and Human Services, Public Health Service, Agency for Health Care Policy and Research, 1994.

Schug SA, Zech D, Dörr U. Cancer pain management according to WHO analgesic guidelines. J Pain Symptom Manage 1990; 5:27–32.

Spross JA, McGuire DB, Schmitt RM. Oncology Nursing Society position paper on cancer pain. Part I. Oncol Nurs Forum 1990; 17:595–614, 751–760, 943–955.

Takeda F. Results of field testing in Japan of the WHO draft interim guidelines on relief of cancer pain. Pain Clin 1986; 1:83–89.

Ventafridda V, Bonezzi C, Caraceni A, et al. Antidepressants for cancer pain and other painful syndromes with deafferentation component comparison of amitryptyline and tradozone. Ital J Neurol Sci 1987; 8:579–587.

Ventafridda V, Caraceni A, Gamba A. Field-testing of the WHO Guidelines for Cancer Pain Relief: summary report of demonstration projects. In: Foley KM, Bonica JJ, Ventafridda V (Eds). Proceedings of the Second International Congress on Pain, Advances in Pain Research and Therapy, Vol. 16. New York: Raven Press, Ltd., 1992, pp 451–464.

Walker VA, Hoskins PJ, Hanks GW, White ID. Evaluation of WHO Analgesic Guidelines for Cancer Pain in a hospital-based palliative care unit. J Pain Symptom Manage 1988; 3:145–149.

Ward SE, Goldberg N, Miller-McCauley V, et al. Patient-related barriers to management of cancer pain. Pain 1993; 52:319–324.

Zech DFJ, Grond SUA, Lynch J, Herterl D, Lehmann KA. Validation of World Health Organization Guideline for cancer pain relief: a 10-year prospective study. Pain 1995; 63:65–76.

Correspondence to: Richard Payne, MD, Department of Neuro-Oncology, University of Texas M. D. Anderson Cancer Center, 1515 Holcombe Blvd., Box 8, Houston, TX 77030, USA. Tel: 713-794-4998; Fax: 713-794-4999; email: rp@utmdacc.mda.uth.tmc.edu.

Part II

Cancer Pain Assessment:
Research and Clinical Issues

Assessment and Treatment of Cancer Pain,
Progress in Pain Research and Management,
Vol. 12, edited by R. Payne, R.B. Patt, and
C.S. Hill, IASP Press, Seattle, © 1998.

3

Culture and Pain Assessment in Hispanic Patients

Guadalupe Palos

Department of Neuro-Oncology, Pain Research Group,
The University of Texas M. D. Anderson Cancer Center, Houston, Texas, USA

Recent changes in demographic trends in the United States, such as the significant increase in the Hispanic population, have prompted clinicians and policy makers to reevaluate the barriers, practice standards, and treatment outcomes related to pain assessment and management in this population. Despite some elements of universality in a person's response to a diagnosis of cancer, each patient represents a cultural background, beliefs, and behaviors that can influence any aspect of the cancer experience for the patient, the family, and the provider, including how cancer pain is expressed, understood, and dealt with.

As early as the 1950s, investigators reported variations in the pain experience between cultural or ethnic groups (Zborowski 1952; Zola 1966; Lipton and Marbach 1984). Despite these early attempts to study this problem, research on these variations and the integration of cross-cultural knowledge in the assessment and management of cancer pain continues to receive limited scientific attention. This chapter will focus on current theories of culture, ethnicity, and acculturation and describe some of the characteristics and values of the Hispanic population that need to be addressed in conducting effective pain assessments. The chapter also will discuss limitations of current theories or research and their influence on methods, tool development, and practice related to pain assessment in Hispanic populations. To conclude, the chapter introduces a model for developing a culturally competent approach to cancer pain management—one that integrates the world views of patients with a biomedical perspective to formulate an ethnorelative approach to cancer pain assessment and management.

WORLD VIEWS, CULTURE, AND ACCULTURATION

We live in a culturally diverse and pluralistic society in which culture does not always apply to race, ethnic background, or country of origin. Culture can be determined by religion or practices related to age—as in the culture of violent adolescent gangs or in the isolation of the elderly. Culture can even be ascertained by gender, sexual preference, or, as noted by the anthropologist Oscar Lewis (1966), by wealth or poverty. A person's cultural roots or heritage can influence behavioral patterns, including pain behavior (Bates 1987; Cleeland 1990; Spector 1991; Edwards 1992). In an effort to explore the factors that influence a person's cultural roots, Kleinman (1980) developed a cultural systems model that explores the overlap and interaction of three social worlds: the professional or contemporary biomedical world, the social-support or popular world, and the ethnic or folk medicine world. He described how behavior, beliefs, relationships, and use or nonuse of health care services are affected when a patient with a particular social support and ethnic medical universe interacts with the biomedical world (Palos 1997). For example, an elderly Hispanic man coming to the pain clinic for an initial visit may arrive about 30–45 minutes after his scheduled time and may be accompanied by many family members. The clinician, whose primary goal is to provide optimum pain relief within a designated time, may not understand the differences in the patient's and provider's meaning of time, the significance of introducing oneself to the patient and the family members before any assessment begins, and the importance of asking about nontraditional methods such as prayers or folk remedies that the patient may be using for pain relief. Clinicians need to understand how the interaction of these worlds can create barriers to effective assessment of pain and to patient compliance with a recommended pain treatment plan.

Understanding begins by learning concepts and terms that are integral to developing cross-cultural knowledge and competency. Table I lists the terms that are relevant to understanding culture. Max Weber and Emile Durkheim reviewed the concept of culture in the early 1900s (COSSMHO, 1995). These social scientists found that non-Western subgroups of European societies do not view the relationship between individuals and their societies in the same manner as do most other Western Europeans or Americans. They proposed that some of the major cultural foundations of groups should be viewed as norms evolving from a dominant family value that varies from culture to culture. Weber and Durkheim showed that culture functions as a framework or a "seamless web" that provides an understanding or way of seeing the world or a set of values that aids in determining response to various stimuli. Other researchers have found that culture has a functional

Table I
Key terms relevant to cross-cultural theory

Ancestry
Refers to a person's specific nationality or group, or the country in which the person, their ancestors, or their parents resided before migrating to the person's current nation (Spector 1991).

Culture
The sum total of socially inherited characteristics of a human group that comprises everything which one generation can tell, convey, or hand down to the next (Fejos 1959).

Learned patterns of living, including health beliefs and behaviors, that have been handed down from generation to generation (Endelman and Mandel 1986).

Ethnicity
A subset of a larger cultural system, incorporating a sense of belonging to a specific group (Bates and Edwards 1992).

---

purpose that provides either a set of rules or framework needed for a group to survive, or an integrative purpose that permits individuals to form a sense of identity (Bates and Edwards 1992; Kawaska-Singer 1994). Some definitions, such as those posed by Fejos (1959) and Endelman and Mandel (1986), imply that human groups must exist for a sufficiently long time to develop their own cultural world. However, current societal changes require a definition that addresses certain demographic characteristics or personal preferences including, age, gender, economic status, sexual preference, or even geographic residence, such as urban or rural settings. Thus, the definition proposed by Bates and Edwards (1992) seems more appropriate for current trends in societal values in which culture is "patterned ways in which humans have learned to think about and act in their world."

Culture, ethnicity, and ancestry have also been regarded as interchangeable terms; yet, the definitions listed in Table I show the different meanings associated with each one. Spector suggests that ancestry refers to a person's specific nationality or country in which the person, ancestors, or parents lived before migrating to the United States. Bates and Edwards (1992) suggest that ethnicity develops a sense of belonging to a specific group. According to Kawaska-Singer (1994), culture tends to refer to a single group while ethnicity refers to a multicultural context or a social/political construct. Used in this context, ethnicity may create barriers to understanding, communication, and practice. For example, a study of ethnic differences has shown ethnicity to be a factor in pain management in the emergency room for patients with bone fractures (Todd et al. 1993). The study found that Hispanics were twice as likely to receive inadequate pain management compared to their white counterparts. Although the researchers did not iden-

dementia. It has been estimated that as many as 15% of elderly patients may have some cognitive impairment. Among nursing home residents, over 50% may have substantial dementia or psychological illness. These patients typically have deficits in memory, attention, visual spatial skills, and language (aphasia). Behavioral problems are not uncommon.

Despite these potential barriers, Parmelee et al. (1993) found no evidence of "masking" of pain complaints by cognitive impairment among subjects in a study of 758 nursing home residents from a single long-term care facility in Philadelphia (Parmelee et al. 1993). The authors of this study concluded that although elderly patients slightly underreported pain, their reports were no less valid than those of cognitively intact patients. Findings from our studies suggest that most cognitively impaired elderly patients in pain can respond to available pain intensity scales if they are administered in a manner sensitive to the patients' disabilities (Ferrell et al. 1995). These patients often require time to assimilate questions about pain and respond appropriately. They have limited attention spans and are easily distracted. It is helpful to provide visual cues in large print and prepare these patients by providing adequate ambient light and hearing devices when necessary.

Despite these issues, most cognitively impaired patients appear able to reliably report current pain. The extent to which they are able to accurately report pain in the last week or in the last month remains unknown. Clinical experiences suggest that cognitively impaired patients will likely require frequent assessment of current pain to ensure effectiveness of management strategies (Ferrell et al. 1995). It is also clear that much additional work is needed to establish methods for pain evaluation among those who are mute or who have more profound impairment.

PAIN MANAGEMENT STRATEGIES IN THE ELDERLY

Pain in the elderly is most commonly treated with oral analgesic medications. The analgesic drugs of choice for elderly patients are those with the lowest side-effect profiles. Adverse effects are more common in the elderly including drug-drug interactions, drug-induced disease, and untoward drug reactions. Thus, several factors should be considered in prescribing analgesic drugs for elderly patients.

Acetaminophen is the most often prescribed analgesic in nursing homes (Ferrell et al. 1990, 1995). It appears to be reasonably safe and effective for mild and moderate pain complaints in this population. Alternatives to acetaminophen, most commonly nonsteroidal anti-inflammatory drugs (NSAIDs), must be weighed against their known side-effect profiles.

NSAIDs often work well for elderly persons whether given alone or in combination with opioid analgesics for inflammatory conditions and metastatic bone pain. However, the risk of peptic ulcer disease, renal injury, and bleeding diathesis is much higher in the elderly compared to younger persons. Among the frail elderly, these drugs occasionally cause constipation, cognitive impairment, and headaches (Ferrell 1995).

A recent review noted that older persons have generally been omitted from clinical trials of NSAIDs (Rochon et al. 1993). Between 1987 and 1990, 83 randomized trials involving almost 10,000 patients included only 203 patients over age 65 and none over age 85. This situation is particularly disturbing given the high incidence of gastric bleeding associated with NSAIDs in elderly persons. Griffin and colleagues estimated that the relative risk of peptic ulcer disease associated with NSAIDs in the elderly was more than four-fold higher (relative risk 4.1; 95% confidence interval 3.5 to 4.7) compared to elderly persons who did not use them (Griffin et al. 1991). Moreover, the relative risk increases with dose from 2.8 among the lowest dosage to 8.0 for the highest dosage.

Although opioid analgesic drugs will be discussed in more detail elsewhere, some opioids require special mention. Propoxyphene is a controversial drug that is probably overprescribed for elderly persons. Reports suggest an efficacy no better than aspirin or acetaminophen, and it has a potential for dependency and renal injury with long-term use. Pentazocine should be avoided because it frequently causes delirium and agitation in elderly persons. Meperidine is also particularly hazardous in the elderly, especially for patients with renal impairment. The active metabolite normeperidine is particularly prone to accumulate and cause delirium and seizure activity. Methadone should be used with caution because of its long half-life and propensity to accumulate. Finally, transdermal fentanyl is an extremely potent drug that, because of its unique transdermal delivery system and prolonged half-life, is particularly dangerous in opiate-naive persons (Ferrell 1993, 1995).

Adjuvant analgesic drugs, such as antidepressants, neuroleptics, and some systemically administered local anesthetic drugs, may be helpful in some patients with recalcitrant pain syndromes. Of concern are their frequent high side-effect profiles in the elderly, who are particularly sensitive to the anticholinergic effects of amitriptyline and other antidepressants. Elderly patients are also particularly sensitive to the central nervous system side effects of neuroleptic and local anesthetic drugs. In general, these drugs should probably be reserved for patients with severe pain and disability when other treatments have failed (Ferrell 1995).

Many nonpharmacologic pain management strategies are effective in elderly persons, especially when combined with drug strategies. Most nondrug

In the United States, close to two million elderly persons reside in almost 20,000 nursing homes (Ouslander et al. 1991). This is almost triple the number of acute care hospitals and double the number of hospital beds. It is estimated that about 5% of elderly persons reside in nursing homes. However, this figure is somewhat misleading. Among those 65–74 years of age, less than 2% live in nursing homes. The figure rises to about 7% for those aged 75–84, while almost 20% of those over age 85 live in nursing homes. Longitudinal studies in the United States suggest that persons 65 years of age and older a have better than 40% chance of spending some time in a nursing home before they die. Of those who enter nursing homes, 55% will spend at least one year there and over 20% will spend more than five years. Nursing homes are needed not simply because of disease and functional disabilities, but also due to a lack of social support. Many nursing home patients have outlived close family or the family becomes exhausted after caring for a patient for a long time. Among the most disturbing symptoms that result in early family fatigue are incontinence and behavioral problems such as wandering or disruptive actions often associated with dementia and Alzheimer's disease (Ouslander 1989; Ouslander et al. 1991).

Patients in alternative care settings such as nursing homes and those confined to their homes present substantial challenges to medical care and pain management (Ferrell 1994, 1995, in press). In these settings evaluation and treatment are more difficult due to logistical barriers such as the lack of availability of laboratory, radiographic, and pharmaceutical services that have the capacity to respond rapidly. Many physicians do not see patients at home or in nursing homes and those who do frequently provide substandard care. These patients are often sent to distant clinics or the emergency department, where they are evaluated by personnel who are generally not familiar with their baseline status and goals of care, and who lack training or interest in the care of frail and dependent elderly patients (Ferrell 1995).

For these patients, physicians have a responsibility to help establish a plan of care that is reasonable given the resources and skills available. Medication regimens and treatment strategies need to be simple so that compliance is maximized and need for nighttime monitoring is minimized. Long-acting analgesics should be used to provide longer duration of action and fewer doses for caregivers to administer. Pain must be acknowledged, anticipated, and prevented by using routine around-the-clock dosing whenever appropriate. Short-acting analgesics should be prescribed and available for breakthrough pain or for pain associated with moving about, bathing, or other potentially painful activities. It is important to remember that most nursing homes and home care settings have limited access to pharmacy resources. Contingency plans for pain management must be anticipated so that delays do not occur during medication changes or dosage adjustments. State regulatory requirements for multiple-copy prescriptions may be a substantial barrier to effective pain management in this setting; careful planning is the only solution.

SUMMARY AND FUTURE DIRECTIONS

Pain is a common problem among a growing segment of the population that can be considered elderly. This frail population is substantially different compared to younger adults, with unique physiology, sociology, and medical care needs. Physicians, nurses, and other health care professionals must understand the constellation of multiple disease possibilities and interrelationships that influence how older persons behave when they are ill. Moreover, professionals must be aware of their own attitudes and beliefs regarding aging and death and how these views influence the delivery of care to the elderly. The multitude and complexity of medical, psychological, and social problems that often affect elderly patients require that professionals cooperate to provide a team approach to care.

Substantial research is desperately needed to further our understanding of pain and its management among elderly persons. More valid and reliable pain measures, function scales, and behavior scales should be established in this population. New drugs with milder side-effect profiles are urgently needed. Nondrug strategies require further investigation. And, comparative studies using long-term outcomes should be conducted. As the need for health systems for elderly people continues to grow, our most important obligation is to provide comfort and effective pain control for these patients during their remaining time.

REFERENCES

Abrass IB. Biology of aging. In: Wilson JD, Braunwald E, Isselbacher KJ, et al. (Eds). Principles of Internal Medicine, 12th ed. New York: McGraw-Hill, 1991.

Baime MJ, Nelson JB, Castell DO. Aging of the gastrointestinal system. In: Hazzard WR, Bierman EL, Blass JP, Ettinger WH Jr, Halter JB (Eds). Principles of Geriatric Medicine and Gerontology. New York: McGraw Hill, 1994, pp 665–681.

Cakour MC, Gibson SJ, Bradbeer M, Helme RD. The effect of age on Aδ- and C-fiber thermal pain perception. Pain 1996; 64:143–152.

Coleman PD, Flood DG. Neuron numbers and dendritic extent in normal aging and Alzheimer's disease. Neurobiology of Aging 1987; 8:521.

Crook J, Rideout E, Brown G. The prevalence of pain complaints among a general population. Pain 1984; 18:299–314.

Davis MA. Epidemiology of osteoarthritis. Clin Geriatr Med 1988; 4(2):241–255.

Egbert AM, Parks LH, Short LM, Burnett ML. Randomized trial of postoperative patient controlled analgesia vs intramuscular narcotics in frail elderly men. Arch Intern Med 1990; 150:1897–1903.

Ettinger WH, et al. A randomized trial comparing aerobic exercise and resistance exercise with a health education program in older adults with knee osteoarthritis: The Fitness Arthritis and Seniors Trial (FAST). JAMA 1997; 277(1):25–31.

Ferrell BA. Pain management in elderly people. J Am Geriatr Soc 1991; 39:64–73.

Ferrell BA. Pain. In: Yoshikawa TT, Cobbs EL, Brummel-Smith K (Eds). Ambulatory Geriatric Care. St. Louis: Mosby, 1993, pp 382–390.

Ferrell BA. Pain evaluation and management. In: Katz P, Kane RL (Eds). Quality Care in Geriatric Settings. New York: Springer, 1995a, pp 195–209.

Ferrell BA. Pain evaluation and management in the nursing home. Ann Intern Med 1995; 123:681–687.

Ferrell BA. Home care. In: Cassel CK, et al. (Eds). Geriatric Medicine, 3rd ed. New York: Springer Verlag, 1997, pp 109–118.

Ferrell BA, Ferrell BR, Osterweil D. Pain in the nursing home. J Am Geriatr Soc 1990; 38:409–414.

Ferrell BA, Ferrell BR, Rivera L. Pain in cognitively impaired nursing home patients. J Pain Symptom Manage 1995; 10:591–595.

Ferrell BA, Josephson KR, Pollan AM, Loy S, Ferrell BR. A randomized trial of walking versus physical methods for chronic pain management. Aging: Clinical and Experimental Research, in press.

Ferrell BR, Rhiner M, Cohen MZ, Grant M. Pain as a metaphor for illness. Part 1: Impact of cancer pain on family caregivers. Oncol Nurs Forum 1991; 18:1303–1309.

Foley K. Pain in the elderly. In: Hazzard WR, Bierman EL, Blass JP, Ettinger WH Jr, Halter JB (Eds). Principles of Geriatric Medicine and Gerontology. New York: McGraw Hill, 1994.

Fulop T, Worum I, Csongor J, Foris G, Leavey A. Body composition in elderly people. Gerontology 1985; 31:6–14.

Gordon RS. Pain in the elderly. JAMA 1979; 241:2191–2192.

Griffin MR, Piper JM, Dougherty JR, Snowden M, Ray WA. Nonsteroidal antiinflammatory drug use and increased risk for peptic ulcer disease in elderly persons. Ann Intern Med 1991; 114.257–263.

Harkins SA. Pain perceptions in the old. Clin Geriatr Med 1996; 12(3):435–459.

Hazzard WR, Bierman EL, Blass JP, Ettinger WH Jr, Halter JB (Eds). Principles of Geriatric Medicine and Gerontology. New York: McGraw Hill, 1994.

Lakatta EG. Changes in cardiovascular function with aging. Eur Heart J 1990; 11(Suppl C):22–28.

Lindeman RD, Tobin J, Shock NW. Longitudinal studies of the rate of decline in renal function with age. J Am Geriatr Soc 1985; 33:278–285.

Manton KG. Epidemiological, demographic and social correlates of disability among the elderly. Milbank Q 1989; 67:13.

Miller RA. The biology of aging and longevity. In: Hazzard WR, Bierman EL, Blass JP, Ettinger WH Jr, Halter JB (Eds). Principles of Geriatric Medicine and Gerontology. New York: McGraw Hill, 1994, pp 3–18.

Nishikawa ST, Ferrell BA. Pain assessment in the elderly. Clinical Geriatrics and Issues in Long Term Care 1993; 1:15–28.

Ouslander JG. Medical care in the nursing home. JAMA 1989; 262:2582–2590.

Ouslander GJ, Osterweil D, Morley J. Medical Care in the Nursing Home, New York: McGraw-Hill, 1991, pp 3–19.

Parmelee PA, Smith B, Katz IR. Pain complaints and cognitive status among elderly institution residents. J Am Geriatr Soc 1993; 41:517–522.

Perneger TV, Whelton PK, Klag MJ. Risk of kidney failure associated with use of acetaminophen, aspirin, and nonsteroidal antiinflammatory drugs. N Engl J Med 1994; 331:1675–1679.

Province MA, Hadley EC, Hornbrook MC, et al. The effects of exercise on falls in elderly patients. A preplanned meta-analysis of the FICSIT Trials. Frailty and injuries: Cooperative studies of intervention techniques. JAMA 1995; 273:1381–1383.

Rochon PA, Fortin PR, Dear KB, Minaker KL, Chalmers TC. Reporting of age in data in clinical trials of arthritis. Arch Intern Med 1993; 153:243–248.

Short P, Leon J. Use of home and community services by persons aged 65 and older with functional disabilities. National Medical Expenditure Survey Findings 5, DHHS Publication no. (PHS) 90-4366. Rockville, MD: US Department of Health and Human Services, Public Health Service, Agency for Health Care Policy and Research, 1990.

Stone R, Cafferata GL, Sangl J. Caregivers of frail elderly: a national profile. Gerontologist 1987; 27:616.

Turk DC, Melzack R (Eds). Handbook of Pain Assessment. New York: Guilford Press, 1992.

Wedon M, Ferrell BR. Professional and ethical considerations in the use of high tech pain management. Oncol Nurs Forum 1991; 18:1135–1143.

Williams ME. Clinical management of the elderly patient. In: Hazzard WR, Bierman EL, Blass JP, Ettinger WH Jr, Halter JB (Eds). Principles of Geriatric Medicine and Gerontology. New York: McGraw Hill, 1994, pp 195–201.

Correspondence to: Bruce A. Ferrell, MD, Sepulveda VA Medical Center (11E), 16111 Plummer St., Sepulveda, CA 91343, USA.

Assessment and Treatment of Cancer Pain,
Progress in Pain Research and Management,
Vol. 12, edited by R. Payne, R.B. Patt, and
C.S. Hill, IASP Press, Seattle, © 1998.

5

Radiological Imaging in the Cancer Patient with Back Pain

Norman E. Leeds and Ashok J. Kumar

*Department of Radiology, The University of Texas
M. D. Anderson Cancer Center, Houston, Texas, USA*

In imaging the spine in cancer patients who are experiencing pain, the structures to target are the osseous components, vertebrae, posterior elements, transverse and spinous processes and intervertebral disks, the components within the spinal canal, the spinal cord, nerve roots and surrounding dura mater and leptomeninges, the adjacent paravertebral soft tissues, and the brachial and lumbosacral plexuses. The objective is to determine the cause of back pain in the cancer patient and whether the pain is produced by metastases or from its mimics.

OSSEOUS SPINAL STRUCTURES

A bone scan is often the first procedure in the examination of the osseous spinal structures in cancer patients. The bone scan does not often show marrow-replacement disease, but it does frequently indicate osseous disease. Spinal fractures are not usually visible on the bone scan during the first 48 hours after the injury, but ensuing scans will show the fractures for up to one year (Wiener et al. 1989).

It is important to avoid potential pitfalls in discriminating between benign and malignant lesions that cause a collapse of the vertebral bodies. A review of 659 autopsies of cancer patients with collapsed vertebral bodies revealed benign lesions in at least one-third of the vertebral bodies (Fornasier and Czitron 1979). Benign lesions that must be differentiated from malignant disease include degenerative disease of the spine, acute fractures, insufficiency fractures, hemangiomas, Paget's disease, radiation-induced osteitis, and inflammatory lesions.

DEGENERATIVE SPINAL DISEASE

A radionuclide bone scan that reveals increased uptake may be due to degenerative disk disease or spondylosis and may require magnetic resonance imaging (MRI) to exclude the possibility of metastasis. For example, a patient with a liver neoplasm who was experiencing back pain was examined at an outside facility. A radionuclide bone scan suggested metastatic disease. The scan showed diffuse uptake in the lumbar region, which is more characteristic of spondylosis than metastasis (Evan-Sapir et al. 1993) (Fig. 1A). A subsequent MRI scan revealed no radiological manifestations of metastasis, but rather degenerative disk disease with marrow preservation (Fig. 1B). No abnormal enhancement was observed after contrast administration. The characteristics observed were marrow preservation without signal changes except for those adjacent to the disk space, e.g., the presence of fatty infiltration, spur formation, granulation tissue, or fibrosis (Modic et al. 1988).

RADIATION-INDUCED CHANGES

Patients who have received radiation treatment are at risk for osseous abnormalities. These abnormalities include radiation-induced insufficiency fractures (particularly of the sacrum), osteitis of the vertebral body, and neoplasms.

Bluemke et al. 1994 observed abnormalities in bone growth in patients with radiation-induced osteitis as a consequence of damage to osteoblasts, which results in deformations of the bony matrix. The response to this type of pathophysiological change is an attempt to repair the resultant damage by bone deposition in unaffected trabeculae in the area. The authors observed varying patterns of osteopenia, foci of coarse trabeculation, and zones of increased bone density (Bluemke et al. 1994). Fat deposition also occurred in the damaged marrow six weeks after therapy. These findings may mimic metastasis. A prior history of radiation therapy in the affected region may be helpful in making the correct diagnosis.

Patients with pelvic neoplasms often receive irradiation to control or eradicate cancer. However, radiation therapy may alter the bony matrix. Consequent to this structural damage, the residual bone may be unable to withstand the accompanying stress and strain of bearing weight. Fractures may develop, particularly in the sacrum (Boldly et al. 1993). These fractures are uncommon in premenopausal women but occur in postmenopausal women after pelvic irradiation (Blomlie et al. 1993). For example, the MRI scan of a patient with pelvic pain revealed a fracture of the sacrum and well-defined

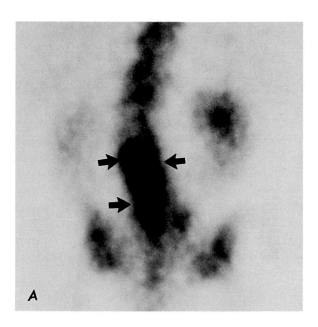

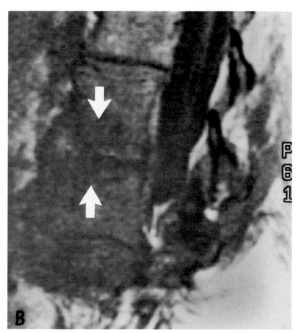

Fig. 1. Degenerative spondylosis. **A.** Bone scan reveals diffuse, abnormal uptake of radionuclide (arrows) in the lower lumbar region. **B.** Sagittal T1-weighted MRI scan. The disk space at L4–L5 level is markedly narrowed with band-like, low signal intensity involving the L4 and L5 vertebral bodies (arrows) paralleling the disk space.

zone of low signal intensity within the left sacral ala (Fig. 2). The diminished signal intensity on the T1-weighted axial image was caused by edema. The bright signal in the ilium reflects marrow fat replacement secondary to irradiation. The factor that differentiates a post-irradiation insufficiency fracture from metastatic disease is the presence of a focal lesion with well-defined margins (Blomlie et al. 1993; Baker and Siegal 1994). Lesions caused by edema are hypointense on T1-weighted images owing to increased accumulation of water, and at times may reveal fractures. Computed tomography (CT) scans will often clearly delineate a fracture that may not be apparent on the MRI scan. Another cause of insufficiency fractures is steroid treatment, particularly in postmenopausal women.

A 32-year-old man with melanoma and a mediastinal mass treated with radon-seed implants experienced ill-defined thoracic pain. MRI scan of the mid-thoracic region showed vertical bands of decreased intensity in the anterior aspect of adjacent vertebral bodies just behind the mediastinal mass (Fig. 3A). Intravenous contrast administration demonstrated localized contrast enhancement in these areas (Fig. 3B). The fast spin-echo T2-weighted sequence used with fat saturation technique produced a hyperintense signal (Fig. 3C). Radiation-induced osteitis was suspected in this case given the appropriate history and the localized lesions juxtaposed to the treated

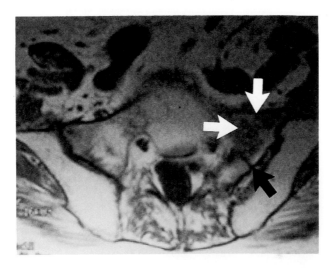

Fig. 2. Radiation-induced insufficiency fracture simulating bony metastasis. Axial T1-weighted MRI scan of the sacrum. Following radiation therapy for a pelvic tumor, the patient experienced severe pelvic pain necessitating an MRI scan to rule out metastasis. A radiation-induced fracture of the left sacrum (black arrow) is associated with well-demarcated low signal intensity of the ala adjacent to the sacrum (white arrows) caused by edema, not to be mistaken for a metastatic lesion.

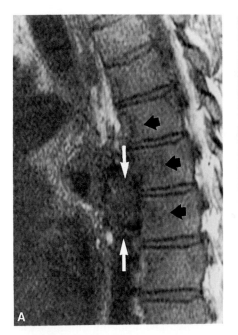

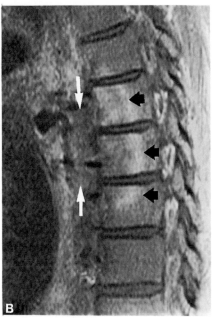

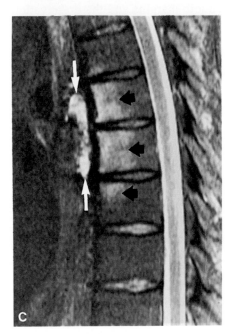

Fig. 3. Radiation-induced osteitis of thoracic vertebral bodies simulating metastasis. A 32-year-old patient with mediastinal metastatic lymphadenopathy from melanoma treated with an interstitial radonseed implant followed by administration of external beam radiation for five weeks. After the patient developed shooting pain in the left upper thorax, an MRI scan was performed to exclude bony metastasis and cord compression. T1-weighted sagittal MRI scan of the thoracic spine reveals bands of low signal intensity in the anterior portion of the adjacent vertebral bodies (black arrows in **A**), abnormal contrast enhancement in postcontrast T1-weighted image (black arrows in **B**) and increased signal intensity in fast spin echo T2-weighted sequence with fat saturation (black arrows in **C**). Mediastinal lymphadenopathy is marked by white arrows.

mediastinal adenopathy. These lesions were atypical of metastases. Radiation-induced lesions, like pelvic insufficiency fractures, are usually sharply demarcated and located within the radiation field. Radiation-induced sarcomas have a prolonged latency and may occur four to 55 years after therapy (Bluemke et al. 1994).

NONMALIGNANT AND MALIGNANT FRACTURES OF THE VERTEBRAL BODIES

The separation of acute metastatic fractures from those that are nonmetastatic is important because of the difference in therapy. Among patients with known primary neoplasms who have vertebral fractures, one-third will have nonmetastatic lesions (Fornasier and Czitron 1978). Krishnamurthy and colleagues (1977) demonstrated that the vertebral body was affected in 39% of patients with metastatic disease and that it was the most common osseous site affected.

In the patient with nonmetastatic nontraumatic fracture, the lesion is usually band-like with preservation of marrow. The imaging findings that suggest a nonmetastatic lesion include smooth margins and the preservation of marrow because the abnormality is the result of a loss of bone substance while the marrow remains intact. The affected vertebral body in patients with nonmetastatic fractures will often revert to a normal signal in one to three months (Yuh et al. 1989). In an MRI study of benign versus metastatic fractures, An and colleagues (1995) reported high sensitivity (85–92%) and specificity (79–100%) with two experienced readers. They also reported that malignant lesions were not missed if contrast enhancement was used.

Although a paraspinal mass is more common with malignant lesions, it can be observed with benign processes (Yuh et al. 1989; An et al. 1995; Cuénod et al. 1996). The paraspinal mass tends to be diffuse in benign lesions and focal in malignant lesions. In patients with benign lesions, Cuénod et al. (1996) reported the presence in the lesions of bone fragments from the superior portion of the vertebral body, smooth margins around a compressed zone, and four patterns (of band-like lesions) in the sagittal plane of the MRI scan. They also observed that signal intensity remains normal in the nonaffected portion of the vertebral body (preserved marrow).

Cuénod et al. (1996) emphasized the following observations pertinent to the patient with a malignant lesion: retropulsion of the posterior portion of the vertebral body, pedicle involvement, nonhomogeneous signal intensity in all or part of the vertebral body, a round or irregular lesion within a noncollapsed vertebral body, and the presence of epidural soft-tissue components that are rare in nonmalignant fractures. Whether focal or diffuse, a paraspinal soft tissue mass can occur in benign fractures but is much more common in malignant lesions (Yuh et al. 1989).

Yuh et al. made two important points that aid in the differentiation of malignant and nonmalignant lesions. One point is that a malignant lesion invariably leads to a fracture when marrow replacement by the tumor occupies the entire vertebral body. The second is that the trabecular cortex is destroyed in malignant lesions.

A patient with carcinoma of the lung developed severe back pain. The MRI scan revealed sharply demarcated, band-like lesions in the L2 and L3 vertebral bodies with preservation of the remainder of the marrow, a characteristic of benign disease (Figs. 4A–C). The patient also had acute and chronic benign fractures in the thoracic spine (Figs. 4D–F). A bone scan revealed nonspecific uptake in the spine (Fig. 4G). Another patient had

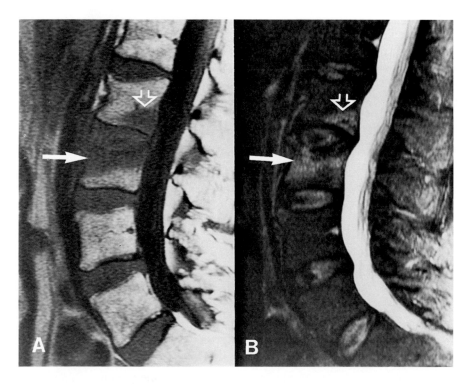

Fig. 4. Benign nontraumatic osteopenic fractures. A patient with carcinoma of the lung developed severe back pain necessitating an MRI scan of the spine to rule out metastasis. **A.** Sagittal T1-weighted MRI scan of the lumbar spine. The L3 (white arrow) and L2 (open arrow) vertebral bodies demonstrate band-like areas of low signal intensity. **B.** Increased signal in the fast spin-echo T2-weighted sequence with fat saturation.

Fig. 4. C. Abnormal enhancement following intravenous contrast administration due to end-plate collapse. **D.** T1-weighted MRI scan of the thoracic spine revealed an acute osteopenic fracture of the inferior end plate of a midthoracic vertebral body with low signal intensity (white arrow). Open arrows point to several chronic fractures. **E.** Increased signal intensity in the fast spin-echo T2-weighted sequence with fat saturation (white arrow).

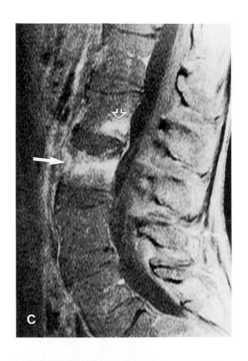

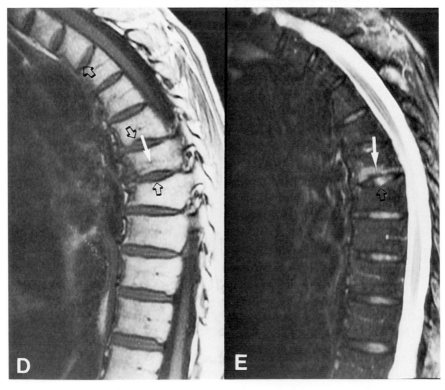

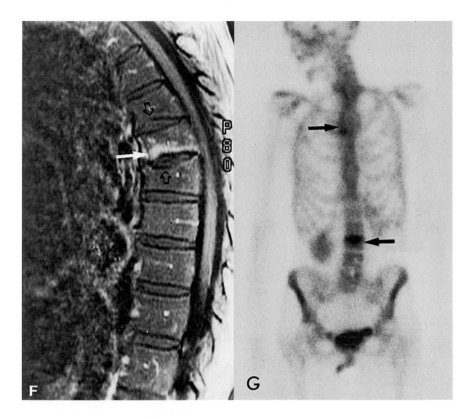

Fig. 4. F. Abnormal contrast enhancement in the postcontrast image (white arrow). **G.** A bone scan revealed nonspecific uptake in the thoracic and lumbar spine.

acute and chronic fractures in the thoracic and lumbar spine, and metastatic disease in the fourth lumbar vertebral body without a fracture (Fig. 5).

In metastatic disease in the vertebral body, lesions may be single or multiple and may demonstrate the following characteristics: retropulsion of the posterior portion of the vertebral body (Fig. 6); pedicle involvement and a nonhomogeneous pattern of involvement of the entire body (without a fracture) (Fig. 6); epidural mass (Fig. 6); or focal, paravertebral soft-tissue mass (Fig. 7) (Cuénod et al. 1996). Mehta et al. 1995 stressed the value of short-angle inversion recovery, fast spin-echo T2-weighted images, and inversion-recovery with fast spin-echo in evaluating vertebral-body metastasis. They also observed that inversion-recovery sequences, although not good in visualizing the epidural component, were better for demonstrating the marrow replacement changes.

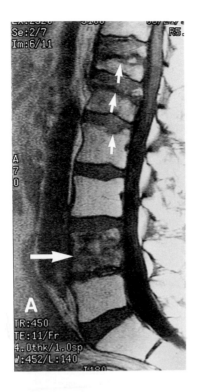

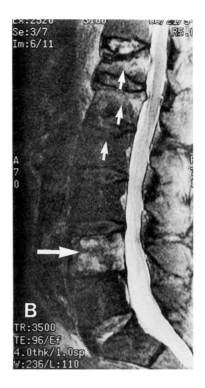

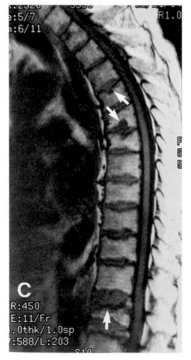

Fig. 5. Osteopenic fracture and a metastatic lesion. A sagittal MRI scan of the lumbar and thoracic spine was obtained in a patient with breast cancer. Nonmetastatic, osteopenic compression fractures of the L1 and L2 vertebral bodies and several thoracic vertebral bodies were noted (small white arrows in **A–C**). In addition, a diffuse nonhomogeneous, abnormal signal is seen at L4 both in the T1-weighted pulse sequence (large arrow in **A**) and in the fast spin-echo T2-weighted fat saturation pulse sequence (large arrow in **B**), characteristic of a metastatic lesion.

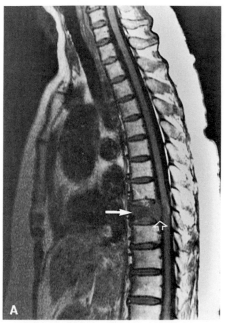

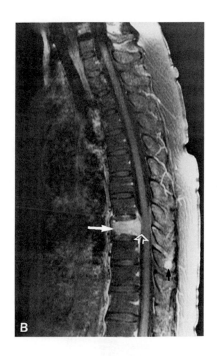

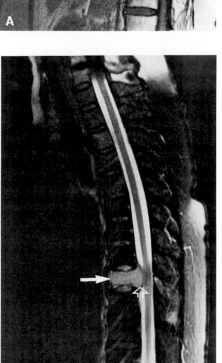

Fig. 6. Metastasis to a thoracic vertebral body. **A.** Classical appearance of metastasis to a thoracic vertebral body with low signal intensity in a T1-weighted pulse sequence (white arrow). **B.** Abnormal enhancement in post-contrast T1-weighted image (white arrow). **C.** Increased signal intensity in a fast spin-echo T2-weighted sequence with fat saturation (white arrow). Retropulsion of the posterior portion of the vertebral body and epidural tumor is also shown (open arrow); this resulted in compression of the adjacent spinal cord. A small bony metastasis (black arrows) to the spinous process of an adjacent vertebral body (B, C) is also observed.

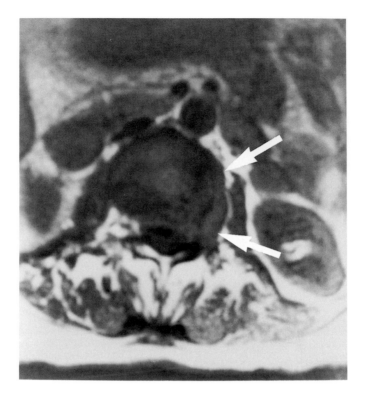

Fig. 7. Bony metastasis from lung carcinoma associated with a localized, left paravertebral soft-tissue mass (arrows).

INFLAMMATORY LESIONS

Inflammatory lesions may simulate metastatic disease (Hovi et al. 1994). Patients with inflammatory lesions often have acute onset of back pain. The development of disk-space involvement, even in the cancer patient, should prompt consideration of an inflammatory process (Darouiche et al. 1992). The lumbar vertebral bodies are the most common site of inflammatory lesions. The lesions usually arise from infections within the pelvis and then spread via epidural veins to the lumbar vertebral bodies. The usual imaging findings include involvement of two adjacent vertebral bodies and the intervening disk space. The lesions are hypointense on T1-weighted images, and often produce a diffuse, paravertebral and epidural mass (Figs. 8, 9B). On T2-weighted images, the intervertebral disk will appear hyperintense, a characteristic that should raise the suspicion of an inflammatory lesion (Fig. 9A) rather than a metastasis.

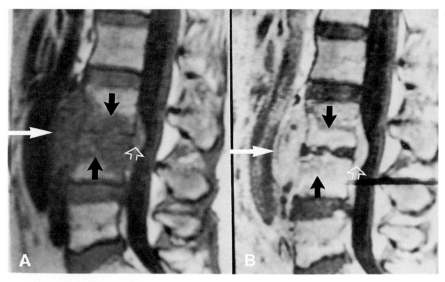

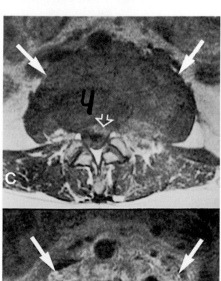

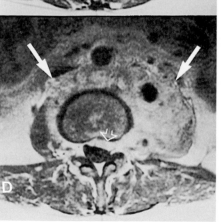

Fig. 8. Osteomyelitis of L3 and L4 vertebral bodies produced by brucella infection. The infected L3 and L4 vertebral bodies show horizontal bands of low signal intensity in a sagittal T1-weighted pulse sequence (black arrows in **A**). The bodies demonstrate intense enhancement following intravenous contrast administration (black arrows in **B**). The disc space between L3 and L4 is narrowed with irregular end plates. Infection of the spine is associated with large prevertebral (white arrows in **A** and **B**) and paravertebral masses on the axial, precontrast, T1-weighted image (white arrows in **C**), with enhancement in the postcontrast study (white arrows in **D**). An epidural abscess compresses the thecal sac (open arrows in **A–D**).

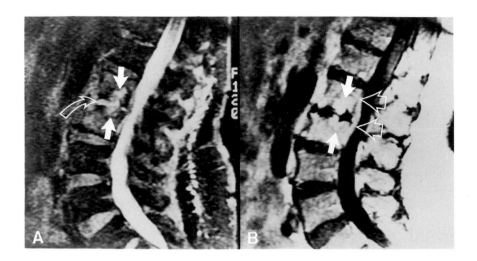

Fig. 9. Osteomyelitis affecting L2 and L3 vertebral bodies. **A.** Sagittal MRI scan using the fast spin-echo T2-weighted fat saturated pulse sequence demonstrates increased signal intensity of diseased vertebral bodies (white arrows) and the disc space between L2–L3 (open curved arrow).**B.** An epidural abscess compressing the thecal sac is observed in a sagittal, postcontrast image (open arrows).

LEPTOMENINGEAL DISEASE

Other potential pathological abnormalities in patients with metastatic disease that may result in back pain and neurological findings are the presence of leptomeningeal disease and involvement of the nerve-root ganglia. Symptoms that may be observed include polyradiculopathy featuring radicular pain, sensory loss, lower motor neuron weakness, and areflexia (Stübgen 1995). In most cases, leptomeningeal seeding is secondary to the shedding of cells from intracranial metastases (Fig. 10). Metastases may occur in the nerve-root ganglia because a blood-spine barrier does not exist at the level of the ganglia (Fig. 11).

BRACHIAL PLEXUS

Involvement of the roots of the brachial plexus is another source of pain in cancer patients that may require investigation. It is important to also examine the cervical spine because the nerve roots that comprise the brachial plexus originate from the cervical spinal cord, specifically the ventral roots originate from C5 through C8. The nerve roots descend between the anterior and middle scalene muscles and enter the supraclavicular fossa;

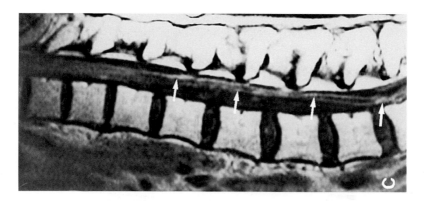

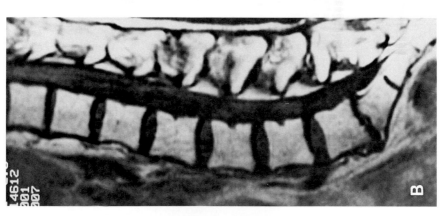

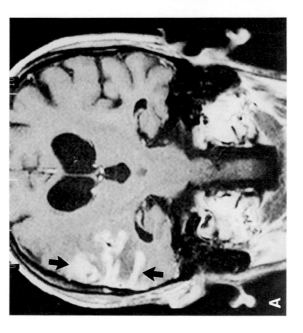

Fig. 10. Leptomeningeal tumor seeding the lumbar subarachnoid space in a patient with lung carcinoma who presented with back pain. **A.** Postcontrast coronal MRI scan of the brain reveals leptomeningeal tumor infiltration of the right frontotemporal operculum (black arrows). Precontrast (**B**) and postcontrast sagittal T1-weighted (**C**) MRI scans of the lumbar spinal canal reveal leptomeningeal dropped metastasis to the lumbar nerve roots (arrows in **C**).

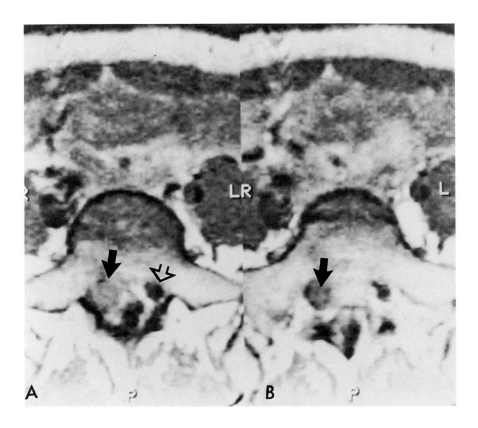

Fig. 11. Breast cancer patient with lumbar radiculopathy suggesting a herniated disc. Postcontrast axial MRI scans of the lumbosacral junction. **A.** The black arrow indicates metastatic involvement of the nerve-root ganglia, and the open arrow indicates normal left S1 nerve root at the neural foramen. **B.** The black arrow indicates metastatic involvement of the nerve root exiting the right neural foramen

they can be identified paralleling and lying just above and posterior to the subclavian artery. The plexus is composed of three trunks, six divisions and three cords (Fig. 12) (Posniak et al. 1993; Russell and Windebank 1994; Iyer et al. 1996). Fat-saturation images should be avoided because the low-intensity nerve roots are best visualized in contrast with the brightness of the surrounding fatty tissue on T1-weighted images (Fig. 13).

Solid tumors spread to the lateral group of axillary nodes, which are in close contact with the lower portion of the plexus (Stübgen 1995). Upper plexus involvement suggests epidural extension of a neoplasm (Stübgen 1995). Symptoms often develop insidiously, with increasing severity followed by progressive weakness (Russell and Windebank 1994). A primary neoplasm is usually present in such cases. Apical neoplasms of the lung

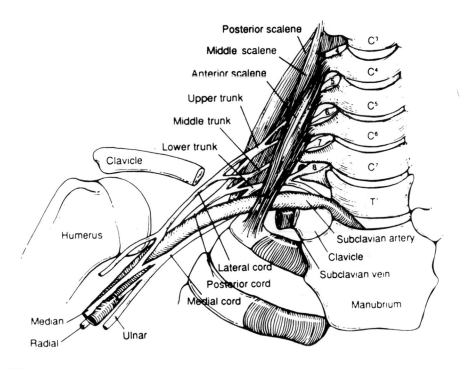

Fig. 12. Anatomy of the brachial plexus (coronal anatomical drawing) (Posniak et al. 1993).

usually affect nerve roots of C8 and T1. Thus, clinical manifestations of solid tumors are often related to direct invasion of nerve roots by tumor or to lymph node involvement (Posniak et al. 1993; Stübgen 1995).

Radiation-induced plexopathy tends to occur when a dose greater than 60 gray (60 Gy) has been administered. Paresthesia and swelling of the extremity are more common than pain (Stübgen 1995). These changes are observed three months to 26 years after treatment (Stübgen 1995). The pathological changes result from perineural fibrosis with obliteration of the nervi vasorum (Posniak et al. 1993). The nerves are usually unaffected because they are resistant to radiation therapy (Posniak et al. 1993). Radiation-induced fibrosis may be unilateral (Fig. 13) or bilateral (Fig. 14), depending upon the treatment portal. In patients with radiation-induced fibrosis, diffuse thickening of the nerve roots can be visualized on T1-weighted images in the coronal plane. On the unaffected side, thin nerve roots can be clearly delineated by the surrounding fat; while on the pathological side, nerve roots are markedly thickened in comparison (Fig. 13) or may be thickened bilaterally (Fig. 14). In a patient with metastasis from a primary lung neoplasm, the metastasis within the lung is recognized invading right side of the neural foramen and the brachial plexus (Fig. 15).

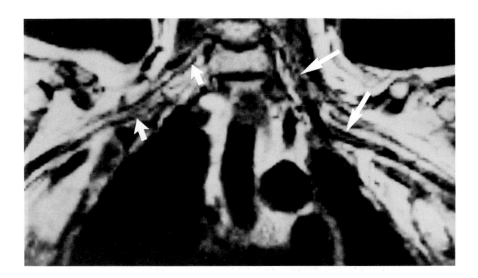

Fig. 13. Radiation-induced fibrosis of the left brachial plexus. Coronal T1-weighted MRI scans of the lower neck outlining the normal right brachial plexus (small arrows) and contrasting with the bright signal intensity of surrounding fat. The markedly thickened left brachial plexus (large arrows) is secondary to radiation-induced fibrosis.

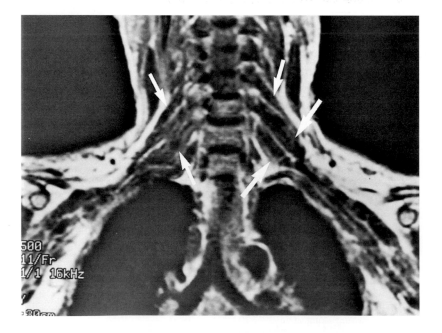

Fig. 14. Radiation-induced fibrosis of the brachial plexus noted bilaterally. Radiation-induced fibrosis producing marked thickening of the brachial plexus is well shown on this coronal T1-weighted MRI scan of the lower neck (arrows).

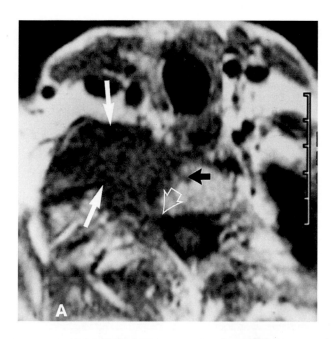

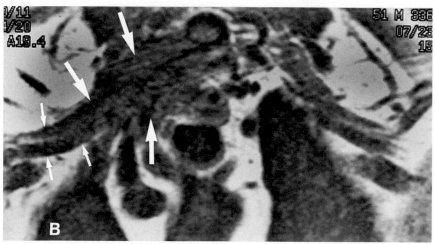

Fig. 15. Carcinoma of the right apical lung invading the adjacent brachial plexus. **A.** Axial T1-weighted MRI scan of the lower neck reveals carcinoma arising within the apex of the right lung (white arrows) extending into the neural foramina (open arrow) and partially destroying the T1 vertebral body (black arrow). **B.** Coronal T1-weighted MRI scan of the lower neck and upper thorax reveals tumor invading the brachial plexus (large white arrows) and extending along the cords (small white arrows).

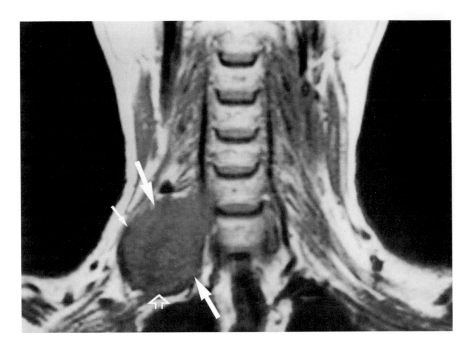

Fig. 16. Coronal T1-weighted MRI scan of the lower neck. A neurofibroma involving the middle trunk of the right brachial plexus (large arrows) and displacing the upper trunk (small white arrow) and lower trunk (open arrow) of the brachial plexus.

Neurofibroma is the most common tumor affecting the cervical nerve roots and brachial plexus. Neurofibromas may be recognized as single or multiple mass lesions arising from a cervical nerve root; they may extend to the brachial plexus (Fig. 16).

LUMBOSACRAL PLEXUS

The lumbar plexus is composed of nerve roots arising from vertebrae L1 through L4 with a branch from T12. The nerves originating from this segment of the plexus include the lateral anterior nerve of the thigh and the iliohypogastric, ilioinguinal, femoral, and obturator nerves (Russell and Windebank 1994). The lumbosacral trunk (Fig. 17) includes the L5 vertebra, a portion of the anterior rami of the vertebra, L4 and the anterior rami of the vertebra from S1 through S3, and a portion of the ventral roots of the vertebra S4. This portion of the lumbosacral plexus includes the tibial and peroneal nerves, which join to form the sciatic nerve, and the superior gluteal, inferior gluteal, posterior femoral cutaneous, and pudendal nerves (Russell and Windebank 1994).

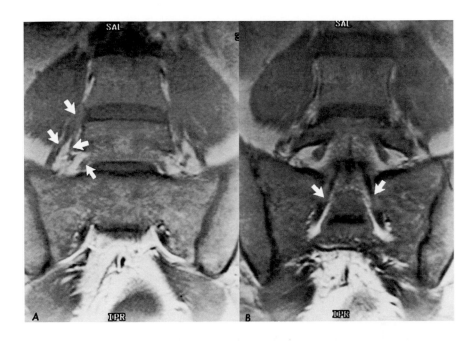

Fig. 17. Normal lumbosacral plexus. Coronal T1-weighted images of the lower lumbar nerve roots (arrows in **A**), sacral nerves (arrows in **B**), and lumbosacral plexus (arrows in **C**).

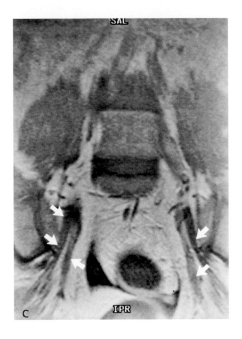

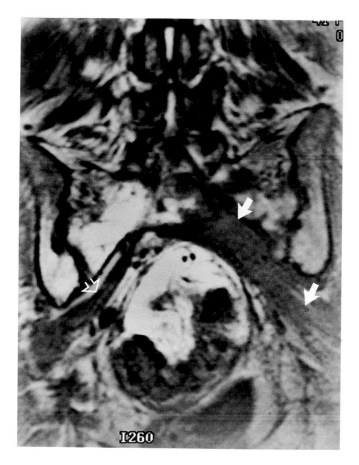

Fig. 18. A patient with carcinoma of the cervix presented with back and leg pain and lumbosacral plexopathy. Coronal T1-weighted MRI scan of the pelvis reveals diffuse tumoral infiltration and thickening of the lumbosacral plexus (white arrows), which was identified as a source of the patient's pain. The right plexus is normal (open arrows).

The lumbosacral plexus is affected by direct extension from neoplasms in the pelvis in approximately 75% of cases (Evans and Watson 1985; Jaeckle et al. 1985; Stübgen 1995). Plexus involvement has an insidious onset with slow progression. Pain occurs early and is a frequent symptom (Evans 1981; Stübgen 1995). Weakness may develop afterward (Evans 1981). Incontinence is uncommon, as is bilateral disease. (Stübgen 1995). Radiological imaging using CT and MRI scans may reveal involvement of the lumbosacral plexus by a pelvic mass involving the nerve roots and often the pelvic wall. These tumors usually originate from either the cervix or the colorectal region (Fig. 18). As in the brachial plexus, neurofibroma is the most common tumor to affect the lumbar plexus (Fig. 19).

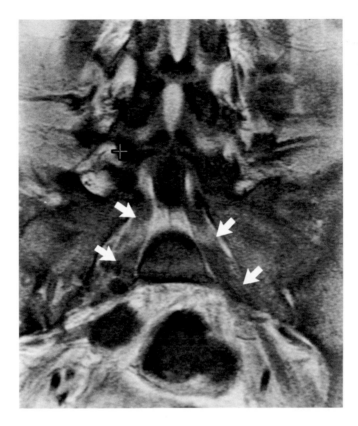

Fig. 19. Plexiform neurofibroma involving lumbosacral plexus bilaterally. Coronal T1-weighted MRI scan of the pelvis reveals involvement of the lumbosacral plexus bilaterally (arrows) by plexiform neurofibroma.

SUMMARY

Magnetic resonance imaging plays a significant role in identifying the cause of back pain in the patient with cancer. It also helps in distinguishing several benign mimics of metastatic disease to avoid unnecessary cancer therapy.

REFERENCES

An HS, Andreshak TG, Nguyen C, et al. Can we distinguish between benign versus malignant compression fractures of the spine by magnetic resonance imaging? Spine 1995; 20:1776–1782.

Baker RJ Jr, Siegel A. Sacral insufficiency fracture: half of an "H." Clin Nucl Med 1994; 19:1106–1107.

Blomlie V, Lien HH, Iversen T. Radiation-induced insufficiency fractures of the sacrum: evaluation with MR imaging. Radiology 1993; 188:241–244.

Bluemke DA, Fishman EK, Scott WW Jr. Skeletal complications of radiation therapy. Radiographics 1994; 14:111–121.

Cuénod CA, Laredo JD, Chevret S, et al. Acute vertebral collapse due to osteoporosis or malignancy: appearance on unenhanced and gadolinium-enhanced MR images. Radiology 1996; 199:541–549.

Darouiche RO, Hamill RJ, Greenberg SB, et al. Bacterial spinal epidural abscess. Review of 43 cases and literature survey [review]. Medicine 1992; 71:369–385.

Evans BA. Lumbosacral plexus neuropathy. Neurology 1981; 31:132–133.

Evans RJ, Watson CPN. Lumbosacral plexopathy in cancer patients. Neurology 1985; 35:1392–1393.

Even-Sapir E, Martin RH, Barnes DC, et al. Role of SPECT in differentiating malignant from benign lesions in the lower thoracic and lumbar vertebrae. Radiology 1993; 187:193–198.

Fornasier V, Czitron A. Collapsed vertebral: a review of 659 autopsies. Clin Orthop 1978; 131:261–265.

Hovi I, Lamminen A, Salonen O, et al. MR imaging of the lower spine. Differentiation between infectious and malignant disease. Acta Radiol 1994; 35:532–540.

Iyer RB, Fenstermacher NMJ, Libshitz HI. MR imaging of the treated brachial plexus [pictorial essay]. Am J Roentgenol 1996; 167:225–229.

Jaeckle KA, Young DE, Foley KH. The natural history of lumbosacral plexopathy in cancer. Neurology 1985; 35:8–15.

Krishnamurthy GT, Tubis M, Hiss J, et al. Distribution pattern of metastatic bone disease: a need for total body skeletal image. JAMA 1977; 237:2504–2506.

Mehta RC, Marks MP, Hinks RS, et al. MR evaluation of vertebral metastases: T1-weighted short-inversion-time inversion recovery, fast spin-echo and inversion-recovery fast spin-echo sequences. Am J Neuroradiol 1995; 16:281–288.

Modic MT, Steinberg PH, Ross JS, et al. Degenerative disk disease: assessment of changes in vertebral body marrow with MR imaging. Radiology 1988; 166:193–199.

Posniak HV, Olson MC, Dudiak CM, et al. MR imaging of the brachial plexus. Am J Roentgenol 1993; 161:373–379.

Russell JW, Windebank AJ. Brachial and lumbar neuropathies. Bailliere's Clin Neurol 1994; 3:173–191.

Stübgen JP. Neuromuscular disorders in systemic malignancy and its treatment. Muscle Nerve 1995; 18:636–648.

Wiener SN, Neumann DR, Rzeszotarski M. Comparison of magnetic resonance imaging and radionuclide bone imaging of vertebral fractures. Clin Nucl Med 1989; 14:666–670.

Yuh WTC, Zachar CK, Barloon TJ, et al. Vertebral compression fractures: distinction between benign and malignant causes with MR imaging. Radiology 1989; 172:215–218.

Correspondence to: Norman E. Leeds, MD, University of Texas M. D. Anderson Cancer Center, Diagnostic Radiology - 057, 1515 Holcombe Blvd., Houston, TX 77030, USA. Tel: 713-745-0562; Fax: 713-745-0848.

Assessment and Treatment of Cancer Pain,
Progress in Pain Research and Management,
Vol. 12, edited by R. Payne, R.B. Patt, and
C.S. Hill, IASP Press, Seattle, © 1998.

6

Medical Decision Making: Application to Pain Assessment and Treatment

Scott B. Cantor

*Ambulatory and Supportive Care Oncology Research Program,
Section of General Internal Medicine, Department of Medical Specialties,
The University of Texas M. D. Anderson Cancer Center, Houston, Texas, USA*

This chapter is an introduction to the field of medical decision making and its potential application to pain assessment and treatment, the theme of this volume. This chapter will cover the following points:

- Why should pain specialists be interested in medical decision making?
- How might medical decision making be applied to pain assessment and treatment?
- What are the research challenges and opportunities?

Many methods of pain assessment are available (Turk 1992; Cherney and Portenoy 1993). One tool is the Brief Pain Inventory, with which we can evaluate the *severity* of pain and its effect on the patient (Serlin et al. 1995). We can evaluate the sensory and temporal *characteristics* of pain to determine its location and frequency. It is important to know if the pain is acute or chronic. Finally, we can evaluate the *effect* of pain by administering quality of life measures, such as the Functional Assessment of Cancer Therapy (FACT), which includes questions on pain (Cella 1995).

One missing piece in pain assessment is how the patient feels about the presence and intensity of pain and willingness to pursue specific measures for pain relief. The following questions are not included in the standard methods of pain assessment: What changes in pain levels would be most meaningful to the patient? Do a priori measurements of pain consider the uncertainty of the outcomes associated with treatments for pain? What can the patient and the physician expect given differences in the natural history of painful conditions, especially those associated with chronic medical illnesses such as cancer? Do the measurements incorporate preferences regarding trade-offs in length of life and quality of life, if these are relevant or appropriate considerations? And from an economic perspective, are the treatment interventions "worth it," i.e., are the treatments "cost effective?"

CLINICAL DECISION ANALYSIS

Clinical decision analysis, or medical decision making, is a set of tools and methods that can evaluate such questions (Cantor 1995). Medical decision making is an analytical approach to making individual clinical and public policy decisions under uncertain conditions. This interdisciplinary field integrates tools from various fields including clinical medicine, clinical epidemiology, probability and statistics, computer science, psychology, economics, and ethics. Clinical decision analysis has been a recognized discipline for approximately 20 years, but has seen relatively few applications for pain assessment and treatment.

Substantial research in medical decision making focuses on the prescriptive aspects of clinical decisions. The word *prescriptive* refers to the recommended clinical course of action. What *should* we do for our patients? Assuming a prescriptive approach to clinical decision making, we can then analyze clinical problems from two perspectives: clinical and economic.

The clinical perspective focuses on the individual—typically the patient. We attempt to answer questions such as: How can we maximize life expectancy? How can we maximize or improve quality of life? By combining the two questions, we might ask: How can we improve *quality-adjusted* life expectancy? From an economic perspective, we attempt to answer a different set of questions by using a more global perspective, for example: How can society best allocate scarce health care dollars to improve quality of life or life expectancy of a population? How can a health care organization best spend its dollars in the most cost-beneficial manner?

Decision analysis is a "divide and conquer" methodology that breaks down a clinical problem in the following way:

- Who is the decision maker? Is the decision maker a patient? Or is the decision maker a larger entity, such as a health care maintenance organization? Or are we interested in the societal perspective?
- What are the choices to be made? What are the various clinical strategies that are available to approach the problem?
- What are the various outcomes of the alternative clinical strategies and their likelihood of occurrence?
- How do we evaluate these outcomes?

- How do we synthesize all this information to determine the best decision for the patient, provider, or society?
- If we are uncertain about some of the assumptions, what strategies can we employ to feel more confident about our conclusions?

One of these components, the evaluation of outcomes, is the focus of the first part of this chapter. The information contained in the evaluation of outcomes will then be useful for considering the economic evaluation of clinical strategies, the focus of the second part of this chapter.

THE EVALUATION OF CLINICAL OUTCOMES USING UTILITIES

One way to evaluate outcomes is to understand a concept called utility. A utility is a quantitative numerical measure of the attractiveness of a potential outcome that explicitly incorporates preferences. In clinical decision making, the potential outcomes are called "health states." Typically, a health state is described in explicit detail before the subject or patient determines the utility for that health state. In this way some aspect of the quality of life is evaluated, but with an important difference—the person determining the utility incorporates feelings, attitudes, and preferences into the evaluation of that health state.

In the literature on clinical decision analysis, the utility of a health state is typically evaluated on a scale that is anchored by "perfect health" at one end and "death" at the opposite end. Health states that are considered "worse than death" can be evaluated by using utility assessment procedures (Patrick et al. 1994); however, for the purposes of this discussion, we will assume that health states can be considered equivalent to perfect health or death or fall somewhere in between. [See Editor's Comment.]

A utility is a comprehensive measure that can evaluate physical, emotional, sensory, cognitive, and self-care functions (Goodwin 1991). It combines all these attributes into one scale rather than separating them out into different items, as might be done with a multidimensional quality of life instrument. Because utilities can be combined into a single scale, they can be generalized across different health states and evaluations. Thus, it is possible to consider different kinds of health problems and compare utilities from different clinical situations.

The preference is evaluated from the perspective of the person or entity being studied. For example, if we were interested in a patient-based study for clinical decision making, we should elicit preferences from patients. If we were interested in an economic analysis from the societal perspective so as to allocate health care resources, we should assess utilities from the perspectives of members of the community and not necessarily of patients.

Thus, it is theoretically possible to evaluate health states by utility assessment without necessarily experiencing the health states directly, an approach that is an important area of controversy. It might be argued that people cannot reasonably and accurately evaluate health states that they have not experienced. However, those who have experienced health states may have too great a personal stake in the outcome to objectively determine the utilities of specific health states. For example, patients may feel that an "inferior" health state, never previously experienced, "isn't as bad as they thought it would be"; alternatively, the health state may be even worse than they had originally imagined once they actually experience it!

Finally, utilities are useful in that they combine morbidity and mortality in a single outcome measure—the quality-adjusted life year (QALY). This outcome measure incorporates a quality of life component, the utility measure, and the length of life. Quality-adjusted life years are used for two purposes. For clinical decision making for patients, we can choose a strategy or clinical intervention that maximizes quality-adjusted life expectancy. For decisions from an economic perspective, we can incorporate quality-adjusted life expectancy into a cost-effectiveness analysis that uses dollars per quality-adjusted life year as the outcome measure. The latter part of this chapter will review the economic applications of quality-adjusted life years. [See Editor's Comment.]

THE EVALUATION OF PAIN HEALTH STATES

A most critical issue in utility assessment for clinical decision making in pain management is to define what pain health states might be evaluated. For example, as part of a larger study Rabin et al. (1993) evaluated health states based on various levels of pain assumed to have a one-year duration. The five levels were: "no pain," "slight pain," "moderate pain," "severe pain," and "agonizing pain." The subjects, who were university students, were asked to evaluate these health states even though many had never experienced them.

One measure to evaluate the pain or discomfort level of a patient is the EuroQol instrument (EuroQol Group 1990), which assesses three levels of pain: "no pain and discomfort," "moderate pain," and "extreme pain." The limitation of the Rabin et al. study and the EuroQol instrument is that patients or subjects may not clearly understand what they are evaluating in the utility assessment. In these examples, the health state descriptions are not detailed. The simple adjectives of "slight," "moderate," and "severe" may

Table I
Pain levels from Torrance's Health Utilities Index

Level 1	Free of pain and discomfort.
Level 2	Occasional pain. Discomfort relieved by nonprescription drugs or self-control activity without disruption of normal activities.
Level 3	Frequent pain. Discomfort relieved by oral medicines with occasional disruption of normal activities.
Level 4	Frequent pain; frequent disruption of normal activities. Discomfort requires prescription narcotics for relief.
Level 5	Severe pain. Pain not relieved by drugs and constantly disrupts normal activities.

Source: Torrance 1986.

have little meaning or have wide interpretation, especially to a person who has never experienced pain.

It is important to describe health states for utility assessment as completely and fairly as possible. In studies with utility assessment as the central component, much more sophisticated descriptions of health states are typically presented. These descriptions can be in paragraph or bullet-point format, may be presented in the first, second, or third person, and may be enhanced by multimedia equipment to more accurately depict the health state of interest.

For example, the health states shown in Table I were developed by Torrance (1986) as part of his Health Utilities Index, a multiattribute utility evaluation, i.e., an evaluation of health states based on many features of the condition. As can be seen in the table, the descriptions contain slightly more detail than do the typical quality of life measures. However, more description may be necessary to give an improved picture of what happens to a person living in this health state. With a detailed description of a health state, researchers can then elicit preferences for that health state with more confidence than is the case with simple adjectival descriptions.

UTILITY ASSESSMENT: THE PROCESS

The three standard methods of utility assessment are the standard gamble, the time trade-off, and the visual analog scale. This section explains the general assessment for each method and gives a specific example of how the utility assessment is done by using the example of "moderate pain for one year," with the assumption that we have a detailed description for that health state.

STANDARD GAMBLE

The standard gamble method is the ideal one for utility assessment as it is based on the axioms of expected utility theory (von Neumann and Morgenstern 1944). This theory is based on a normative model in which optimal decisions will be made when the choice that maximizes the expected utility is selected. However, the standard gamble method is the most complicated method of utility assessment.

Fig. 1 presents a simplified diagram of a decision tree showing two options for a subject or patient to consider. The first option is Choice A, to be in a chronic health state for the rest of one's life. The second option is Choice B, which is a gamble between two health states: with probability p to be in perfect health for the rest of one's life; and with probability $1 - p$ to succumb to an immediate death. In the standard gamble method of utility assessment, the objective is to find the indifference probability p^* such that the subject is indifferent between Choice A, the sure thing, and Choice B, the gamble.

To begin the process to find the indifference probability p^*, the interviewer might start with the value $p = 0.50$; in other words, the subject is asked to select a preference—to be in Health State A for the rest of the life expectancy, or to take Choice B, the gamble, with probability 0.5 to be healthy for the rest of one's life and probability 0.5 to immediately die. Based on the preference, the probabilities are then adjusted until the break-even point is found where the subject is indifferent between the chronic health state and the gamble.

For example, let's assume that we are interested in assessing the utility for the chronic health state of severe angina. If in Fig. 1, the probability p is

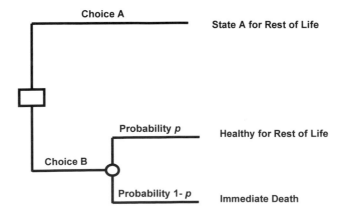

Fig. 1. Standard gamble method for assessing the utility of a generic chronic health state.

set equal to 1, then the choice would simplify to selecting "severe angina for the rest of one's life expectancy" (Choice A) versus a state of perfect health for the rest of one's life expectancy (Choice B). Clearly, Choice B would be the better choice. However, if the probability of being "in perfect health for the rest of one's life expectancy" was zero, leaving a probability of 1 for "immediate death," then clearly Choice A would be preferred. So by varying the probability p, at some point the subject will be indifferent between Choice A (the sure thing) and Choice B (the gamble). At that point, at probability p^* between 0 and 1, we set the utility of the chronic health state "severe angina for the rest of one's life expectancy" for this patient.

Now, let us apply this method to evaluate the health state "moderate pain for one year." (Fig. 2). Obviously the one-year duration is arbitrary, but may be an appropriate length of life to evaluate for patients with some cancer-related pain problems such as bone metastases. In this case, "moderate pain for one year of life expectancy" becomes Choice A, the "sure thing." Choice B is a gamble between choosing an intervention that would provide a health state that is either "pain free" for one year or immediate death. The initial question in the utility assessment process might be to set the probability p equal to 0.50 and ask if the subject would prefer Choice A to Choice B; the initial gamble is a 50% chance of being pain free for one year and a complementary 50% chance of immediate death. If the subject prefers the sure thing, then the interviewer increases the probability of being pain free to 75% and asks the preference question again. This iterative process continues until the break-even point is found. This process, though complicated, can be done with trained interviewers and with a knowledgeable subject who must have a basic understanding of probability.

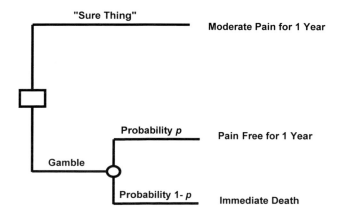

Fig. 2. Standard gamble method for assessing the utility of the health state "moderate pain for one year."

TIME TRADE-OFF METHOD

The time trade-off method was developed primarily because the standard gamble method, although theoretically rigorous, has the disadvantage of complexity. The time trade-off method eliminates the uncertainty from the utility assessment, so the results from the assessment cannot be considered "true" utilities—they may be considered as approximations, or can be transformed into utilities by using the results of additional research (O'Leary et al. 1995).

In Fig. 3, subjects or patients are asked to determine the number of years of perfect health that they are willing to "trade off" for a longer time in an intermediate health state. Let's apply the time trade-off method to the health state "severe angina for 40 years of life expectancy," which becomes Choice A. The initial question in the time trade-off method might be whether Choice A is preferred to 20 years of "perfect health." Again, based on the response, the number of years in perfect health is varied until the subject is indifferent between the two options. At that point, the utility approximation can be made: the utility is set equal to the number of years in perfect health considered equivalent to the longer time of the intermediate health state divided by the number of years of life expectancy. In this example, if 30 years of perfect health are considered equivalent to 40 years of "severe angina," then the utility of the health state "severe angina" is set equal to 0.75 (30/40).

The time trade-off method can be applied to evaluating pain health states in the following example (Fig. 4). To evaluate the health state "moderate pain for one year," it may be easier to describe the health state as "moderate pain for 12 months." Here, equivalence needs to be found for "moderate pain for 12 months" and "pain free for x months," where x is

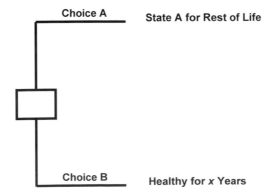

Fig. 3. Time trade-off method for assessing the utility of a generic chronic health state.

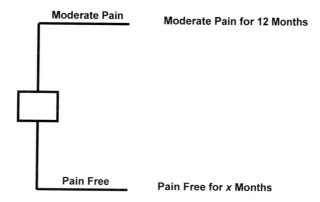

Fig. 4. Time trade-off method for assessing the utility of the health state "moderate pain for one year."

some number less than 12. For example, the subject can be asked, "Would you prefer to have moderate pain for 12 months or to be pain free for six months?" We then can vary the number of pain-free months to determine at what point the subject views these two choices as equivalent.

VISUAL ANALOG (RATING) SCALE

The third method of utility assessment is the visual analog or rating scale technique. This method has the least validity as it does not explicitly incorporate uncertainty or trade-offs in the evaluation process. However, it is sometimes used as an approximation for utilities, especially after an appropriate transformation (see, e.g., Torrance et al. 1982). It is the easiest of the three utility assessment techniques for subjects and patients to understand.

Fig. 5 shows a visual analog scale for a generic chronic health state. The subject is asked to identify a point for the health state to be evaluated between immediate death (with utility 0) and perfect health for remaining life expectancy (with utility 1) at which the relative distance between the point represents a strength of preference for the health states. The approximated utility is then simply equal to the number between 0 and 1 that the subject assigns to the health state.

Similarly, to perform utility assessment using the visual analog scale for the health state "one year in severe pain," the two anchors would be "immediate death" and "pain free for one year" (Fig. 6). The subject or patient marks the line based on the relative strength of preference among the three health states. This point on the 0 to 1 line becomes the approximated utility for the assessed health state. [See Editor's Comment.]

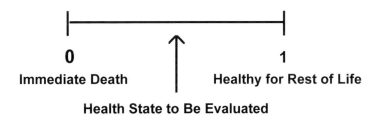

Fig. 5. Visual analog scale method for assessing the utility of a generic chronic health state.

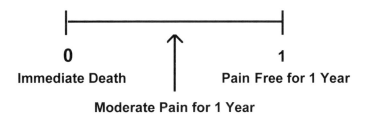

Fig. 6. Visual analog scale method for assessing the utility of the health state "moderate pain for one year."

ECONOMIC EVALUATION OF HEALTH CARE PROGRAMS

As discussed earlier, utilities are useful to determine the number of quality-adjusted life years (QALYs) that an intervention is expected to yield. By itself, the quality-adjusted life expectancy can be used as a criterion for determining the optimal clinical management based on informed patient preferences that incorporate knowledge of the risks and benefits of specific treatments. But when combined with economic data, we can determine both the expected costs and expected benefits in a cost-effectiveness analysis, the subject for the next portion of this chapter.

Several methods are available to evaluate the economic costs and health benefits of health care interventions (Detsky and Naglie 1990):

- Cost-minimization analysis determines which intervention has the minimum cost under the assumption that all interventions yield the same clinical outcome.
- Cost-benefit analysis incorporates and converts all outcomes into dollars. Thus, in a cost-benefit analysis paradigm, interventions are considered cost effective if the sum total of the benefits is greater than the sum total of the costs. Cost-benefit analysis is controversial because it forces an answer to the question: How many dollars is a human life worth?

- Cost-consequence analysis uses the outcome measure dollars per unit of clinical outcome, such as dollars per millimeter of blood pressure change or dollars per life year gained. Cost-consequence analysis does not allow for direct comparison among programs that have different denominators; for example, we cannot compare a program that costs $5,000 to detect a case of colorectal cancer with another program that costs $25,000 to treat a case of early-stage prostate cancer.
- Cost-utility analysis is the method of economic evaluation of health care programs that incorporates utilities for health states. Cost-utility analysis is evaluated in dollars per quality-adjusted life year. This method explicitly demonstrates the potential trade-offs between dollars and quality-adjusted life expectancy, the latter of which incorporates both length of life and quality of life in the evaluation of health benefits. For the purposes of this chapter, we will refer to cost-utility analysis as cost-effectiveness analysis.

When comparing two or more interventions in a cost-effectiveness analysis, we are typically given the expected costs, expressed in dollars, and the expected benefits, expressed in quality-adjusted life years. If we have an intervention that both saves money and improves health (as measured in quality-adjusted life expectancy), then we have an obvious choice —we would prefer that option. Comparing two interventions becomes difficult if one intervention costs money and improves health; then the question becomes, "Is it worth it?" This question leads to the concept of cost-effectiveness. How can we determine the clinical strategy that has the most "bang for the buck" for a specific patient or a specific clinical condition?

The key concept in economic evaluation is incrementalism. In particular, to properly evaluate a health care intervention, we need to know its alternative. At that point, we perform an incremental cost-effectiveness analysis by determining the additional cost that is necessary to obtain additional benefit. In health care policy decisions, the incremental cost-effectiveness ratio is defined as the difference in costs of two interventions divided by their differences in quality-adjusted life expectancy.

We can use these concepts to evaluate pain treatments. These concepts are still valid even though pain treatments are not likely to increase life expectancy in a clinical condition such as metastatic cancer. With the process of utility assessment, we can estimate the gains of quality-adjusted life expectancy using new pain treatments compared to the standard of care. By incorporating the relevant costs, we can then calculate the incremental cost-effectiveness ratio, as expressed in dollars per quality-adjusted life year, of the new innovation compared to the current practice. The incremental cost-effectiveness ratio for the new treatment can then be compared to previously

Table II
League table of health care interventions

Health Care Intervention	Cost per Quality-Adjusted Life Year (adjusted to 1996 dollars)	Reference
Smoking cessation for man	1,500	Cummings et al. 1989
Interferon alpha for chronic myelo-genous leukemia	22,000	Kattan et al. 1996
Adjuvant chemotherapy for early breast cancer	23,000	Hillner and Smith 1991
Treatment of mild hypertension for 40-year-old man	42,000	Stason and Weinstein 1977
Estrogen therapy for postmenopausal woman	60,000	Weinstein 1980
Autologous bone marrow transplan-tation for metastatic breast cancer	116,000	Hillner et al. 1992
Prophylactic intravenous immuno-globulin for chronic lymphocytic leukemia	7,230,000	Weeks et al. 1991

performed cost-effectiveness analyses that have evaluated health care interventions using the same cost per QALY as the yardstick for evaluation. However, this type of analysis may be biased against pain interventions occurring in terminal conditions such as cancer and AIDS because of the patients' short life expectancy.

Table II is a sample of health care interventions that have been previously analyzed, commonly known as a "league table." Most of the interventions used no treatment or no screening as the strategy for comparison. All these interventions have some degree of health benefit. An intervention can be cost saving—smoking cessation for pregnant women leads to both cost savings and increased health benefits because of the significant costs incurred due to the detrimental effects to smoking to newborns. On the other extreme, interventions can be expensive—prophylactic intravenous immunoglobulin for chronic lymphocytic leukemia provides some minute benefits at a hefty price—seven million dollars per QALY is an expensive intervention. There are no formal "cutoffs" for when a health care intervention becomes "cost effective;" however, these league tables are useful simply for purposes of comparison.

CHALLENGES OF APPLYING MEDICAL DECISION MAKING TO PAIN ASSESSMENT AND TREATMENT

Many of the challenges for applying medical decision making methods to pain assessment and treatment are not unique to this clinical area. However, the challenges for applying utility assessment to pain assessment and treatment may be greater because of the limited amount of published research.

The *stability* of preferences is a question of critical importance. A major controversy in the research literature is whether preferences change over time (Llewellyn-Thomas et al. 1993), and if they do, then how should preferences be incorporated in clinical decision analysis? As asked earlier in this chapter, do patients become accustomed to inferior health states, or are they even worse than they had originally imagined?

The feasibility of utility assessment is often questioned. One criticism of the standard gamble method is that people are risk averse; patients may be in an undesirable health state but still be unwilling to risk any possibility of shortening their life. A potential problem with the time trade-off method is that the investigator must predict the subject's life expectancy accurately. A utility assessment procedure that is not framed properly might raise fear if the patient misunderstands or misinterprets the concept of life expectancy.

Another challenge is that the process of utility assessment is inherently complicated and patients experiencing pain may not be fully cooperative or attentive at a time when their preferences are being assessed. Is it feasible to elicit preferences through a complicated utility assessment while a patient is enduring pain? Patients with advanced cancer can have various kinds of pain. How can we evaluate them all? Pain can be chronic or temporary. A current challenge for researchers is how to adapt utility assessment methods to evaluate short-term health states.

Finally, an interesting feature of pain assessment is cultural variation—an issue that researchers are just beginning to address in respect to utility assessment. Although the effect of pain may be similar for persons from different cultures, their preferences for pain treatments may vary enormously as a consequence of their culture (Cleeland et al. 1996). Thus, any conclusions from studies about the evaluation of pain health states must include information about the racial and ethnic makeup and some knowledge of the cultural preferences of the population sampled.

SUMMARY

The many challenges to utilities assessment mentioned above can be met. The methodology of medical decision making can provide a useful, structured framework for evaluating pain and its potential treatments. The use of patient preferences can help clinicians understand how their patients feel about pain health states that they are experiencing, have experienced, or may experience in the future. After collecting appropriate clinical outcomes data, researchers can evaluate the risks and benefits of pain management strategies for clinical decision making. With the collection of cost data, we can use information from the assessment of patient preferences for cost-effectiveness analyses, which will be useful for health policy decisions.

ACKNOWLEDGMENTS

I thank Michael W. Kattan, PhD, for his contributions, which enhanced the quality of this manuscript.

REFERENCES

Cantor SB. Decision analysis: theory and application to medicine. Prim Care 1995; 22:261–270.

Cella DF. Measuring quality of life in palliative care. Semin Oncol 1995; 22:73–81.

Cherney NI, Portenoy RK. Cancer pain management: current strategy. Cancer 1993; 72:3393–3415.

Cleeland CS, Nakamura Y, Mendoza TR, et al. Dimensions of the impact of cancer pain in a four country sample: new information from multidimensional scaling. Pain 1996; 67:267–273.

Cummings SR, Rubin SM, Oster G. The cost-effectiveness of counseling smokers to quit. JAMA 1989; 261:75–79.

Detsky AS, Naglie IG. A clinician's guide to cost-effectiveness analysis. Ann Intern Med 1990; 113:147–154.

EuroQol Group. EuroQol—a new facility for the measurement of health-related quality of life. Health Policy 1990; 16:199–208.

Goodwin PJ. Economic evaluations of cancer care: incorporating quality-of-life issues. In: Osoba D (Ed). Effect of Cancer on Quality of Life. Boca Raton, FL: CRC Press, Inc., 1991, pp 125–136.

Hillner BE, Smith TJ. Efficacy and cost-effectiveness of adjuvant chemotherapy in women with node-negative breast cancer: a decision analysis model. N Engl J Med 1991; 324:160–168.

Hillner BE, Smith TJ, Desch CE. Efficacy and cost-effectiveness of autologous bone marrow transplantation in metastatic breast cancer: estimates using decision analysis while awaiting clinical trial results. JAMA 1992; 267:2055–2062.

Kattan MW, Inoue Y, Talpaz M, et al. Cost-effectiveness of alpha-interferon compared to conventional chemotherapy in chronic myelogenous leukemia. Ann Intern Med 1996; 125:541–548.

Llewellyn-Thomas HA, Sutherland HJ, Thiel EC. Do patients' evaluations of a future health state change when they actually enter that state? Med Care 1993; 31:1002–1012.

O'Leary JF, Fairclough DL, Jankowski MK, Weeks JC. Comparison of time-tradeoff utilities and rating scale values of cancer patients and their relatives: evidence for a possible plateau relationship. Med Decis Making 1995; 15:132–137.

Patrick DL, Erickson P. Health Status and Health Policy. New York: Oxford University Press, 1993.

Patrick DL, Starks HE, Cain KC, Uhlmann RF, Pearlman RA. Measuring preferences for health states worse than death. Med Decis Making 1994; 14:9–18.

Rabin R, Rosser RM, Butler C. Impact of diagnosis of utilities assigned to states of illness. J Royal Soc Med 1993; 86:444–448.

Serlin RC, Mendoza TR, Nakamura Y, Edwards KR, Cleeland CS. When is cancer pain mild, moderate or severe? Grading pain severity by its interference with function. Pain 1995; 61:277–284.

Smith TJ, Hillner BE, Desch. Efficacy and cost-effectiveness of cancer treatment: rational allocation of resources based on decision analysis. J Natl Cancer Inst 1993; 85:1460–1474.

Stason WB, Weinstein MC. Allocation of resources to manage hypertension. New Engl J Med 1977; 296:732–739.

Torrance GW. Measurement of health state utilities for economic appraisal: a review. J Health Econ 1986; 5:1–30.

Torrance GW, Boyle MH, Horwood SP. Application of multi-attribute utility theory to measure social preferences for health states. Oper Res 1982; 30:1043–1069.

Turk DC, Melzack RC (Ed). Handbook of Pain Assessment. New York: The Guilford Press, 1992.

von Neumann J, Morgenstern O. Theory of Games and Economic Behavior. Princeton: Princeton University Press, 1944.

Weeks JC, Tierney MR, Weinstein MC. Cost-effectiveness of prophylactic intravenous immune globulin in chronic lymphocytic leukemia. N Engl J Med 1991; 325:81–86.

Weinstein MC. Estrogen use in postmenopausal women: costs, risk and benefits. New Engl J Med 1980; 303:308–316.

Correspondence to: Scott B. Cantor, PhD, The University of Texas M. D. Anderson Cancer Center, Department of Medical Specialties, Section of General Internal Medicine, 1515 Holcombe Blvd., Box 40, Houston, TX 77030-4095, USA. Tel: 713-745-4516; Fax: 713-745-3674; email: sbcantor@mdanderson.org.

Editor's Comment on Chapter 6: Medical Decision Making: Application to Pain Assessment and Treatment

Richard Payne, MD

The chapter by Scott B. Cantor describing health utilities in medical decision making and their application to pain assessment and treatment is quite provocative, especially if applied to patients with terminal illnesses such as cancer and AIDS. Medical decision making is a new field, but its core principles are becoming increasingly important in the evaluation of individual patient outcomes and for the analysis of health policy decisions regarding pain therapies and their reimbursement. Dr. Cantor referred to the paper by Patrick et al. measuring preference for health states worse than death (Patrick D, Starks HE, Cain KC, et al. Measuring performance for health states worse than death. Med Decis Making 1994; 14:9–18). In this study, these authors used methods similar to those described in the Cantor chapter, such as the standard gamble approach and time trade-off, to evaluate health preferences for states deemed worse than death in 40 well adults living at home and 41 nursing home residents. Somewhat surprisingly, these adults evaluated several hypothetical but terrifying health states such as being in "constant pain for the rest of your life" as being a state that was not worse than death. However, in this study dementia and coma were more likely to be considered equal to or worse than death. Conventional wisdom would suggest that patients with terminal illnesses might evaluate severe constant pain as a state worse than death, as this health state is usually given as a reason for patients advocating physician assistant suicide and euthanasia. It would be interesting to evaluate similar preferences in patients with terminal illnesses such as advanced cancer and AIDS.

Some pain researchers have raised moral objections to using approaches such as standard gamble and time trade-off when evaluating patients with pain and terminal illness. Is it morally acceptable to ask a patient with an terminal illness to "trade off" pain relief for more days of life? It is also true that the interpretation of the terms "the risk of immediate death" vs. "perfect health," which are used as anchors in these health state assessments, have different meanings to patients with terminal illness. For example, when evaluating the possible adverse outcomes of pharmacotherapy, anesthetic or neurosurgical procedures to relieve pain, the risk of "immediate death" is usually very small relative to the risk of death from the underlying disease. These issues must be further explored and clarified if this method of analysis is to be used appropriately to assess pain health states and terminally ill patients.

Finally, the appropriateness of the concept of the quality-adjusted life year (QALY) analysis as described by Cantor is also questioned when applied to populations with terminal illnesses. The following example gives an indication of this.

The pain and symptom management service at The University of Texas M. D. Anderson Cancer Center recently evaluated a 46-year-old uninsured woman with widely advanced endometrial carcinoma. She had severe bone and pelvic visceral pain, graded at 10/10 in intensity on a numerical rating scale. She was in the midst of a "pain crisis" and had not slept for almost 48 hours prior to consultation by our service. On evaluation she was sitting upright in a soft chair rocking continuously in an attempt to ease pain. Physical examination revealed a large pelvic mass and neurological findings consistent with a lumbosacral plexopathy as the causes of her pain. Prior to pain consultation she was being managed with intravenous doses of morphine titrated to the dose-limiting side effects of nausea, myoclonus, and sedation. In the next three days, she was switched to intravenous fentanyl and titrated to dose-limiting toxicity—sedation and nausea. She still experienced inadequate pain relief, and, therefore, an epidural catheter was placed for administration of epidural fentanyl and bupivacaine. Despite this, her pain was still uncontrolled, and she underwent subarachnoidal neurolysis, which could now be justified because of loss of bowel and bladder control secondary to progressive tumor growth in the sacral plexus. Following this procedure, she was pain free, but died less than 24 hours later.

In the last week of her life, many thousands of dollars were spent to control her pain and to allow her to die without pain. A QALY calculation would far exceed those values listed on Table II, given the small denominator that is essentially unchangeable because we were treating a patient at the end of life, when life-prolonging therapy was not possible, or even desirable. How can we evaluate the cost effectiveness of palliative care approaches in comparison to the traditional medical procedures and treatments typically measured in such analysis? The challenge of understanding better these issues will require the active collaboration of palliative care clinicians and medical decision scientists.

Assessment and Treatment of Cancer Pain,
Progress in Pain Research and Management,
Vol. 12, edited by R. Payne, R.B. Patt, and
C.S. Hill, IASP Press, Seattle, © 1998.

7

Psychological Interventions for Pain: Potential Mechanisms

C. Richard Chapman

*Departments of Anesthesiology, Psychiatry, and Behavioral Sciences,
University of Washington School of Medicine, Seattle, Washington, USA*

It is now clear that nondrug psychological interventions can play a significant role in the multidisciplinary management of pain in patients with cancer and other medical disorders. Although the literature on such interventions for addressing pain in these populations is still sparse, results thus far available indicate that (1) psychological interventions can complement pharmacological and other medical therapies, and (2) the most beneficial ones are brief, cost effective, and suitable for use by a wide variety of health care professionals (Roth-Roemer et al. 1996). Although psychological approaches can help patients live with pain, they can also reduce pain (Syrjala et al. 1995).

What constitutes a psychological intervention? At present such treatments fall into three main groupings: (1) cognitive-behavioral interventions such as hypnosis, relaxation, and coping skill training; (2) educational interventions such as those that allay patient fears about opioid drugs or foster compliance with medical treatments; and (3) group support for cancer patients with pain or other symptoms. These interventions exist in the pain field only because clinical researchers have noted their success in other areas and applied them to pain patients.

A widely accepted theoretical basis for how psychological interventions may work for pain is lacking. This is of concern because lack of theory inhibits the development of new approaches and the refinement of existing methods. Conventional Cartesian theories of pain are ill suited for explaining how psychological interventions might work. They posit a passive nervous system in which pain is an automatic response to an injurious event. Moreover, such theories construe pain as the product of nociceptive or neuropathic signaling in the periphery, and the brain as a repository that registers

tissue trauma information from the periphery. Intervention consists of blocking or gating signals so that they do not reach the brain. From the behavioral
perspective, this model is more a barrier to explanation than an asset. Psychologists see pain as the end product of a complex process that has emotional and cognitive as well as sensory aspects. Moreover, pain is a coherent
experience that involves the whole person and not simply a noxious sensation intruding into the awareness of the person. In short, pain is the dynamic
creation of a complex and active brain that produces and emits emotion as
well as registers sensory information. Psychological interventions address
the patient's active, dynamic nervous system, and guide and assist the patient in achieving goals. This position requires a theoretical basis for pain
that can accommodate the assumption of an active nervous system.

To date, researchers concerned with basic mechanisms of pain have
addressed sensory processing almost exclusively. Why pain is disturbing
and compels the individual to seek relief remains a mystery. This chapter
argues that pain is in part an emotional phenomenon and that emotion is a
key element in understanding the mechanisms of psychological interventions for pain. Literature on the neurophysiology of emotion and the neuro-
endocrinology of stress, both rich sources of literature, suggest approaches
for studying the affective component of pain. Moreover, psychological research and theory in these areas also provide a valuable resource and a fresh
perspective. By bringing knowledge from these fields together with knowledge about the sensory features of pain, we have the potential to build a
comprehensive perspective that will allow the development of theory about
psychological interventions.

This chapter proposes that tissue trauma: (1) excites both spinoreticular
and spinothalamic pathways; (2) generates concomitant affective and sensory processes that subserve complementary adaptive functions; (3) activates predominantly noradrenergic limbic structures to produce the affective
dimension of pain; and (4) the hypothalamically mediated stress response is
an important feature of pain and a mechanism of its emotional dimension. In
addition, the chapter briefly reviews current concepts of emotion, certain
pertinent aspects of emotional behavior, and the relevant central neuroanatomy
and endocrinology of negative emotion, and suggests a model that accounts
for emotional arousal in the experience of pain. This approach may help
clarify how psychological interventions can work alone and together with
medical treatments to help control pain and prevent suffering in cancer
patients.

EMOTION: ITS FUNCTIONS AND EXPRESSIONS

DEFINITIONS OF EMOTION

To entertain the concept of emotion as a component of pain, we need a clear notion of what emotion is. This seemingly simple matter poses a major barrier to developing the concept of emotion in the study of pain. Despite a large literature on the psychophysiology of emotion, little consensus exists on a formal definition for emotion; theorists have suggested myriad meanings for the term. In fairness, the concept of emotion encompasses a wide range of animal and human phenomena, but the problem extends beyond this complication. For example, Rolls (1986, p. 126) stated, "Emotions can be usefully defined as states elicited by reinforcing stimuli." Fonberg (1986, p. 302) contended that "Emotion is the nervous process that determines what kind of stimuli coming from the inner and outer environments are desirable for the organism and what are not." Averill (1980, p. 312) asserted that "An emotion is a transitory social role (a socially constituted syndrome) that includes an individual's appraisal of a situation and that is interpreted as a passion rather than as an action." For Kosslyn and Koenig (1992, pp. 437–438), emotion is "a type of information stored in memory." Such seemingly unrelated definitions of the term reflect the divergent theoretical frameworks within which emotion researchers work, and as a result focus on markedly different subjective, behavioral, or social phenomena.

The problem of defining emotion has been a source of contention since ancient times; the Greeks debated issues that persist today. One such issue is whether a few fundamental emotions exist, from which all others derive. Several contemporary theorists argue for this assumption. For example, Plutchik (1980) listed eight basic emotions. The subjective feeling, associated behaviors, and sociobiological functions associated with these emotions are listed in Table I.

None of these affects correspond to pain precisely, but, given that Plutchik views emotions as cognitively mediated and future focused, the basic emotion most closely approximating pain may be fear.

Lazarus, who sees emotions as feelings linked to thoughts (and pain as a sensation), holds that people appraise events and persons that they encounter and that the emotions they produce represent personal significance (Lazarus 1993). He postulates 15 basic emotions. Of these, four are positive feelings: happiness, love, pride, and relief. Another nine are negative: anger, anxiety, disgust, envy, fright, guilt, jealousy, sadness, and shame. Two others that represent mixed hedonic qualities may qualify for the list of basic feeling states: hope and compassion. Each emotion characterizes a relationship

Table I
The eight basic emotions and associated
feelings, behaviors, and sociobiological functions

Feeling	Behavior	Function
fear	escape	protection
anger	attack	destruction
joy	mate	reproduction
sadness	cry	reintegration
acceptance	groom	incorporation
disgust	vomit	rejection
expectation	map	exploration
surprise	stop	orientation

Source: Adapted from Plutchik 1980.

between the person and the environment and signifies the person's way of adapting to the environment.

In contrast, MacLean (1990) postulated three classes of affects: basic, general, and specific. Basic affects derive from needs such as hunger, the urge to urinate, or sexual expression. General affects are complex feelings aroused by situations, other people, or things. Specific affects correspond to specific sensory experiences such as smells or sounds. Pain falls into this class of experience because we experience it as a bodily sensation. Ictal aura phenomena often provide striking examples of emotions in this class, and MacLean noted many instances of ictal emotions involving bizarre pain states.

These striking differences in theory typify the lack of consensus about basic emotions. We could belabor this point by citing many other lists of fundamental feelings from the literature, but this will yield little additional insight. The basic point is clear: many theorists contend that basic emotions exist, but cannot agree on what these are, which undermines their contention. Some theorists contest the assumption that basic emotions exist at all (Ortony and Turner 1990).

Despite a lack of consensus on basic concepts, mainstream emotion researchers appear to strongly agree on the following points:

1. Emotional phenomena evolved to foster survival of the individual and the species, and emotional responses to stimuli and emotional expression foster biological adaptation.

2. Emotions impute positive or negative hedonic qualities to a stimulus in accordance with the biological importance and meaning of that stimulus.

3. The central neuroanatomy for emotion corresponds to the limbic brain.
   - Emotions activate—they produce impulses to act or to express the self.
   - Emotions communicate, and the negative emotional expression of one person will tend to produce negative emotion in another.
4. Human cognitions and emotions function interdependently. What we think influences what we feel, and the reverse also holds true.

These points of agreement help to clarify what current science means by emotion, but a conclusive, consensual definition for emotion remains elusive, and in its absence our definition of pain remains incomplete.

I advocate a sociobiological (evolutionary) framework for the emotional aspect of pain that interprets feeling states, related physiology, and behavior in terms of adaptation and survival. Nature has equipped human beings with the capability for negative emotion for a purpose; bad feelings are not simply accidents of human consciousness. By understanding the emotional dimension of pain from this perspective, we may gain some insight about how to prevent or control emotions that foster suffering. Implementation of this approach as a "world view" of pain requires dispensing with conventional language habits that describe pain as a transient sensory event. Instead, I argue that we construe pain as a state of the individual that has as its primary defining feature awareness of, and homeostatic adjustment to, tissue trauma.

ADAPTIVE FUNCTIONS OF EMOTION

Emotions and the emotional dimension of pain characterize mammals exclusively and appear to foster mammalian adaptation. MacLean (1990, p. 425) contends that emotions "impart subjective information that is instrumental in guiding behavior required for self-preservation and preservation of the species. The subjective awareness that is an affect consists of a sense of bodily pervasiveness or by feelings localized to certain parts of the body." This view relates closely to that of Kosslyn and Koenig (1992), who see emotion as information stored in memory. Emotion colors memories and may determine the "priority" of stored facts. As emotion has evolved to facilitate adaptation and survival, negative emotion comes to play an important defensive role. The ability to impute threat to certain types of environmental events protects against life-threatening injury.

Within consciousness threat manifests as a feeling state, and in humans threatening events that are not immediately present can exist as emotionally colored somatosensory images. We can react emotionally to the mental image of a painful event before it happens (e.g., venipuncture), or for that matter we can respond adversely to the sight of another person's tissue trauma. The emotional intensity of such a feeling marks the adaptive significance of the event that produced the experience. The threat of a minor injury normally provokes less intense feeling than one that incurs a high risk of death. The emotional magnitude of a pain, therefore, is the internal representation of the threat associated with the event that produced the pain. The key point is that the strength of emotional arousal indicates, and expresses, perceived threat to the biological integrity of the individual.

EMOTIONS AND BEHAVIOR

Emotions compel action and also expression through vocalization, posture, variations in facial musculature patterns, and alterations of activity. This process enhances communication and social support, and thus contributes to survival. Darwin (1872), observing animals, noted that emotions enable communication through vocalization, startle, posture, facial expression, and specific behaviors. Contemporary investigators who study emotions and human or animal social behavior emphasize that communication is a fundamental adaptive function of emotion (Ploog 1986). Social mammals, including humans, use one another or their social group as resources for adaptation and survival. The emotional expression of pain in the presence of supportive persons is socially powerful; it draws upon a fundamental sociobiological imperative, communicates threat, and summons assistance.

CENTRAL NEUROANATOMY OF EMOTION

The limbic brain represents an anatomical common denominator across mammalian species (MacLean 1990, p. 257), which suggests that emotion represents a common feature in consciousness for all mammals. Early investigators focused on the role of olfaction in limbic function. Papez (1937) linked the limbic brain to emotion, and stated that: "It is proposed that the hypothalamus, the anterior thalamic nuclei, the gyrus cinguli, the hippocampus and their interconnections constitute a harmonious mechanism which may elaborate the functions of central emotion, as well as participate in emotional expression." Emotion may have evolutionary roots in olfactory perception.

MacLean introduced the term "limbic system" four decades ago and characterized its functions (MacLean 1952). More recently, he identified three main subdivisions of the limbic brain: amygdala, septum, and thalamocingulate (MacLean 1990). Fig. 1 illustrates three main subdivisions of the limbic brain. These represent sources of afferents to parts of the

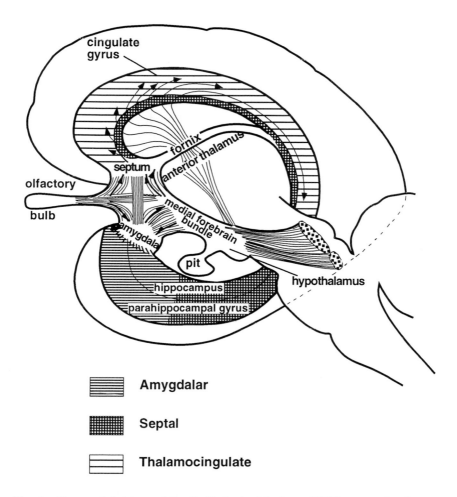

Fig. 1. Three subdivisions of the limbic brain. MacLean (1990) proposed a three-part grouping of limbic structures and functions: amygdalar, septal, and thalamocingulate subdivisions. These groupings appear as shadings. The figure, derived from MacLean's illustration (1990, p. 315), portrays the hippocampus as an upright arch joining the septum at one end and the amygdala at the other.

limbic cortex. He also postulated that the limbic brain responds to two basic types of input: interoceptive and exteroceptive, which refer to sensory information from internal and external environments, respectively.

Pain research has yet to address the links between nociception and limbic processing. However, anecdotal evidence implicates limbic structures in distress associated with pain. Radical frontal lobotomies, once performed upon patients for psychosurgical purposes, typically interrupt pathways projecting from hypothalamus to cingulate cortex and putatively relieved the suffering of intractable pain without destroying sensory awareness (Fulton 1951). Such neurosurgical records help clarify recent positron emission tomographic and magnetic resonance imaging observations of human subjects receiving painful cutaneous heat stimulation: noxious stimulation activates the contralateral anterior cingulate and the primary and secondary somatosensory cortex (Talbott et al. 1991).

EMOTION IN LEARNING AND MEMORY

Organisms that can learn readily from experience have adaptive advantages over those that cannot. That which promotes learning promotes survival. The affective component of pain contributes to both operant (instrumental) learning and classical conditioning (learning by association). Operant learning requires reinforcers, and reinforcers are events accompanied by emotions. Classical conditioning represents the formation of an association between a normally neutral event and the negative emotion associated with the onset of pain. Memory of past events, as with learning, depends heavily upon emotion (Kosslyn and Koenig 1992), and memories of past experience tend to shape expectations for the present and future.

Operant learning can occur in any setting with active patients and reinforcing events. A reinforcer is an event that follows a behavior and alters the future likelihood that the behavior will recur (Fordyce 1990). Events that create pleasant feelings function as rewards (positive reinforcers); events that produce negative feelings are punishments (i.e., they suppress behaviors). The positive or negative nature of reinforcers and their personal significance occur in conscious awareness as feelings (Rolls 1986). Put another way, events that shape behavior are those that are emotionally prominent. Emotion-free events have no reinforcing properties and therefore cannot contribute to adaptive learning.

Fear that accompanies pain can become associated with non-noxious stimuli through classical conditioning. In fear conditioning, the repeated pairing of a neutral stimulus with a noxious one can condition the perceiver so that the neutral stimulus, occurring alone, acts as a trigger to elicit fear. Many people develop fear or frank phobia in dentist's offices through classical conditioning.

Biologically, fear conditioning supports survival by fostering avoidance of potentially dangerous situations. Through conditioning, ordinarily neutral stimuli become warning cues for danger (Staddon 1983). It also helps the person martial a flight or fight response to a challenge after preexposure to it. Osborne et al. (1975) found that MHPG (3-methoxy-4-hydroxyphenylglycol), an indicator of norepinephrine turnover in brain, provided a marker of fear conditioning; exposure to a painful event increased MHPG in a manner that tracked the conditioning process.

Conditioned emotional responses are essentially sensory-affective associations. The amygdala appears to be the key structure that links sensory experience to emotional arousal and for conditioning of negative emotional associations (Gray 1982; Fonberg 1986; LeDoux et al. 1990). It probably contributes to the emotional evaluation of cognitive events (via corticofugal pathways) and sensory events that reach it via the dorsal noradrenergic bundle or sensory thalamus. Aggleton and Mishkin (1986) described the amygdala as a gateway to the emotions for stimuli (simple or complex) in all sensory modalities, both conditioned and unconditioned.

Sensory processing (in the case of pain, spinothalamic processing) can elicit complex, negative emotional processes through Pavlovian conditioning. This cortical association is not "postsensory," but rather a by-product of thalamic processing. LeDoux and colleagues (1988, 1990), working with auditory stimuli, determined that projections from the acoustic thalamus to the amygdala allow the classical conditioning of emotional responses to normally neutral auditory stimuli in experimental animals. To condition animal subjects, they paired tones with footshock and evaluated autonomic responses and emotional behaviors. Their lesion work implicates separate efferent projections from the amygdala in conditioning of autonomic and behavioral responses. Moreover, their work indicates that emotional memories established by conditioning of subcortical systems strongly resist extinction (LeDoux 1993). These and other observations suggest that emotion is a complex process sustained by several mechanisms. Under controlled circumstances individual mechanisms can be independently conditioned.

Fear conditioning almost certainly occurs in patients who experience repeated painful diagnostic or treatment procedures. Fear conditioning can exacerbate the affective dimension of pain in cases where minor pain and intense affective arousal have been paired. Moreover, it can form associations between the environment surrounding a painful event and affective processing of that event so that the environment alone could elicit some elements of the affective dimension of pain. Fear conditioning may contribute to phobic behavior patterns in pediatric patients.

Emotion associated with pain probably influences memory. Memory researchers surmise that both limbic and nonlimbic mechanisms contribute to memory processes (Gabriel et al. 1986). Emotional significance controls at least some and perhaps much memory formation: evidence exists that the brain preferentially stores information that has strong emotional loadings (Bower 1981; Tucker et al. 1990). Heath (1986) proposed that learning and memory are "rooted in feeling and emotion" (p. 6) and identified the hippocampus, cortical medial amygdala, and cingulate gyrus as key areas involved in negative emotions.

To recapitulate, the emotional component of pain seems to support adaptation and survival by facilitating learning, memory, and related cognitive processes. It provides a bridge by which pain can affect the psychological status of the person and behavioral tendencies. Inadvertent conditioning can cause anticipatory anxiety or exacerbate the emotional distress associated with a painful event.

EMOTION AND COGNITION

Negative feelings appear to be much more than reactions to undesirable events; in nature they help an individual to determine that which benefit versus that which threaten survival, and they compel behavior consistent with such evaluations. Moreover, emotional expression allows the individual to communicate this judgment to others and thus set up a group approach or avoidance behaviors. As noted above, MacLean (1990) described emotion as a process that imparts subjective information. In these respects, emotion approximates a crude intelligence. If emotion is a proto-intelligence, then evolutionarily newer structures, namely the later stages of cortical development, should have demonstrable links with limbic structures and functions.

Such interconnections exist. Parts of the frontal lobe (the dorsal trend) appear to have developed from rudimentary hippocampal formation while other parts (the paleocortical trend) originated in olfactory cortex. Although these two areas interconnect anatomically, the former analyzes sensory information while the latter contributes emotional tone to that sensory information (Pandya et al. 1987, pp. 66–67). Pribram (1980), noting that limbic function involves frontal and temporal cortex, offered a bottom-up concept for how cognition relates to feelings: that is, emotion determines cognition. However, the multimodal neocortical association areas project corticifugally to limbic structures (Turner et al. 1980), which suggests that cognitions may drive emotions. Plutchik (1980) argued that cognitions (evaluations) always precede emotions and may be based upon information provided by internal or external stimuli. These points of view may not be as diametrically opposed as they appear. Plutchik has postulated that emotions precede cognitions in evolution and that cognitions have evolved in the service of emotions. The sociobiological purpose of cognition, for Plutchik, is to predict the future. Indeed, theorists agree that human thinking involves intimate interplay with emotions.

CENTRAL MECHANISMS FOR THE EMOTIONAL DIMENSION OF PAIN

NOCICEPTION AND CENTRAL NORADRENERGIC PROCESSING

Central sensory and affective pain processes share common peripheral sensory circuitry: Aδ and C fibers serve as tissue trauma transducers (nociceptors) for both; the chemical products of inflammation sensitize these nociceptors, and peripheral neuropathic mechanisms such as ectopic firing excite both processes. Differentiation of sensory and affective processing begins at the dorsal horn of the spinal cord. Sensory transmission follows spinothalamic pathways, while transmission destined for affective processing occurs in spinoreticular pathways. As others have described sensory processing of nociception well, it need not be reviewed here (Willis 1985; Fields 1987; Peschanski and Weil-Fugacza 1987; Bonica 1990).

Nociceptive centripetal transmission engages both spinoreticular and spinothalamic pathways (Villanueva et al. 1989). The spinoreticular tract contains somatosensory and viscerosensory afferent pathways that terminate at distinct brain stem sites. Spinoreticular axons possess receptive fields that resemble those of spinothalamic tract neurons projecting to medial thalamus, and, like their spinothalamic counterparts, they transmit tissue injury infor mation (Fields 1987; Bonica 1990; Villanueva et al. 1990). Most spinoreticular neurons carry nociceptive signals and many respond preferentially to noxious input (Bowsher 1976; Willis 1985; Abou-Samra 1987; Bing et al. 1990).

The processing of nociceptive signals that influence affect commences in reticulocortical pathways. Four extrathalamic afferent pathways project to the neocortex: (1) the dorsal noradrenergic bundle (DNB) originating in the locus coeruleus (LC); (2) the serotonergic fibers that arise in the dorsal and median raphe nuclei; (3) the dopaminergic pathways of the ventral tegmental tract that arise from substantia nigra; (4) and the acetylcholinergic neurons that arise principally from the nucleus basalis of the substantia innominata (Foote and Morrison 1987). Of these, the noradrenergic pathway is most closely linked to negative emotional states (Gray 1982, 1987). The set of structures receiving projections from this complex and extensive network corresponds to the classic definition of the limbic brain (Papez 1937; Isaacson 1982; Gray 1987; MacLean 1990).

Although other processes governed predominantly by other neurotransmitters almost certainly play important roles in the complex experience of emotion during pain, this chapter emphasizes the role of central noradrenergic processing. This limited focus offers the advantage of simplicity and as such permits the model to tell a well-focused story. Processing involves two central noradrenergic pathways: the dorsal and ventral noradrenergic bundles.

LOCUS COERULEUS AND THE DORSAL NORADRENERGIC BUNDLE

The locus coeruleus (LC), a pontine nucleus, resides bilaterally near the wall of the fourth ventricle. The locus has three major projections: ascending, descending, and cerebellar. The ascending projection, the DNB, is the most extensive and important (Fillenz 1990), as Fig. 2 illustrates. The DNB projects from the LC throughout limbic brain and to the entire neocortex, and accounts for about 70% of all brain norepinephrine (Watson et al. 1986; Svensson 1987). The LC gives rise to most central noradrenergic fibers in the spinal cord, hypothalamus, thalamus, and hippocampus (Levitt and Moore 1979; Aston-Jones et al. 1985) in addition to its projections to the limbic cortex and neocortex. Consequently, this seemingly inauspicious nucleus exerts an enormous influence on brain activity.

The LC reacts to signaling from sensory stimuli that potentially threaten the biological integrity of the individual or signal damage to that integrity.

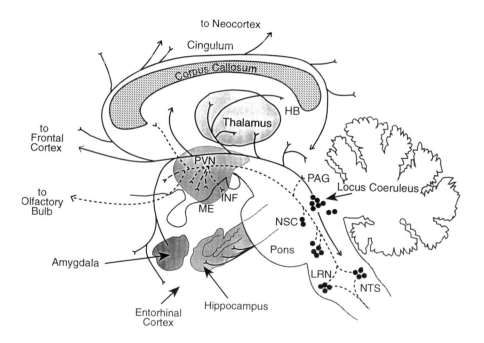

Fig. 2. Central corticipetal noradrenergic transmission in a primate brain (parasagittal view). The cell bodies of neurons that produce norepinephrine appear as black circles. The major projections of these cell bodies are the dorsal noradrenergic bundle (*DNB*) and the ventral noradrenergic bundle (*VNB*). Tissue trauma signals from spinoreticular pathways excite the primarily noradrenergic locus coeruleus (*LC*) and activate the DNB, which extends throughout the limbic brain and to neocortex. *ME:* median eminence; *PAG:* periaqueductal gray; *HB:* habenula; *NSC:* nucleus subcoeruleus; *LRN:* lateral reticular nucleus; *NTS:* nucleus tractus solitarius; *INF:* infundibulum; *PVN:* paraventricular nucleus.

Nociception inevitably and reliably increases activity in neurons of the LC, and LC excitation appears to be a consistent response to nociception (Korf et al. 1974; Stone 1975; Morilak et al. 1987; Svensson 1987). Notably, this process does not require cognitively mediated attentional control because it occurs in anesthetized animals. Foote, Bloom, and Aston-Jones (1983) reported that slow, tonic spontaneous activity at the locus in rats changed under anesthesia in response to noxious stimulation. Experimentally induced phasic LC activation produces alarm and apparent fear in primates (Redmond and Huang 1979; Charney et al. 1990), and lesions of the LC eliminate normal heart rate increases to threatening stimuli (Redmond 1977).

The LC reacts consistently, but does not respond exclusively to noxious sensory input. LC activity increases following nonpainful threatening occurrences such as strong cardiovascular stimulation (Elam et al. 1985; Morilak et al. 1987) and certain visceral events such as distention of the bladder, stomach, colon, or rectum (Elam et al. 1986b; Svensson 1987). Thus, while consistently reactive to nociception, the LC is not a nociceptive-specific nucleus. Rather, it responds to biologically threatening events, of which tissue injury is a significant subset. We can describe the LC as a central analog of the sympathetic ganglia (Amaral and Sinnamon 1977).

Invasive studies confirm the link between LC activity and perceived threat. Direct activation of the DNB and associated limbic structures in laboratory animals produces sympathetic nervous system response and elicits emotional behaviors such as defensive threat, fright, enhanced startle, freezing, and vocalization (McNaughton and Mason 1980). This response indicates that enhanced activity in these pathways corresponds to negative emotional arousal and behaviors appropriate to perceived threat.

Normally, activity in the locus increases alertness; tonically enhanced LC and DNB discharge corresponds to hypervigilance and emotionality (Foote et al. 1983; Butler et al. 1990). The DNB is the mechanism for vigilance and orientation to affectively relevant and novel stimuli. It also regulates attentional processes and facilitates motor responses (Foote and Morrison 1987; Gray 1987; Svensson 1987). In this sense, the LC continually influences the stream of consciousness and readies the individual to respond quickly and effectively to threat when it occurs.

The LC and DNB support biological survival by facilitating global vigilance to threatening and harmful stimuli. Siegel and Rogawski (1988) hypothesized a link between the LC noradrenergic system and vigilance. They focused on rapid eye movement (REM) sleep and noted that LC noradrenergic neurons maintain continuous activity in both normal waking state and non-REM sleep, but that during REM sleep these neurons virtually cease discharge activity. Moreover, an increase in REM sleep ensues after either

lesions of the DNB or following administration of clonidine, an α_2 adreno-
ceptor agonist. Because LC inactivation during REM sleep permits rebuild-
ing of noradrenergic stores, REM sleep constitutes necessary preparation for
sustained periods of high alertness during subsequent waking. Siegel and
Rogawski (1988, p. 226) contended that "a principal function of NE in the
CNS is to facilitate the excitability of target neurons to specific high priority
signals." Conversely, reduced LC activity periods (REM sleep) allow time
for a suppression of sympathetic tone.

These considerations, viewed collectively, suggest that the emotional
dimension of pain shares central mechanisms with vigilance. This biologically important process, intensified by injury signals from within the organism, distressing environmental events from without the organism, or a combination of these, can generate a state that progresses to hypervigilance and
beyond, to panic. As a subjective experience, the emotional quality of pain
represents awareness of immediate biological threat.

THE VENTRAL NORADRENERGIC BUNDLE AND THE
HYPOTHALAMO-PITUITARY-ADRENOCORTICAL (HPA) AXIS

The ventral noradrenergic bundle (VNB) is an ascending noradrenergic
system that enters the medial forebrain bundle (Fig. 2). Neurons in the
medullary reticular formation project to the hypothalamus via the VNB (Sumal
et al. 1983; Bonica 1990). Sawchenko and Swanson (1982) have identified
two VNB-linked noradrenergic and adrenergic pathways to the paraventricular
hypothalamus in the rat and described them using the Dahlström and Fuxe
(1964) designations: the A1 region of the ventral medulla (lateral reticular
nucleus, LRN), and the A2 region of the dorsal vagal complex (the nucleus
tractus solitarius, NTS), which receives visceral afferents. These medullary
neuronal complexes supply 90% of catecholaminergic innervation to the
paraventricular hypothalamus via the VNB (Assenmacher et al. 1987). Regions A5 and A7 make comparatively minor contributions to the VNB.

Because it innervates the hypothalamus, the VNB holds strong implications for pain research. The noradrenergic axons in the VNB respond to
noxious stimulation (Svensson 1987), as does the hypothalamus (Kanosue et
al. 1984). Moreover, nociception-transmitting neurons at all segmental levels of the spinal cord project to medial and lateral hypothalamus and several
telencephalic regions (Burstein et al. 1988). These projections provide the
major necessary neurophysiologic link between tissue injury and the hypothalamic response. Hormonal messengers may also play a part in some circumstances.

The hypothalamic paraventricular nucleus (PVN) serves as the coordinating center for the HPA axis. Neurons of the PVN receive afferent information from several reticular areas including the ventrolateral medulla, dorsal raphe nucleus, nucleus raphe magnus, LC, dorsomedial nucleus, and the nucleus tractus solitarius (Sawchenko and Swanson 1982; Peschanski and Weil-Fugacza 1987; Lopez et al. 1991). Still other afferents project to the PVN from the hippocampus and amygdala. Nearly all hypothalamic and preoptic nuclei send projections to PVN.

In responding to potentially or frankly injurious stimuli the PVN initiates a complex series of events regulated by feedback mechanisms (Fig. 3). These processes ready the organism for extraordinary behaviors that will

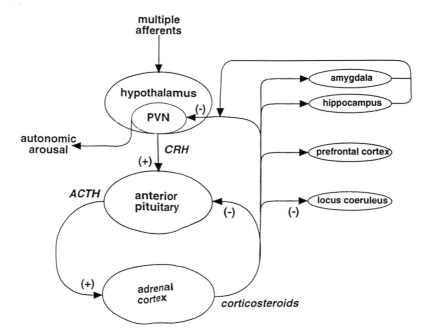

Fig. 3. Schematic representation of feedback-mediated activation in the hypothalamo-pituitary-adrenocortical axis. In response to afferent input including noxious stimulation, the hypothalamic paraventricular nucleus (*PVN*) synthesizes corticotropin releasing hormone (*CRH*) and secretes CRH into the portal circulation, which stimulates the anterior pituitary. This leads sequence leads to neurohypophyseal secretion of several pro-opiomelanocortin-derived neuropeptides including adrenocorticotrophic hormone (*ACTH*) into systemic circulation. ACTH stimulates the adrenal cortex to release corticosteroids such as hydrocortisone and corticosterone. Corticosteroids provide feedback to regulatory processes by inhibiting the anterior pituitary, which represses pro-opiomelanocortin gene expression and thus attenuates further ACTH secretion. Corticosteroid receptors exist on parvocellular PVN neurons, and in addition corticosteroids bind to the amygdala, hippocampus, and prefrontal cortical areas. In binding to hippocampus and amygdala, corticosteroids initiate further inhibitory feedback to the hypothalamic PVN and also restrain the activity of the locus coeruleus. (–) = inhibition, (+) = excitation.

maximize its chances to cope with the threat at hand (Selye 1978). Cannon (1929) described this "flight or fight" capability as an emergency reaction. Contemporary writers such as Henry (1986) and LeDoux (LeDoux et al. 1988) hold that neuroendocrine arousal mechanisms are not limited to emergency situations even though most research emphasizes that such situations elicit them. In complex social contexts, submission, dominance, and other transactions can elicit neuroendocrine and autonomic responses, modified perhaps by learning and memory. This line of thinking suggests that neuroendocrine processes accompany all sorts of emotion-eliciting situations.

Strong links exist between the hypothalamus and autonomic nervous system reactivity (Panksepp 1986). Psychophysiologists hold that diffuse sympathetic arousal reflects, albeit imperfectly, negative emotional arousal (Lacey and Lacey 1970). The PVN invokes autonomic arousal through neural and hormonal pathways. It sends direct projections to the sympathetic intermediolateral cell column in the thoracolumbar spinal cord and the parasympathetic vagal complex, sources of preganglionic autonomic outflow (Krukoff 1990). In addition, it signals release of epinephrine and norepinephrine from the adrenal medulla. ACTH (adrenocorticotrophic hormone) release, while not instantaneous, is quite rapid: it occurs within about 15 seconds (Sapolsky 1992). These considerations implicate the HPA axis in the neuroendocrinologic and autonomic manifestations of emotion during pain states.

In addition to controlling neuroendocrine and autonomic nervous system reactivity, the HPA axis coordinates emotional arousal with behavior (Panksepp 1986). Direct stimulation of hypothalamus can elicit well-organized action patterns, including defensive threat behaviors, accompanied by autonomic manifestations (Hess 1954; Mancia and Zanchetti 1981 Jänig 1985a,b). The existence of demonstrable behavioral subroutines in animals suggests that the hypothalamus plays a key role in matching behavioral reactions and bodily adjustments to challenging circumstances or biologically relevant stimuli. Moreover, at high levels, stress hormones, especially glucocorticoids, may affect central emotional arousal, lower startle thresholds, and influence cognition (Sapolsky 1992). Saphier (1987) observed that cortisol altered the firing rate of neurons in limbic forebrain. Put simply, the HPA axis takes executive responsibility for coordinating behavioral readiness with physiological capability, awareness, and cognitive function.

PAIN AND STRESS

Tissue trauma stimulates the HPA axis and thus produces a complex adaptive stress response involving neural and endocrinologic changes. This process suggests the need for physiological investigation of stress. Concomitantly, the perception of tissue trauma (pain) produces parallel changes in consciousness and behavior. These changes constitute psychological stress and invite study from a psychological perspective. In contrast to the field of emotion, where little consensus exists, physiologists and psychologists agree substantially on the nature of stress, and their theories complement one another. Indeed, these areas overlap. They meet on the common, albeit controversial, scientific ground: emotion research.

Physiologists investigating stress focus on the primarily endocrinologic, feedback-dependent HPA axis. Sapolsky (1992, p. 3), addressing the impacts of acute and chronic stress response on the process of aging, defined the primary concepts of stress research in these terms: "A *stressor* can be defined in a narrow, physiological sense as any perturbation in the outside world that disrupts homeostasis, and the *stress-response* is the set of neural and endocrine adaptations that help reestablish homeostasis." Psychologists, by and large, accept this perspective, but they emphasize psychological rather than physiological reactions to personal threats and injuries that originate in the individual's environment. Both physiological and behavioral perspectives are essential for a comprehensive description of stress.

Lazarus (1993, p. 4) distinguished between physiological and psychological focuses: "What generates physiological stress—that is, what is noxious to tissues—is not the same as what is stressful psychologically." This distinction suggests that the complex psychological dimension of pain requires a different level of inquiry than its underlying physiological processes. In the Lazarus framework, the focus of psychological inquiry must be on personal meaning. Stress depends upon cognitive appraisal of personal harms and threats. Behavior associated with stress is an adaptive effort based on appraisal, and Lazarus calls this coping behavior. If appraisal indicates that the individual can do something to help himself, he engages in *problem-focused coping*. But if there are no apparent ways to engage the problem, *emotion-focused coping* ensues. As I have already noted, the expression of emotion is an active process with potentially significant effects on the social environment.

Taken together, these considerations generate a concept of stress as a *state* of the individual that has both physiological and psychological manifestations. A stressor is any event or circumstance that threatens the biological or psychological integrity of the individual. In nature tissue trauma threatens the biological viability of the individual by definition, and it constitutes a stressor. Physiological stress responses therefore accompany tissue trauma like its shadow, and apart from the first few seconds following injury onset when the body is mobilizing such responses, they coexist with pain.

Psychological responses are complex and involve both cognition and emotion. Most psychological stress involves cognitive mediation, and psychological coping often determines the behavior of a person in pain.

Physiological stress responses interact in complex ways with the sensory qualities of pain and with psychological coping. For example, glucocorticoids released by the HPA axis during stress response diminish inflammation and block the sensitization of nociceptors in injured tissue. This response minimizes peripheral sensitization and attenuates noxious signaling. At the same time, HPA arousal releases ACTH and other pro-opiomelanocortin-derived peptides, including β-endorphin, into the bloodstream (Fig. 3). Conclusive information is not yet available, but evidence suggests that the stress response may concomitantly increase beta endorphinergic activity at the hypothalamic infundibular nucleus and thus centrally modulate the sensory aspect of pain. Such changes could facilitate fight or flight and energize psychological coping.

SUMMARY

In the classical medical perspective on pain and its treatment, negative emotion is a reaction to the presence of pain rather than a part of the pain experience. However, this view is anachronistic. The literature indicates that negative emotional arousal is an integral part of the experience of pain: signals of tissue trauma excite both spinothalamic pathways that convey them to the somatosensory cortex and spinoreticular pathways that lead to limbic areas via extensive noradrenergic projections. In part, the affective aspect of pain involves excitation of central limbic structures involved in vigilance, fear, and panic. It also excites the hypothalamo-pituitary-adrenocortical axis and the feedback-dependent stress response. I propose that, during pain, sensory and affective processing occur simultaneously and in parallel.

The emotional aspect of pain and the intimate link of pain to the structures subserving the stress response help to explain how some aspects of psychological intervention work. Relaxation, for example, engages the limbic brain in a global activity pattern that cannot coexist with fear or negative arousal. If pain cannot displace the patient's sense of relaxation and well-being, then it exists as a nonthreatening sensory awareness rather than a source of suffering.

The therapeutic effect of hypnosis is more difficult to explain than that of relaxation. However, one of the key rules of hypnosis is that the therapist must not express suggestions in negative terms. Negative statements are less likely than positive ones to "take." For hypnosis to work, the hypnotized person needs to achieve a pleasant, comfortable, and positive state of mind. While complex dissociation mechanisms associated with hypnosis may well require further explanation that goes beyond the scope of this chapter, there seems to be a requirement of positive affect. Again, the limbic brain must assume a modus operandi that is mutually exclusive of negative arousal.

Coping skill training may work in part via stress response mechanisms. Many hypotheses about mechanisms of intervention are possible, given that we view pain as an emotional response to tissue trauma that happens to have sensory features. The key concept is that the human brain is an active and autonomous agent that is capable of producing (or preventing) aspects of pain and suffering endogenously. It is not simply a passive register of sensory signaling.

Negative emotion is a complex experience. Feelings of helplessness, a sense of abandonment, loss of treasured activities or roles in society, or fear of an unbearably painful death affect the whole person and set the stage for noxious signals of tissue trauma to evoke strong negative feelings. Pain can elicit a cascade of negative feelings in a patient for whom the present situation holds little hope and many problems or disappointments. Thus, attending to the overall well-being of the cancer or AIDS patient, or providing social support via a structured support group, may contribute significantly to the control of his or her pain and suffering. Correspondingly, controlling pain effectively will tend to relieve depression.

REFERENCES

Abou-Samra AB. Mechanisms of action of CRF and other regulators of ACTH release in pituitary corticotrophs. In: Ganong WF, Dallman MF, Roberts JL (Eds). The Hypothalamic-Pituitary-Adrenal Axis Revisited. Ann NY Acad Sci 1987; 512:67–84.

Aggleton JP, Mishkin M. The amygdala: sensory gateway to the emotions. In: Plutchik R, Kellerman H (Eds). Emotion: Theory, Research and Experience, Vol 3. Orlando: Academic Press, 1986, pp 281–299.

Amaral DB, Sinnamon HM. The locus coeruleus: neurobiology of a central noradrenergic nucleus. Prog Neurobiol 1977; 9:147–196.

Assenmacher I, Szafarczyk A, Alonso G, Ixart G, Barbanel G. Physiology of neuropathways affecting CRH secretion. In: Ganong WF, Dallman MF, Roberts JL (Eds). The Hypo-thalamic-Pituitary-Adrenal Axis Revisited. Ann NY Acad Sci 1987; 512:149–161

Aston-Jones G, Foote SL, Segal M. Impulse conduction properties of noradrenergic locus coeruleus axons projecting to monkey cerebrocortex. Neuroscience 1985; 15:765–777.

Averill JR. A constructivist view of emotion. In: Plutchik R, Kellerman H (Eds). Emotion: Theory, Research, and Experience, Vol 1. New York: Academic Press, 1980, pp 305–339.

Bing Z, Villanueva L, Le Bars D. Ascending pathways in the spinal cord involved in the activation of subnucleus reticularis dorsalis neurons in the medulla of the rat. J Neurophysiol 1990; 63:424–438.

Bonica JJ (Ed). The Management of Pain, 2nd ed. Philadelphia: Lea & Febiger, 1990.

Bower GH. Mood and memory. Am Psychol 1981; 36:129–148.

Bowsher D. Role of the reticular formation in responses to noxious stimulation. Pain 1976; 2:361–378.

Burstein R, Cliffer KD, Giesler GJ. The spinohypothalamic and spinotelecephalic tracts: direct nociceptive projections from the spinal cord to the hypothalamus and telencephalon. In: Dubner R, Gebhart GF, Bond MR (Eds). Proceedings of the 5th World Congress on Pain. New York: Elsevier, 1988, pp 548–554.

Butler PD, Weiss JM, Stout JC, Nemeroff CB. Corticotropin-releasing factor produces fear-enhancing and behavioral activating effects following infusion into the locus coeruleus. J Neurosci 1990; 10:176–183.

Calogero AE, Bernardini R, Gold PW, Chrousos GP. Regulation of rat hypothalamic corticotropin-releasing hormone secretion in vitro: potential clinical implications. Adv Exp Med Biol 1988; 245:167–181.

Cannon WB. Bodily Changes in Pain, Hunger, Fear, and Rage, 2nd ed. New York: Appleton, 1929.

Charney DS, et al. Noradrenergic function in panic disorder. J Clin Psychiatry 1990, 51(Suppl. A):5–11.

Dahlström A, Fuxe K. Evidence for the existence of monoamine-containing neurons in the central nervous system. Acta Physiol Scand 1964; 62:1–55.

Darwin C. The Expression of the Emotions in Man and Animals. London: John Murray, 1872.

Elam M, Svensson TH, Thoren P. Differentiated cardiovascular afferent regulation of locus coeruleus neurons and sympathetic nerves. Brain Res 1985; 358:77–84.

Elam M, Svensson TH, Thoren P. Locus coeruleus neurons and sympathetic nerves: activation by cutaneous sensory afferents. Brain Res 1986a; 366:254–261

Elam M, Svensson TH, Thoren P. Locus coeruleus neurons and sympathetic nerves: activation by visceral afferents. Brain Res 1986b; 375:117–125.

Fields HL. Pain. New York: McGraw-Hill, 1987.

Fillenz M. Noradrenergic Neurons. Cambridge: Cambridge University Press, 1990.

Fonberg E. Amygdala, emotions, motivation, and depressive states. In: Plutchik R, Kellerman H (Eds). Emotion: Theory, Research and Experience, Vol 3. Orlando: Academic Press, 1986, pp 301–331.

Foote SL, Morrison JH. Extrathalamic modulation of corticofunction. Annu Rev Neurosci 1987; 10:67–95.

Foote SL, Bloom FE, Aston-Jones G. Nucleus locus coeruleus: new evidence of anatomical and physiological specificity. Physiol Rev 1983; 63:844–914.

Fordyce WE. Contingency management. In: Bonica JJ (Ed). The Management of Pain, 2nd ed. Philadelphia: Lea & Febiger, 1990, pp 1702–1710.

Fulton JE (Ed). Frontal Lobotomy and Affective Behavior. New York: WW Norton, 1951.

Gabriel M, Sparenborg SP, Stolar N. The neurobiology of memory. In: LeDoux JE, Hirst W (Eds). Mind and Brain: Dialogues in Cognitive Neuroscience. Cambridge: Cambridge University Press, 1986, 215–254.

Gray JA. The Neuropsychology of Anxiety: An Enquiry into the Functions of the Septo-hippocampal System. New York: Oxford University Press, 1982.

Gray JA. The Psychology of Fear and Stress, 2nd ed. Cambridge: Cambridge University Press, 1987.

Heath RG. The neural substrate for emotion. In: Plutchik R, Kellerman H (Eds). Emotion: Theory, Research, and Experience, Vol 3. New York: Academic Press, 1986, pp 3–35.

Henry JP. Neuroendocrine patterns of emotional response. In: Plutchik R, Kellerman H (Eds). Emotion: Theory, Research and Practice, Vol. 3. Orlando: Academic Press, 1986, pp 37–60.

Hess WR. Diencephalon: Autonomic and Extrapyramidal Functions. New York: Grune & Stratton, 1954.

Isaacson RL (Ed). The Limbic System, 2nd ed. New York: Plenum Press, 1982.

Jänig W. The autonomic nervous system. In: Schmidt RF (Ed). Fundamentals of Neurophysiology. New York: Springer-Verlag, 1985a, pp 216–269.

Jänig W. Systemic and specific autonomic reactions in pain: efferent, afferent and endocrine components. Eur J Anaesth, 1985b; 2:319–346.

Kanosue K, Nakayama T, Ishikawa Y, Imai-Matsumura K. Responses of hypothalamic and thalamic neurons to noxious and scrotal thermal stimulation in rats. J Thermobiol, 1984, 9:11–13.

Korf J, Bunney BS, Aghajanian GK. Noradrenergic neurons: morphine inhibition of spontaneous activity. Eur J Pharmacol 1974, 25:165–169.

Kosslyn SM, Koenig O. Wet Mind: The New Cognitive Neuroscience. New York: The Free Press, 1992.

Krukoff TL. Neuropeptide regulation of autonomic outflow at the sympathetic preganglionic neuron: anatomical and neurochemical specificity. Ann NY Acad Sci 1990; 579:162–167.

Lacey JI, Lacey BC. Some autonomic-central nervous system interrelationships. In: Black P (Ed). Physiological Correlates of Emotion. New York: Academic Press, 1970, pp 205–227.

Lazarus RS. From psychological stress to the emotions: a history of changing outlooks. Annu Rev Psychol 1993; 44:1–21.

LeDoux JE. Emotional memory: in search of systems and synapses. In: Crinella FM, Yu J (Ed). Brain Mechanisms. Ann NY Acad Sci, 1993, 702:149–157.

LeDoux JE, Iwata J, Cicchetti P, Reis DJ. Different projections of the central amygdaloid nucleus mediate autonomic and behavioral correlates of conditioned fear. J Neurosci 1988; 8:2517–2529.

LeDoux JE, Farb C, Ruggiero DA. Topographic organization of neurons in the acoustic thalamus that project to the amygdala. J Neurosci 1990; 10:1043–1054.

Levitt P, Moore RY. Origin and organization of the brainstem catecholamine innervation in the rat. J Comp Neurol 1979; 186:505–528.

Lopez JF, Young EA, Herman JP, Akil H, Watson SJ. Regulatory biology of the HPA axis: an integrative approach. In: Risch SC (Ed). Central Nervous System Peptide Mechanisms in Stress and Depression. Washington, DC: American Psychiatric Press, 1991, pp 1–52.

MacLean PD. Some psychiatric implications of physiological studies on frontotemoral portion of limbic system (visceral brain). Electroencephalogr Clin Neurophysiol 1952; 4:407–418.

MacLean PD. The Triune Brain in Evolution: Role in Paleocerebral Functions. New York: Plenum Press, 1990.

Mancia G, Zanchetti A. Hypothalamic control of autonomic functions. In: Morgane JP, Panksepp J (Eds). Handbook of the Hypothalamus: Behavioral Functions of the Hypothalamus, Vol. 3. New York: Dekker, 1981, pp 147–202.

McNaughton N, Mason ST. The neuropsychology and neuropharmacology of the dorsal ascending noradrenergic bundle: a review. Prog Neurobiol 1980; 14:157–219.

Morilak DA, Fornal CA, Jacobs BL. Effects of physiological manipulations on locus coeruleus neuronal activity in freely moving cats. II. Cardiovascular challenge. Brain Res 1987; 422:24–31.

Ortony A, Turner TJ. What's basic about basic emotions? Psychol Rev 1990; 97:315–331.

Osborne FH, Mattingley BA, Redmon WK, Osborne JS. Factors affecting the measurement of classically conditioned fear in rats following exposure to escapable versus inescapable signaled shock. J Exp Psychol 1975; 1:364–373.

Pandya DN, Barnes CL, Panksepp J. Architecture and connections of the frontal lobe. In: Perecman E (Ed). The Frontal Lobes Revisited. Hillsdale, NJ: Lawrence Erlbaum Associates, 1987, pp 41–72.

Panksepp J. The anatomy of emotions. In: Plutchik R, Kellerman H (Eds). Emotion: Theory, Research and Experience, Vol. 3. Orlando: Academic Press, 1986, pp 91–124.

Papez JW. A proposed mechanism of emotion. Arch Neurol Psych 1937; 38:725–743.

Peschanski M, Weil-Fugacza J. Aminergic and cholinergic afferents to the thalamus: experimental data with reference to pain pathways. In: Besson JM, Guilbaud G, Paschanski M (Eds). Thalamus and Pain. Amsterdam: Excerpta Medica, 1987, pp 127–154.

Ploog D. Biological foundations of the vocal expressions of emotions. In: Plutchik R, Kellerman

H (Eds). Emotion: Theory, Research, and Experience, Vol. 3. New York: Academic Press, 1986, pp 173–198.

Plutchik R. A general psychoevolutionary theory of emotion. In: Plutchik R, Kellerman H (Eds). Emotion: Theory, Research, and Experience, Vol 1. New York: Academic Press, 1980, pp 3–33.

Pribram KH. The biology of emotions and other feelings. In: Plutchik R, Kellerman H (Eds). Emotion: Theory, Research, and Experience, Vol. 1. New York: Academic Press, 1980, 245–269.

Redmond DE Jr. Alteration in the functions of the nucleus locus coeruleus: a possible model for studies of anxiety. In: Hannin I, Usdin E (Eds). Animal Models in Psychiatry and Neurology. New York: Pergamon Press, 1977, pp 293–306.

Redmond DE Jr, Huang YG. Current concepts. II. New evidence for a locus coeruleus-norepinephrine connection with anxiety. Life Sci 1979; 25, 2149–2162.

Rolls ET. Neural systems involved in emotion in primates. In: Plutchik R, Kellerman H (Eds). Emotion: Theory, Research, and Experience, Vol 3. New York: Academic Press, 1986, pp 125–144.

Roth-Roemer S, Abrams JR, Syrjala KL. Nonpharmacologic approaches to adult cancer pain management. Bull Am Pain Soc 1996; 6:1–4,9.

Saphier D. Cortisol alters firing rate and synaptic responses of limbic forebrain units. Brain Res Bull 1987; 19:519–524.

Sapolsky RM. Stress, the Aging Brain, and the Mechanisms of Neuron Death. Cambridge: MIT Press, 1992.

Sawchenko PE, Swanson LW. The organization of noradrenergic pathways from the brain stem to the paraventricular and supraoptic neuclei in the rat. Brain Res Rev 1982; 4:275.

Selye H. The Stress of Life. New York: McGraw-Hill, 1978.

Siegel JM, Rogawski MA. A function for REM sleep: regulation of noradrenergic receptor sensitivity. Brain Res Rev 1988; 13:213–233.

Staddon JER. Adaptive Behavior and Learning. London: Cambridge University Press, 1983.

Stone EA. Stress and catecholamines. In: Friedhoff AJ (Ed). Catecholamines and Behavior, Vol. 2. New York: Plenum Press, 1975, pp 31–72.

Sumal KK, Blessing WW, Joh TH, Reis DJ, Pickel VM. Synaptic interaction of vagal afference and catecholaminergic neurons in the rat nucleus tractus solitarius. J Brain Res 1983; 277:31–40.

Svensson TH. Peripheral, autonomic regulation of locus coeruleus noradrenergic neurons in brain: putative implications for psychiatry and psychopharmacology. Psychopharmacology 1987; 92:1–7.

Syrjala KL, Donaldson GW, Davis MW, Kippes ME, Carr JE. Relaxation and imagery and cognitive-behavioral training reduce pain during cancer treatment: a controlled clinical trial. Pain 1995; 63:189–198.

Talbott JD, Marrett S, Evans AC, et al. Multiple representations of pain in human cerebral cortex. Science 1991; 251:1355–1358.

Tucker DM, Vannatta K, Rothlind J. Arousal and activation systems and primitive adaptive controls on cognitive priming. In: Stein NL, Leventhal D, Trabasso T (Eds). Psychological and Biological Approaches to Emotion. Hillsdale, NJ: Lawrence Erlbaum Associates, 1990, pp 145–166.

Turner BH, Mishkin M, Knapp M. Organization of the amygdalopedal projections from modality-specific cortical association areas in the monkey. J Comp Neurol 1980; 19:515–543.

Villanueva L, Bing Z, Bouhassira D, Le Bars D. Encoding of electrical, thermal, and mechanical noxious stimuli by subnucleus reticularis dorsalis neurons in the rat medulla. J Neurophysiol 1989; 61:391–402.

Villanueva L, Cliffer KD, Sorkin LS, Le Bars D, Willis WD Jr. Convergence of heterotopic nociceptive information onto neurons of caudal medullary reticular formation in monkey (Macaca fascicularis). J Neurophysiol 1990; 63:1118–1127.

Watson SJ, Khachaturian H, Lewis ME, Akil H. Chemical neuroanatomy as a basis for biological psychiatry. In: Berger PA, Brodie HKH (Eds). Biological Psychiatry, Vol 8. [of Arieti S (Ed.). American Handbook of Psychiatry, 2nd ed.]. New York: Basic Books, 1986, pp 4–33.

Willis WD Jr (Ed). The Pain System: The Neurobasis of Nociceptive Transmission in the Mammalian Nervous System. New York: Karger, 1985.

Correspondence to: C. Richard Chapman, PhD, Department of Anesthesiology, Box 356540, University of Washington, Seattle, WA 98195-6540, USA. Tel: 206-543-2474; Fax: 206-543-2958.

Part III

Impact of Pain on Survival:
What Do We Know?

Assessment and Treatment of Cancer Pain,
Progress in Pain Research and Management,
Vol. 12, edited by R. Payne, R.B. Patt, and
C.S. Hill, IASP Press, Seattle, © 1998.

8

Pain Kills: Animal Models and Neuro-Immunological Links

Gayle Giboney Page[a] and Shamgar Ben-Eliyahu[b]

*aCollege of Nursing, The Ohio State University, Columbus, Ohio, USA;
and bDepartment of Psychology, Tel Aviv University, Tel Aviv, Israel*

Animal researchers use a variety of painful stimuli to investigate the effects of pain on the nervous, endocrine, and immune systems, and the stress of undergoing and recovering from surgery is prominently included in this literature (e.g., Pollock et al. 1987; Udelsman et al. 1987; Cover and Buckingham 1988). Both human and animal studies have documented a characteristic hormonal and metabolic response to surgery and significant suppression of several immune functions.

The physiological perturbations of surgery occur in multiple systems ranging from local changes brought about by the cutting, stretching, and tearing of tissues to systemic neuroendocrine and immune responses. For example, tissue damage results in the release of a cascade of inflammatory factors such as prostaglandins, substance P, and bradykinin, and various cytokines are released from activated leukocytes that are attracted to the injury site. Together, these factors produce local pain, redness, and swelling (Yaksh 1993). Systemically, surgery-induced neuroendocrine alterations include activation of the sympathetic nervous system and the release of catecholamines. Activation of the hypothalamic-pituitary-adrenal axis initiates the release of pituitary hormones such as opioids and growth hormone, and the adrenocortical release of corticosterone and cortisol. This pattern of hormone discharge results in major metabolic changes, including fat and protein catabolism, and hyperglycemia coupled with poor glucose utilization (Anand 1986; Cousins 1994).

These surgery-induced perturbations do not occur as isolated events; multiple levels of communication link the brain, neuroendocrine, and immune responses to tissue-damaging stressors such as surgery (Ader et al. 1990; Kusnecov and Rabin 1994). For example, the cytokine interleukin-1 has been shown to mediate local hyperalgesia (Schweizer et al. 1988) and illness symptoms such as fever and malaise (Watkins et al. 1995). Prostaglandin E has been shown to both sensitize peripheral afferent fibers (Martin et al. 1987) and suppress natural killer (NK) cell activity (Leung 1989; Ellis et al. 1990). Lymphoid organs are innervated by the sympathetic nervous system and immune cells possess catecholamine receptors (Ader et al. 1990).

Surgery has been shown to suppress some immune functions in both humans (Tønnesen 1989; Pollock et al. 1991) and animals (Tanemura et al. 1982; Pollock et al. 1987). One such function, NK cell activity, is believed to play an important role in controlling tumor development, in particular the development of metastasis. Animal studies have provided convincing and causal evidence of the key role played by NK cells in controlling metastasis. For example, abolishing NK activity by using an antiserum (antiasialo GM_1) or a monoclonal antibody (NKR-P1) selective for large granular lymphocyte (LGL)/NK cells in rats results in a more than 30-fold increase in the number of lung metastases that develop after the intravenous (i.v.) injection of tumor cells (Barlozzari et al. 1985; Ben-Eliyahu and Page 1992). Further, Barlozzari et al. (1985) showed that the adoptive transfer of purified LGL/NK cells into the NK-depleted host before tumor cell injection restored its ability to resist metastasis. Conversely, augmenting NK cell function by using the interferon-γ inducer, polyinosinic-polycytidylic acid significantly reduces the number of lung metastases (Ben-Eliyahu and Page 1992).

Human studies of NK competence and risk for metastasis are consistent with these animal findings. Specifically, persons with higher levels of preoperative NK cell activity were found to be at less risk for disease recurrence after surgery for colorectal (Tartter et al. 1987), pharyngeal (Schantz et al. 1987), and breast (Levy et al. 1985) cancer.

For the studies described herein, we used the MADB106, a model of lung metastasis developed from a chemically induced mammary adenocarcinoma in the inbred Fischer 344 rat. The seeding and colonization of MADB106 tumor cells occurs only in the lungs, and both these metastatic processes are highly controlled by NK cells. Notably, this NK cell control is limited to the first 24 hours after i.v. injection (Barlozzari et al. 1985; Ben-Eliyahu and Page 1992). This time-limited period of NK sensitivity is important in attributing an increase in the number of lung surface metastases to a suppression of NK activity resulting from a specific acute stressful event rather than to some intervening experience the animal may have had during the three weeks necessary to allow tumor colony growth. The 18-hour lung clearance assay provides a measure of the seeding of MADB106 cells in the lungs and indicates the number of metastases that would develop in the ensuing weeks if allowed to grow into colonies (Ben-Eliyahu and Page

1992). Given its NK sensitivity and well-characterized behavior after i.v. injection, we believe the MADB106 tumor model provides an in vivo indicator of both host resistance against metastasis and NK function.

The general purpose of this research is to assess the role of pain in mediating the immunosuppressive and metastatic-enhancing effects of surgery. The possibility that the pain of undergoing and recovering from surgery underlies these potentially life-threatening consequences of surgery is largely uninvestigated. Thus, the objective of this series of studies is to investigate the effects of analgesic doses of morphine on postoperative suppression of NK cell activity and host resistance against metastasis.

METHODS

ANIMALS

Mature male Fischer 344 rats were used for all studies. Animals were maintained in multiple housing on a 12-hour dark:light cycle. All surgeries were completed within the first four hours of dark onset. Food and water were available ad libitum except for the eight hours before surgery when only water was available. The institutional committee for the care and use of animal subjects approved all experimental protocols.

SURGERY AND ANESTHESIA

Surgery animals underwent a standardized abdominal laparotomy while anesthetized with halothane. Briefly, following skin preparation and penicillin prophylaxis, a 4-cm midline abdominal incision was made through the skin and muscle layers, and 10 cm of the small intestine was externalized. After gentle friction was applied between two pieces of gauze, the intestine was covered with saline-soaked gauze for four minutes. After the intestine was returned to the abdominal cavity, the skin and muscle layers were sutured with 5-0 monofilament wire. Anesthesia only animals were anesthetized at the same time and in the same dose as the surgery animals. Control animals remained in their cages throughout this period.

MADB106 TUMOR CELL MAINTENANCE AND PREPARATION

MADB106 tumor cells are maintained in a standard cell medium incubated at 37°C. For the metastatic colonization assay, cells are removed from the flask surface with trypsin 0.25%, washed in phosphate-buffered saline (PBS), and resuspended in PBS for injection. For the lung clearance assay, the DNA of the MADB106 cells is radiolabeled by adding [^{125}I]iododeoxy-uridine to the growing cell culture one day before the experiment. Following removal from the flask surface, cells are washed and resuspended in PBS (Ben-Eliyahu and Page 1992).

For both assays the prepared MADB106 cells were injected into the tail vein. For the metastatic colonization assay, lungs were removed three weeks after tumor cell injection, and the lung surface tumor colonies were counted. For the lung clearance assay, lungs were removed 18 hours after tumor cell injection and their radioactive content was measured in a gamma counter. The percent retention was calculated given the known radioactivity of the injectate.

FINDINGS

THE EFFECTS OF SURGERY ON NK CYTOTOXICITY AND METASTASIS

Surgery resulted in a significant suppression of NK cytotoxic activity, as assessed by a ^{51}Cr release assay with the standard YAC-1 murine target cell, and a significant increase in the number of lung surface metastases. These effects were evident when either blood was taken for the NK assay or when MADB106 cells were injected at five or 24 hours after surgery, but not seven days later (Page 1992; Page et al. 1993). The number of lung metastases increased more than two-fold in the surgery animals compared to the control animals, and anesthesia animals exhibited numbers of metastases that were not significantly different from controls.

Further, the number of lung tumor colonies did not increase if animals underwent surgery at 24 hours after MADB106 tumor cell injection, at a time beyond the NK-sensitive period of the tumor. This finding further confirms the time-limited sensitivity of MADB106 tumor cell metastasis to in vivo NK activity.

THE EFFECT OF ANALGESIC DOSES OF MORPHINE ON SURGERY-INDUCED INCREASES IN METASTASIS

We used both the metastatic colonization and lung clearance assays to explore the possible beneficial effects of providing morphine analgesia on surgery-induced increases in metastasis. To study this issue, we used a simple 2 × 2 experimental design: surgery with anesthesia versus anesthesia only, and morphine versus the morphine vehicle. Morphine was administered in saline 30 minutes before surgery, and postoperatively in an oil emulsion that releases the drug over several hours. Postoperative doses of morphine were administered subcutaneously immediately after the completion of surgery and with MADB106 tumor cell injection at five hours after surgery. The five-hour time point for MADB106 tumor cell injection was decided upon in an effort to capture the postoperative experience of the animal rather than responses to intraoperative events.

We found a significant interaction between the effects of surgery and morphine, such that morphine attenuated the observed surgery-induced increase in both the retention and metastatic colonization of MADB106 cells in the lungs. As we observed previously, surgery resulted in approximately a twofold increase in the number of lung surface tumor colonies, and the administration of morphine almost completely blocked this increase. In the lung clearance assay, tumor cell retention increased more than fivefold in the untreated surgery animals, and morphine administration reduced this effect by more than 50%. Morphine exerted no significant effects in the anesthesia only animals in either assay (Page et al. 1993, 1994).

THE EFFECTS OF PRE- VERSUS POSTOPERATIVE ADMINISTRATION OF MORPHINE ON SURGERY-INDUCED INCREASES IN MADB106 TUMOR CELL RETENTION

To begin to investigate the possibility that the pain-relieving effects of morphine are responsible for its beneficial effect on surgery-induced increases in metastasis, we designed this study to assess the relative importance of the pre- versus postoperative administration of morphine in this paradigm. Animals were assigned to undergo either surgery or anesthesia only and received either morphine or the vehicle at the same three times described above: 30 minutes before surgery, at the completion of surgery, and at time of radiolabeled MADB106 tumor cell injection at five hours after surgery. Anesthesia animals received either morphine or the vehicle at all three times. Surgery animals were assigned to one of five groups: (A) vehicle at all three times, (B) morphine at all three times, (C) morphine before surgery only, (D) morphine after surgery only, and (E) the same as the "D" group except that the preoperative dose of morphine in saline was administered in addition to the postoperative dose in the oil emulsion. Thus, the "E" surgery group received the same total dose as the "B" surgery group, except that all of the morphine was administered postoperatively.

As observed previously, surgery resulted in a large increase in the lung retention of MADB106 tumor cells. All morphine treatment regimens significantly attenuated this effect; however, there appeared to be some differences among the morphine-treated animals in their ability to resist metastasis. Specifically, there was a slightly larger reduction in the surgery-induced increase in tumor cell retention exhibited by the groups receiving morphine preoperatively compared to those receiving morphine only postoperatively. Indeed, only the groups receiving preoperative morphine treatment exhibited levels of tumor cell retention that were not significantly different from the anesthesia/vehicle group (Page et al. 1997).

THE EFFECTS OF ANALGESIC DOSES OF MORPHINE AND SURGERY ON EXPLORATORY BEHAVIOR

We have previously observed both qualitative and quantitative differences in the behavior exhibited by animals undergoing surgery that were treated with morphine versus those who were not (Page et al. 1993). We believe the most salient behavior is rearing, when the animal raises both forepaws off the cage floor to explore his environment. We conducted this experiment to learn whether pre- versus postoperative morphine treatment would affect postoperative exploratory behavior. Rats were placed in individual cages immediately upon awakening from surgery, and for the latter half of each of the first four postoperative hours, each rear was scored.

As we had previously observed, surgery significantly inhibited rearing behavior throughout the first four postoperative hours, and this inhibition was blocked with morphine treatment. However, there was one exception to morphine's enhancing effects on rearing behavior, and that was in the animals receiving both the pre- and postoperative doses of morphine upon the completion of surgery (Group "E" as described above). These animals were laying on their bellies, virtually unmoving until the third postoperative hour (Page et al. 1997).

DISCUSSION

These findings show that surgery is a potent suppressor of both NK cell activity and host resistance against metastasis. The NK-suppressive effects of surgery are evident at five and 24 hours, but not seven days after experimental abdominal surgery (Page 1992). These findings are consistent with those of Toge et al. (1981), who found that laparotomy resulted in suppressed NK cell activity at 24 hours but not seven days after surgery in rats. It appears that more invasive surgery extends the period of significant NK suppression to beyond seven days postoperative as was shown by Toge et al. (1981) in rats after laparothoracotomy and Pollock et al. (1987) in mice after hind limb amputation. Evidence supporting the possibility that the duration and severity of postoperative immune suppression increases with the invasiveness of the operative procedure has been presented in humans (Lennard et al. 1985; Tønnesen 1989), and it has been suggested that these consequences are more pronounced in persons undergoing surgery for cancer (Park et al. 1971; Tønnesen 1989).

In our studies, in association with the period of suppressed NK cell activity, a two- to fourfold increase in susceptibility to metastasis, recorded as either the seeding of tumor cells in the lungs or the development of lung tumor colonies, was observed if MADB106 tumor cells were injected during the first 24 hours after surgery. The pre- and postoperative administration of an analgesic dose of morphine significantly reduced the metastatic-enhancing effects of surgery. This pattern of findings was replicated on five different occasions using the metastatic colonization assay (Page et al. 1993), and more than four different occasions in the lung clearance assay (Page et al. 1994, 1997). Further, morphine administration significantly reversed the inhibition of rearing behavior that was observed in surgery animals not treated with morphine. In fact, morphine-treated surgery animals exhibited similar levels of rearing behavior as was observed in control animals.

The beneficial effect of perioperative treatment with analgesic doses of morphine supports the premise that pain plays a role in surgery-induced suppression of NK activity and resistance against metastasis. Support for this suggestion derives from several findings. First, morphine provided its beneficial effects only in the context of surgery; and in fact, our morphine administration regimen in the anesthesia only animals resulted in a small increase in metastasis. Second, morphine attenuated the surgery-induced inhibition of exploratory behavior exhibited by the unmedicated surgery animals. This finding supports the suggestion that morphine provided comfort to the animals recovering from surgery. Finally, the finding that the preoperative dose of morphine was equally efficient as the pre- and postoperative administration of morphine in ameliorating the metastatic-enhancing effects of surgery is consistent with its having prevented, or preempted, postoperative pain by interfering with the establishment of a prolonged hypersensitive state in the central nervous system (Woolf and Chong 1993). In humans, the provision of opiate preoperative medication has increased the time to first postoperative pain medication request (Kiss and Kilian 1992) and reduced both postoperative pain medication consumption via patient-controlled analgesia and pain sensitivity around the incision (Richmond et al. 1993).

These findings are not sufficient to conclude that it is the pain of undergoing and recovering from surgery that mediates the observed increase in susceptibility to metastasis. Indeed, many avenues must be explored before such an assertion can be made. For example, it is important to investigate interventions directed at the possible involvement of specific pain mechanisms such as the local and spinal transmission of nociceptive impulses in surgery-induced increases in metastasis.

In conclusion, these findings of surgery-induced enhancement of metastatic processes in the whole animal provide an indicator of the biological consequences of NK suppression. The administration of analgesic doses of morphine significantly ameliorate this life-threatening consequence of undergoing and recovering from surgery. If these relationships exist in humans, given the current surgical treatment modalities for the removal of tumors with metastatic potential and the possibility of cancer cell embolization with tumor manipulation, the surgery itself becomes a risk factor for metastasis. Adequate management of postoperative pain becomes not only a matter of providing comfort, but a matter of promoting survival.

ACKNOWLEDGMENTS

We dedicate this chapter to the late Dr. John C. Liebeskind, our mentor and friend. The early studies described were supported by National Institutes of Health Grant NS07628 and an Unrestricted Pain Research Grant from the Bristol-Myers Squibb Company. The later research was supported by NIH Grant NR03915.

REFERENCES

Ader R, Felten D, Cohen N. Interactions between the brain and immune system. Annu Rev Pharmacol Toxicol 1990; 30:561–602.

Anand KJS. The stress response to surgical trauma: from physiological basis to therapeutic implications. Prog Food Nutr Sci 1986; 10:67–132.

Barlozzari T, Leonhardt J, Wiltrout RH, Herberman RB, Reynolds CW. Direct evidence for the role of LGL in the inhibition of experimental tumor metastases. J Immunol 1985; 134:2783–2789.

Ben-Eliyahu S, Page GG. The in vivo assessment of natural killer cell activity in rats. Prog Neuroendocrinimmunol 1992; 5:199–214.

Cousins M. Acute and postoperative pain. In: Wall PD, Melzack R (Eds). Textbook of Pain, 3rd ed. Edinburgh: Churchill Livingstone, 1994, pp 357–385.

Cover PO, Buckingham JC. Effects of selective opioid-receptor blockade on the hypothalamo-pituitary-adrenocortical responses to surgical trauma in the rat. J Endocrinol 1988;121:213–220.

Ellis NK, Duffie GP, Young MR, Wepsic HT. The effects of 16,16-dimethyl PGE_2 and phosphodiesterase inhibitors on con A blastogenic responses and NK cytotoxic activity of mouse spleen cells. J Leukoc Biol 1990;47:371–377.

Kiss IE, Kilian M. Does opiate premedication influence postoperative analgesia? A prospective study. Pain 1992; 48:157–158.

Kusnecov AW, Rabin BS. Stressor-induced alterations of immune function: mechanisms and issues. Int Arch of Allergy Immunol 1994; 105:107–121.

Lennard RWJ, Shenton BK, Borzotta A, et al. The influence of surgical operations on components of the human immune system. Br J Surg 1985; 72:771–776.

Leung KH. Inhibition of human NK cell and LAK cell cytotoxicity and differentiation by PGE_2. Cell Immunol 1989; 123:384–395.

Levy SM, Herberman RB, Maluish AM, Schlien B, Lippman M. Prognostic risk assessment in primary breast cancer by behavioral and immunological parameters. Health Psychol 1985; 4:99–113.

Martin HA, Basbaum AI, Kwiat GC, Goetzl EJ, Levine JD. Leukotriene and prostaglandin sensitization of cutaneous high-threshold C- and A-delta mechanonociceptors in the hairy skin of rat hindlimbs. Neuroscience 1987; 22:651–659.

Page GG. The impact of surgery on natural killer cell cytotoxicity and tumor metastasis in rats. Dissertation. University of California Los Angeles, 1992.

Page GG, Ben-Eliyahu S, Yirmiya R, Liebeskind JC. Morphine attenuates surgery-induced enhancement of metastatic colonization in rats. Pain 1993; 54:21–28.

Page GG, Ben-Eliyahu S, Liebeskind JC. The role of LGL/NK cells in surgery-induced promotion of metastasis and its attenuation by morphine. Brain Behav Immun 1994; 8:241–250.

Page GG, Ben-Eliyahu S, McDonald JS. The attenuating effects of morphine on the metastatic and hormonal sequelae of surgery in rats. In: Jensen TS, Turner JA, Wiesenfeld-Hallin Z (Eds). Proceedings of the 8th World Congress on Pain. Progress in Pain Research and Management, Vol. 8. Seattle: IASP Press, 1998, pp 815–823.

Park SK, Brody JI, Wallace HA, Blakemore WS. Immunosuppressive effect of surgery. Lancet 1971; 7688:53–55.

Pollock RE, Lotzová E, Stanford SD, Romsdahl M. Effect of surgical stress on murine natural killer cell cytotoxicity. J Immunol 1987; 138:171–178.

Pollock RE, Lotzová E, Stanford SD. Mechanism of surgical stress impairment of human perioperative natural killer cell cytotoxicity. Arch Surg 1991; 126:338–342.

Richmond CE, Bromley LM, Woolf CJ. Preoperative morphine preempts postoperative pain. Lancet 1993; 342:73–75.

Schantz SP, Brown BW, Lira E, Taylor DL, Beddingfield N. Evidence for the role of natural immunity in the control of metastatic spread of head and neck cancer. Cancer Immunol Immunother 1987; 25:141–145.

Schweizer A, Feige U, Fontana A, Müller K, Dinarello CA. Interleukin-1 enhances pain reflexes: mediation through increased prostaglandin E2 levels. Agents Actions 1988; 25:246–251.

Tanemura H, Sakata K, Kunieda T, et al. Influences of operative stress on cell-mediated immunity and on tumor metastasis and their prevention by nonspecific immunotherapy: experimental studies in rats. J Surg Oncol 1982; 21:189–195.

Tartter PI, Steinberg B, Barron DM, Martinelli G. The prognostic significance of natural killer cytotoxicity in patients with colorectal cancer. Arch Surg 1987; 122:1264–1268.

Toge T, Hirai T, Takiyama W, Hattori T. Effects of surgical stress on natural killer activity, proliferative response of spleen cells and cytostatic activity of lung macrophages in rats. Gann 1981; 72:790–794.

Tønnesen E. Immunological aspects of anaesthesia and surgery—with special reference to NK cells. Dan Med Bull 1989; 36:263–281.

Udelsman R, Goldstein MD, Loriaux DL, Chrousos GP. Catecholamine-glucocorticoid interactions during surgical stress. J Surg Res 1987;43:539–545.

Watkins LR, Goehler LE, Relton JK, et al. Blockade of interleukin-1 induced hyperthermia by subdiaphragmatic vagotomy: evidence for vagal mediation of immune-brain communication. Neurosci Lett 1995; 183:27–31.

Woolf CJ, Chong M. Preemptive analgesia-treating postoperative pain by preventing the establishment of central sensitization. Anesth Analg 1993; 77:362–379.

Yaksh TL. New horizons in our understanding of the spinal physiology and pharmacology of pain processing. Semin Oncol 1993; 20:6–18.

Correspondence to: Gayle Giboney Page, RN, DNSc, Ohio State University, 1585 Neil Ave., Columbus, OH 43210-1289, USA. Tel: 614-292-8341; Fax: 614-292-4948; email: page.69@osu.edu.

Assessment and Treatment of Cancer Pain,
Progress in Pain Research and Management,
Vol. 12, edited by R. Payne, R.B. Patt, and
C.S. Hill, IASP Press, Seattle, © 1998.

9

The Pain–Mortality Link: Unraveling the Mysteries

Peter S. Staats

Division of Pain Medicine, Departments of Anesthesiology and Critical Care Medicine and Oncology, The Johns Hopkins University School of Medicine, Baltimore, Maryland, USA

After a long legacy of undertreatment, the management of pain in patients with terminal diseases has garnered widespread acceptance over the past decade. Activities initiated by numerous professional societies, governmental organizations such as the World Health Organization, and investigators from various disciplines have helped identify the importance of optimal treatment for this previously underserved patient population. Proponents have not only argued that treating pain in patients with terminal diseases has intrinsic value, but have demonstrated that pain relief can be achieved in nearly 90% of patients with the application of relatively straightforward approaches. As priorities in contemporary health care have shifted, pain control has become cost-effective both in cancer and noncancer populations (Ferrell 1996; Turk 1996). In the population of patients with nonmalignant pain, a variety of outcomes have been used to establish the efficacy of treatment including return to work, closure of disability claims, decreased health care utilization, and improved functional status. However, another compelling reason to provide optimal pain treatment in patients with terminal diseases is mounting evidence that pain can kill.

A literature review suggests that patients with pain may indeed die sooner than their counterparts without pain, an effect that appears to be operant in a variety of disease states. This proposed relationship has received surprisingly little attention in the medical and pain communities, perhaps due to failure to recognize correlations between pain and mortality or because it is difficult to definitively prove a direct link between these multifactorial phenomena. Heightened morality may be simply viewed as a

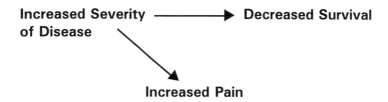

Fig. 1. In the unidirectional model, pain is ephemeral and does not affect survival.

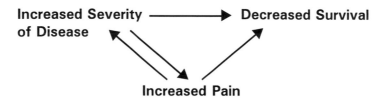

Fig. 2. In this model, increased severity of disease affects pain and survival, and pain, in turn, adversely affects survival.

natural consequence of increasing severity of underlying disease and therefore unworthy of further study (Fig. 1).

However, it is possible that a simple unidirectional model is insufficient and that pain and its sequelae contribute to reduced survival (Fig. 2). Data from investigations in animals and indications from the clinical literature support the thesis that stress and pain lead to higher mortality. This chapter will address the correlations in the clinical literature between pain and mortality and, where possible, correlations between pain relief and physiologic end points, including survival. Cardiac pain, AIDS-related pain, sickle cell–related pain, and cancer pain all show a positive correlation between pain and mortality. This chapter will present a framework for understanding how the severity of disease can affect pain, and how pain consequently affects the severity of disease. Indeed, pain may be more than an index of disease, but also an important determinant of survival.

PAIN AND SURVIVAL: ANGINA AS A MODEL

Chest pain related to angina is an ideal starting place for the development of an interactive pain model. The pathophysiologic relationship between pain and angina (i.e., that persons with ischemia experience pain) is well understood. A decrease in blood supply can result in abnormalities of perfusion and ischemia which, in turn, lead to pain that may initiate a vicious cycle. Unchecked, ischemia also increases infarct size and increases subsequent mortality. This model suggests that it would be unwise to mask pain with opioids or anesthesia, as pain serves a *protective* function by keeping the organism from overexerting itself and further perturbing the oxygen supply-demand ratio. This unfavorable oxygen supply-demand ratio results in ischemia—interpreted first as pain and resulting eventually in infarction. In this traditional unidirectional model, pain serves a teleologic function, warning the organism to slow down.

The relationship described above is probably far oversimplified. We now better understand the relationship between the stress response and ischemia. The stress response includes direct and indirect adrenergic stimulation of the coronary vasculature, which in turn results in vasospasm and reduced oxygen supply. While it is understood that pain elicits a stress response, it is far less certain that pain serves an exclusively protective function. It is possible that sympathetically mediated changes associated with pain directly and indirectly affect outcome adversely (Fig. 3). Some lines of evidence support such a hypothesis. During angina, 75% of cases of arteriosclerotic coronary stenosis behave in a dynamic fashion and respond to sympathetic stimulation (Gould 1980; Brown 1981). Constriction of the coronary luminal area occurs with activation of the sympathetic nervous system induced either by performing an isometric hand grip or using the cold pressor test (Raizner et al. 1980; Brown 1985). The resultant decrease in myocardial oxygen supply-demand ratio increases ischemia, and consequently pain. Increased pain elicits further central and peripheral stress responses, which lead to more ischemia. Thus, in this model a viscous cycle develops and rather than serving a protective role, pain may increase the severity of the underlying disease and may adversely affect outcomes.

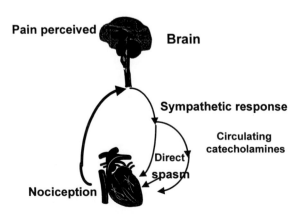

Fig. 3. The interactive nature of pain and angina.

Increased sympathetic tone may adversely effect myocardial ischemia in several ways. First, it can cause a further increase in the constriction of intraluminal diameter with a resultant decrease in blood flow distal to a left anterior descending artery (LAD) stenosis and an increase in left ventricle (LV) wall dyskinesia with subsequent increased ST elevation (Uchaida and Murao 1975). Second, serotonin, which is carried by platelets and is released during early platelet aggregation, causes considerable coronary vasoconstriction when combined with adrenergic stimulation. This sympathetic activation can also trigger cyclic platelet accumulation in areas of disease. Finally, serotonin in concentrations lower than those observed in circulating platelets is known to increase aortic blood pressure and thus myocardial oxygen demand (James et al. 1975; Cohen 1985; Cohen et al. 1987; Folts 1991). Moreover, blood flow is redistributed away from the endocardium to the epicardium during sympathetic stimulation, with resultant decreases in diastolic perfusion pressure (Uchaida and Ueda 1975; Schwartz and Stone 1977) and decreased myocardial oxygen supply to ischemic myocardium. In addition, ischemic myocardium is more sensitive to dysrhythmias as a result of catecholamines released during sympathetic nervous system stimulation.

Assessment of this scenario in human models has revealed that the duration of chest pain correlates with infarct size and with poor long-term prognosis. In 1985, Ledwich and Wong commented, "If the aggressive treatment of pain in patients with acute myocardial infarction, with a consequent reduction in the duration of pain, results in a corresponding reduction in the size of the infarct and an improvement of long term prognosis, the foundation for a successful therapeutic approach to the management of acute myocardial infarction would have been laid" (Ledwich and Wong 1985).

Toward this end, significant work has looked at methods of providing analgesia and minimizing the stress response associated with ischemia. Early neurosurgical approaches included stellate ganglionectomy, with the thought that it may be possible to denervate the heart's sympathetic innervation. Unfortunately, this approach had a relatively high operative mortality and lost favor with the advent of more sophisticated medical approaches (Lindgren 1950). More recently, anesthesiologists have placed thoracic epidural catheters to administer local anesthetics and provide analgesia by blocking sympathetic afferents (and tone) to the diseased myocardium. In these models, sympathectomy resulted in a 20–25% decrease in coronary vascular resistance and was associated with a decreased incidence of dysrhythmias, reduced angina, increased exercise tolerance, and higher endocardial to epicardial blood flow ratio in animals treated with sympathetic analgesia. Animal

studies have also demonstrated that thoracic epidural analgesia reduces myocardial infarct size after coronary occlusion in dogs. The infarcts were 46%
smaller in dogs that received lidocaine for thoracic epidural analgesia compared to controls that received saline.

Several studies have assessed the importance of thoracic epidural analgesia in providing adequate analgesia for patients with status angina. Most
important has been a series of studies by Blomberg and colleagues that
assessed the importance of thoracic epidural analgesia on coronary arteries
and arterioles in patients with severe coronary artery disease. In 27 patients,
pain control was not only more effective with thoracic epidural analgesia
than with traditional methods, but during thoracic epidural analgesia the
intraluminal diameter of the stenotic segments increased from 1.34 ± 0.11 mm
to 1.56 ± 0.13 mm ($P < 0.002$) while the intraluminal diameter of nondiseased
segments remained unchanged (Blomberg et al. 1990). Thus, there appear to
be several advantages to providing epidural analgesia during status angina
(Staats and Panchal, in press). Although the groundwork has been laid,
further clinical studies are needed to document the efficacy of pain control
(and reduced sympathetic discharge) on life expectancy in patients with
coronary artery disease.

PAIN AND SURVIVAL IN PATIENTS WITH AIDS

It is still too early to determine whether patients with AIDS-related pain
have a higher mortality that do those without pain, and in particular whether
a causal relationship exists. Preliminary studies have begun to assess this
correlation. A study from Italy in which 458 patients were seen between
1985 and 1989 determined that 71 (15%) had severe abdominal pain and,
notably, its presence was associated with a reduced survival (Parente et al.
1994). The estimated survival for patients with severe abdominal pain was
180 days as compared to 540 days for controls. Although laparoscopies
were frequently performed in the patients with pain, they were not performed in those without pain. We thus do not have a clear picture of the
severity of disease in the patients with and without pain. Obviously, those
with more severe disease would be expected to have a higher mortality, but
that factor has not been assessed in the only study outlining the correlation
between pain and survival in patients with AIDS. Further studies need to be
performed to discern the importance of pain and pain relief on survival in
patients with AIDS.

MORTALITY IN SICKLE CELL DISEASE

Correlations between pain and mortality have also been demonstrated for patients suffering from sickle cell disease. A recent study reporting on 3764 patients noted that a large proportion of patients who died had no overt chronic organ failure, but expired during an episode of pain. In fact, 78% of these patients who died had pain, chest syndrome, or both at the time of death. While, we cannot assume a causal relationship between death and pain severity, as it could be a manifestation of the severity of disease (Platt et al. 1994), a correlation clearly exists, and the question "could the pain be affecting survival in this population?" warrants further study.

Sickle cells have an abnormal cell structure and a decreased oxygen carrying capacity. During stress (acidosis, hypothermia, etc.) cells undergo further morphologic changes that lead to further reductions in oxygen carrying capacity. Patients with chest syndrome frequently hypoventilate due to pain. Splinting and hypoventilation can in turn predispose to hypercarbia and acidosis, which *may* exacerbate the severity of disease and contribute to further sickling. It was originally postulated that chest syndrome arises from infarcts of the primary pulmonary vasculature in patients without pneumonia or pulmonary embolus. More recently, Gelfand and colleagues have postulated that chest syndrome originates with microbony infarcts, and subsequent rib pain, soft tissue reaction, and pleurisy (Ruscknagel et al. 1991). Rib pain also leads to splinting and hypoventilation, which in turn are responsible for the radiographic features of chest syndrome. This model posits pain as the inciting morbid event. This hypothesis is supported by a recent case of a three-year-old child who was struck in the chest by a baseball bat, which led to ipsilateral pain and splinting and a fulminant chest syndrome on that side (Zuckerberg 1996). Presumably epidural analgesia that blunts the afferent pain transmission would favorably affect the course of such a disorder. Additional studies that assess the importance of the analgesic regimen for sickle cell pain and particularly chest syndrome are badly needed.

PAIN AND SURVIVAL IN PATIENTS WITH CANCER

Although literature support for a correlation between pain and mortality in patients with cancer is somewhat robust, again the relationship is not entirely clear. It seems intuitive and logical that increased pain would correlate with decreased survival due to more advanced disease, more tumor burden, and other factors. In this model, though, pain could simply be a coexisting phenomenon and may not have a direct effect on survival. However, the literature is supportive of a distinct pain-mortality correlation in patients with cancer. Kalser et al. assessed 393 patients with pancreatic cancer and found several independent variables that correlated with survival. While patients with less pain survived longer (Kalser et al. 1985), they also had less severe disease, which confounded the interpretation of this phenomenon.

Data was collected on 14 preoperative and two operative variables in a retrospective survey of 337 patients who had pulmonary resection for bronchial carcinoma. After multiple regression analyses, investigators found that four variables—weight loss, *pain*, tumor size, and cell type—had significant *independent* effects on survival (Clee et al. 1984). The difference in survival between patients with and without pain was highly statistically significant ($P < .005$). While this study also revealed a relationship between pain and weight loss, elevated erythrocyte sedimentation rate (ESR), central location and pneumonectomy, the multiple regression analyses only confirmed tumor size, weight loss, and pain as independent predictors of significantly reduced survival. Thus, in this study pain, independent of the tumor aggressiveness, adversely predicted survival.

Reporting on colon cancer in blacks, Bumper et al. noted a relationship between age at presentation and survival in patients with pain. This study reviewed medical records over a 10-year period in which patients were divided into Group 1 (patients between the ages of 29 and 49) and Group 2 (patients between the ages of 52 and 93). A significantly greater percentage of Group I patients (45%) experienced abdominal pain as compared to Group II (23%). Life expectancy in Group 1 was nearly 23 months while survival for Group 2 averaged about 64 months. Although subjects in Group 1 had greater pain and mortality, investigators raised the possibility that they may have had a more aggressive form of the disease, which would account both for increased pain and shortened survival. However, this study also suggests a relationship between shortened survival and pain in cancer patients (Bumper et al. 1994).

DOES ADEQUATE PAIN RELIEF IMPROVE LIFE EXPECTANCY?

Answering the question of whether adequate pain relief improves human life expectancy is difficult. There are important theoretical reasons to believe that patients with increased disease severity have more pain that may, in turn, further influence the severity of disease and thus survival. How do we prospectively assess whether controlling a person's pain will affect their survival? Animal analgesic-survival studies may provide preliminary answers. Unfortunately, pain relief is such an important outcome measure that withholding analgesia to study survival is unethical. It is, however, ethical and possible to assess the effects of different types of interventions and approaches on comfort, quality of life, and life expectancy.

An ideal example of this type of study was performed by Lillimoe et al. (1993) in a double-blind, placebo-controlled randomized trial designed to assess pain control after intraoperative chemical splanchnicectomy in patients with pancreatic cancer (Lillimoe et al. 1993). Between February 1987 and 1991, the investigators at Johns Hopkins Hospital administered a standardized preoperative questionnaire to 371 patients with pancreatic cancer. The study subsequently excluded 232 patients who had complete tumor resection. In two other patients, the surgeon was unable to perform a splanchnicectomy due to tumor encasement at the level of the celiac axis. The remaining 139 eligible patients were randomized to receive an intraoperative block with 20 cc of either 50% alcohol or normal saline injected on each side of the celiac plexus. In this paradigm the surgeon was handed the syringe without knowledge of whether it contained alcohol or saline. The patients were followed with a questionnaire every two months until death. These two groups were further randomized to patients with minimal pain who had a visual analogue scale (VAS) pain score of less than three, or significant pain, as indicated by a VAS score greater than three. Patients (with and without preoperative pain) who were randomized to the alcohol block were pain-free for a longer time. They also had a larger decrease in the opioid requirement and a lower incidence of pain at death.

Statistical analysis revealed a significant increase in survival and mood in the group receiving the alcohol block (Staats et al. 1997). When patients with pain were followed until death, statistical analysis revealed a marked increase in survival in the group receiving the alcohol celiac plexus block. This finding suggests the possibility that improved analgesia with celiac plexus blockade may improve survival in patients with pancreatic cancer.

EXPLANATIONS FOR THE PAIN-MORTALITY LINK

Why would patients with increased pain have decreased survival? A unidirectional explanation would suggest that increased virulence of disease or more advanced disease occurs in patients with pain. However, bidirectional explanations may also implicate independent influences of pain on sympathetic tone, mood, diet, activities of daily living, and immunologic status—variables that, in turn, affect survival.

PAIN AND MOOD

A new theory of pain focusing on psychological behaviorism proposes that pain and emotions are centrally and inextricably linked. Pain is conceived as a type of negative emotional response that is affected by a variety of biological and psychological factors, and which, in turn, affect behavior. Individuals with more pain experience a lower mood (i.e., depression) that affects behavior (Staats et al. 1996). Patients who are depressed may actively participate in behaviors that shorten their life (suicide) or may simply refrain from activities that may lead to a longer life. Such behaviors can include compliance with medical regimens, decreased oral intake, and sedentary life style. Decreased nutritional status and, probably secondarily, a depressed immunological status, may be by-products of such behaviors. In addition, mood may have direct effects on the immune system or on activities of daily living. A recent study of the efficacy of celiac plexus block (CPB) in patients with pancreatic cancer randomized patients to receive nonsteroidal anti-inflammatory drugs (NSAIDs) plus morphine or a CPB (with NSAIDs plus morphine) as treatment for uncontrolled pain (Kawamata et al. 1996). Investigators detected less deterioration in quality of life (of which mood was one index) in the group receiving CPB. Interestingly, although this small study had high variability in survival time between groups, it also revealed a clear trend toward increased survival in the CPB-treated group.

Spiegel et al. (1989) performed an early study assessing the role of mood and psychosocial treatment on survival. In this study, 86 patients with metastatic breast cancer received one year of interventional psychotherapy, including self-hypnosis for pain control. Subsequently, patients were followed and assessed for 10 years. Interestingly, the researchers observed a divergence in survival among subjects at 20 months after entering into the study (or eight months after completion of the psychotherapy). Patients receiving the psychotherapy package had almost twice the survival rate as those who did not. Other investigators are attempting to replicate these profoundly important findings.

METABOLIC ABNORMALITIES IN PATIENTS WITH CANCER

Physiologic effects of cancer may also affect mood and survival. Patients with a sedentary life-style may have increased calcium levels. Stress (as may occur with poorly controlled pain) can result in increased release of catecholamines and corticosteroids, which deplete magnesium. Elevations in calcium with low levels of magnesium are correlated with an increased risk of cardiovascular damage, arrhythmias, sudden cardiac death, and a hyper-coagulable state. These factors may translate to a higher incidence of deep venous thrombosis in patients with cancer. Further, patients with a depressed mood may also have inadequate oral intake, which may further deplete magnesium levels (Seelig 1994).

IMMUNE FUNCTION AND PAIN

Numerous animal studies indicate that immune function can be modified by pain and by opioid use. Yeager and Colacchio (1991) assessed these phenomena in rats inoculated with colon cancer cells, and demonstrated that daily opioids decreased the growth of tumor cells associated with surgical stress. Lewis et al. (1983) found that both stress and morphine deleteriously affected survival in rats challenged with mammary ascites tumor. In this study, Lewis suggested that both stress and morphine similarly affected the cytotoxicity of natural killer (NK) cells. However, as early as 1986, Simon and Arbo injected Walker 256 tumor cells intravenously to produce pulmo-nary metastases. They found that the number of metastases could be in-creased by pretreatment with morphine and that this increase could be blocked by treatment with naloxone. This finding suggests that morphine has a direct immunologic suppressant effect on NK cell activity (Simon and Arbo 1986). More recently, however, Paige et al. (1993) found that analgesic doses of morphine blocked surgery-induced increases in metastasis without affecting the metastasis in unoperated animals. They argue that pain depresses NK cell activity, and that blunting the pain preserves it. Accordingly, treating pain should minimize tumor growth and metastatic spread.

CONCLUSION

There are strong suggestions in the literature of clear, positive correla-tions between increased pain and increased mortality in multiple disease states. It is not as clear that increased pain *causes* increased mortality in human trials, but when clinical correlates are considered in the context of animal studies, theoretical work, and the small number of clinical studies that support a direct relationship between pain relief and survival, it be-comes clear that uncontrolled pain could result in greater mortality. Accord-ingly, it is increasingly important that patients with pain be aggressively treated, not only because of ethical and moral imperatives, but because of the likelihood that uncontrolled pain contributes to a shortened life expectancy. Physicians still avoid prescribing sufficient doses of strong analgesics in ill-advised efforts to avoid tolerance. Although the reasoning underlying this practice is flawed for several reasons, it may also contribute to an earlier demise in some patients.

Much work needs to be done to confirm the preliminary findings of animal research, basic science investigations, theoretical modeling, and early clinical trials that suggest that controlling pain in patients with certain medical diseases improves life expectancy. The next generation of analgesic studies may assess not only the efficacy of various analgesic regimens on pain control and quality of life, but also survival.

REFERENCES

Blomberg S, Emanuelsson H, Kvist H, et al. Effects of thoracic epidural anesthesia on coronary arteries and arterioles in patients with coronary artery disease. Anesthesiology 1990; 73:840–847.

Brown BG. Coronary vasospasm: observations linking the clinical spectrum of ischemic heart disease to the dynamic pathology of coronary artery after sclerosis. Arch Intern Med 1981; 141:716–722.

Brown BG. Response of normal and diseased epicardial coronary arteries to vasoactive drugs: quantitative arteriographic studies. Am J Cardiol 1985; 56:23E–29E.

Bumper HL, Williams WL, Hassett JM. Colon cancer in blacks: age-related presentation and survival within a similar socioeconomic group. J Nat Med Assoc 1994; 86:216–218.

Clee MD, Hockings NF, et al. Bronchial carcinoma: factors influencing postoperative survival. Br J Dis Chest 1984; 78:225.

Cohen RA. Platelet-induced neurogenic coronary arterial contractions due to accumulation of the false neurotransmitter 5-hydroxytryptamine. J Clin Invest 1985; 75:286–292.

Cohen RA, Zitnay KM, Weisrod RM. Accumulation of 5-hydroxytryptamine leads to dysfunction of adrenergic nerves in canine coronary artery following intimal damage in vivo. Circ Res 1987; 61:829–833.

Ferrell BR. How patients and families pay the price of pain. In: Cohen MJM, Campbell JN (Eds). Pain Treatment Centers at a Crossroads: A Practical and Conceptual Reappraisal. Seattle: IASP Press, 1996, pp 229–239.

Folts JD. An in vivo model of experimental arterial stenosis, intimal damage, and periodic thrombosis. Circulation 1991; 83 (Suppl IV):IV3–14.

Gould KL. Dynamic coronary stenosis. Am J Cardiol 1980; 45:286–292.

James TN, Isobe JH, Urthaler F. Analysis of components in a hypertensive cardiogenic chemoreflex. Circulation 1975; 52:179.

Kalser MH, Barkin J, et al. Pancreatic cancer: assessment of prognosis by clinical presentation. Cancer 1985; 56:397–402.

Kawamata M, Ishitani K, et al. Comparison between celiac plexus block and morphine treatment on quality of life in patients with pancreatic cancer. Pain 1996; 64:597–604.

Ledwich JR, Wong CJ. Duration of chest pain associated acute myocardial infarction: a predictor of long-term prognosis. Can Med Assoc J 1985; 132:Feb. 1.

Lewis JW, Shavit Y, et al. Stress and morphine affect survival of rats challenged with a Mammary Ascites Tumor (MAT 13762B). Nat Immun Cell Growth Regul 1983,1984; 3:43–50.

Lillimoe KD, et al. Chemical splanchnicectomy in patients with unresectable pancreatic cancer: a prospective randomized trial. Ann Surg 1993; 217:447–457.

Lindgren I. Angina pectoris: a clinical study with special reference to neurosurgical treatment [thesis]. Acta Med Scand 1950, pp 1–141.

Page GG, Ben-Eliyahu S, Yirmiya R, Liebskind JC. Morphine attenuates surgery-induced enhancement of metastatic colonization in rats. Pain 1993; 54:21–28.

Parente F, Cernuschi M, Anitonori S. Severe abdominal pain in patients with AIDS: frequency and clinical aspects, causes and outcomes. Scand J Gastro 1994; 29:511–515.

Platt OF, Brambilla DJ, Rosse WT. Mortality in sickle cell disease: life expectancy and risk factors for early death. N Engl J Med 1994; 330:1639–1644.

Raizner AE, Chahine RA, Hisahimori T, et al. Provocation of coronary artery spasm by the cold pressor test: hemodynamic, arteriographic, and quantitative angiographic observations. Circulation 1980; 62:925–932.

Ruscknagel DL, Kalinyak KA Gelfand MJ. Rib infarcts and acute chest syndrome in sickle cell diseases. Lancet 1991; 337:831.

Schwartz P, Stone H. Tonic influence of the sympathetic nervous system on myocardial reactive hyperemia and on coronary blood flow distribution in dogs. Circ Res 1977; 41:51–58.

Seelig MS. Consequences of magnesium deficiency on the enhancement of stress reactions: preventive and therapeutic implications (a review). J Am Coll Nutr 1994; 13:429–446.

Simon RH, Arbo TE. Morphine increases metastatic tumor growth. Brain Res 1986; 16:363–367.

Spiegal D, et al. Effect of psychosocial treatment on survival of patients with metastatic breast cancer. Lancet 1989; 2:888–891.

Staats PS, Panchal SJ. Epidural anesthesia for status angina in the coronary care unit: the evolving roles of the anesthesiologist. Journal of Cardiovascular and Thoracic Anesthesia 1997; 11:105–108.

Staats PS, Hekmat H, Sauter P, Lillimoe K. The effects of alcohol, negative mood, and postoperative pain on life expectancy in patients with pancreatic cancer. Presented at the American Pain Society Annual Meeting, New Orleans, October 1997.

Staats PS, Hekmat H, Staats AW. The psychological behaviorism theory of pain: a basis for unity. Pain Forum 1996; 3:194–207.

Turk DC. Efficacy of multidisciplinary pain centers in the treatment of chronic pain. In: Cohen MJM, Campbell JN. Pain Treatment Centers at a Crossroads: A Practical and Conceptual Reappraisal. Seattle: IASP Press, 1996, pp 257–274.

Uchaida Y, Murao S. Sustained decrease in coronary blood flow in excitation of cardiac sensory fibers following sympathetic stimulation. Jpn Heart J 1975; 16:265–279.

Uchaida Y, Ueda H. Non-uniform myocardial blood flow caused by stellate ganglion stimulation. Jpn Heart J 1975; 16:162–73.

Yeager MP, Colacchio TA. Effect of morphine on growth of metastatic colon cancer in vivo. Arch Surg 1991; 126:454–456.

Correspondence to: Peter S. Staats, MD, Johns Hopkins Hospital, Division of Pain Medicine, 550 Bldg., Rm. 201, 600 N. Wolfe St., Baltimore, MD 21287, USA. Tel: 410-955-7246; Fax: 410-550-6730.

Part IV

Clinical Assessment and Management of Cancer Pain

Assessment and Treatment of Cancer Pain,
Progress in Pain Research and Management,
Vol. 12, edited by R. Payne, R.B. Patt, and
C.S. Hill, IASP Press, Seattle, © 1998.

10

Neuropathic Pain:
Mechanisms and Clinical Assessment

Robert R. Allen

*Department of Neuro-Oncology, The University of Texas M. D. Anderson
Cancer Center, Houston, Texas, USA*

Neuropathic pain, the perception of pain due to a dysfunctional nervous system, remains a clinical challenge. Reviews of neuropathic pain in cancer patients are rare (Portenoy 1993), although several common syndromes are recognized (Table I). In addition to tumor-associated compression of somatic and visceral structures, cancer patients are exposed to unique therapies that may cause neural injury. Consequently, cancer patients frequently have multiple nociceptive and non-nociceptive mechanisms contributing to their pain. We need to ask a fundamental question: Is neuropathic pain in patients with cancer different than that in patients with a noncancer diagnosis? Although history (Table II) and examination (Table III) show common clinical features, the concurrent diagnosis of cancer adds a dimension that becomes an important part of the clinical assessment over time. Assessing the various components of pain and inferring mechanisms based on history, examination, and response to therapy is clinically challenging; whether this process has any bearing on therapeutic choices remains speculative.

This chapter presents a selection of the *theoretical mechanisms* (Table IV) of neuropathic pain and *assessment strategies* with an emphasis on the cancer patient. Data were largely obtained through personal clinical experience and continuing human clinical trials at The University of Texas M. D. Anderson Cancer Center.

CANCER VS. NONCANCER POPULATIONS

There are several important distinctions between patients with neuropathic pain who have cancer and those who have noncancer disorders

Table I
Common clinical syndromes of neuropathic pain in the cancer patient

Toxic neuropathies: chemotherapy: cisplatin, vincristine, paclitaxol

Postsurgical pain: post-thoracotomy, post-mastectomy, post-amputation

Postradiation pain: myelotomy, plexopathy

Paraneoplastic pain: sensory neuronopathy, ganglionopathy

Infections: postherpetic neuralgia

Note: These syndromes, in addition to tumor-related compression of neural structures, may occur anywhere along the neural axis in cancer patients.

such as painful diabetic neuropathy or postherpetic neuralgia. Making these distinctions is most important when dealing with the treatment-related neuropathic pain syndromes. First, many patients and clinicians make informed or uninformed choices regarding therapies that are potentially life saving, but that can cause pain or dysfunction due to neural injury. Many common syndromes (Table I) are the result of such clinical choices; many specific chemotherapies may be continued despite painful symptoms. Second, my experience with noncancer pain centers is that opioids usually are medications of "last resort" for the "nonmalignant" pain syndromes. Although opioids have are effective in both noncancer (Rowbotham et al. 1991) and cancer (Cherney et al. 1994) neuropathic pain syndromes, their chronic use outside a cancer setting remains controversial. In patients with active cancer and pain resulting from multiple mechanisms, opioids coupled with a tricyclic antidepressant, anticonvulsant, or antiarrhythmic agent often produce great success. Patients with treatment-related pain but without active disease begin to look much like patients without malignancy, and opioids are still used with frequent success. Third, the assessment and reassessment of a cancer patient with pain presents the consistent possibility of cancer recurrence and a significant, potentially life-ending, illness. For most patients with cancer

Table II
Common clinical features of neuropathic pain from patient history

Localization of pain in an *area of sensory deficit*

Temporal features
    Spontaneous pain with paroxysms at rest, i.e., unprovoked
    Delay or change in pain character from the time of injury

Quality of pain described as *burning, sharp,* or *shooting*

Note: Features are meant to be specific for neural dysfunction independent of a known cause (such as tumor compression of nerve, or neural hypersensitivity as the result of regional inflammation or swelling).

Table III
Common clinical features of neuropathic pain from sensory examination

---

Positive sensory features in the absence of any clinically evident swelling or regional inflammation.

Allodynia with pain in response to normally innocuous stimuli such as light touch and temperature.

Hyperalgesia with a lowered threshold of pain in response to normally painful stimuli such as pin-prick, temperature, or pressure.

Dynamic rather than static allodynia with evoked pain worse with light brushing than with pressure, or pain relieved by pressure.

Hyperpathia with an increase in the threshold of pain in response to normally painful stimuli such as pin-prick or extreme temperatures with reported summation, spread, and/or prolonged pain after sensation.

---

there is the *fear* and realistic possibility that recurrent cancer is the major reason for pain. This issue becomes clinically important given the high incidence of cancer recurrence coupled with the possible delay in pain following neural injury in common syndromes such as breast cancer with postmastectomy pain syndrome or lung cancer and postthoracotomy pain syndrome.

Understanding some of these differences between cancer and noncancer patients can provide a base for the education of patients, their families, and health professionals involved in their care. Consideration of these issues may influence pain evaluation approaches and could significantly affect therapeutic strategies and outcome.

Table IV
Neuropathic pain mechanisms

Mechanism	Reference
Ectopic impulses	Wall and Devor 1983
Neurogenic inflammation	LaMotte et al. 1991
Gene regulated c-*fos* changes	Basbaum et al. 1992
Neuropeptide changes	Levine et al. 1993
Ephaptic connections	Jänig 1988
Sympathetic dysfunction	Roberts 1988
Neuronal sprouting: peripheral	Inbal et al. 1987
Neuronal sprouting: central	Woolf et al. 1992
Central sensitization	Woolf and Thompson 1991
Thalamic LTS* bursts	Lenz 1991; Jeanmonod et al. 1996
Nervi nervorum†	Asbury and Fields 1984

*LTS = low-threshold calcium spike.
†Pain due to neural compression by a noxious stimulus may be referred to as nociceptive neuropathic pain.

MECHANISMS OF NEUROPATHIC PAIN

It is impossible to discuss mechanisms without discussing therapies. The list of theoretical mechanisms to explain neuropathic pain (Table IV) at times seems endless, with pathophysiologic evidence supporting peripheral and central processes (Fields and Rowbotham 1994). Much of the recent work explaining neuropathic pain comes from animal models of defined neural injury and observed behavior (Zeltser and Seltzer 1994); the relevance of these findings to human conditions remains speculative. Human studies in which administration of intradermal capsaicin has produced patterns of pain and hyperalgesia similar to some neuropathic pain states have provided considerable insight (La Motte et al. 1991; Torebjörk et al. 1992). More recent surgical studies in humans with neuropathic pain suggest that the medial thalamic nuclei may play an important role in these syndromes (Jeanmonod et al. 1996). Still, none of these experimental conditions are representative of the patient with cancer, neural injury, and pain. Such clinical models remain to be developed.

ABNORMAL SODIUM CHANNELS

Early theories of neuropathic pain mechanisms that have stood the test of time include the theory of *ectopic neural activity* due to neuroma formation, with spontaneous neural activity originating at the site of injury and in the dorsal root ganglia (Wall and Devor 1983). Abnormal or dysfunctional sodium channels have been implicated by several groups (Devor et al. 1989; England et al. 1991) as the cause of this ectopic activity and may explain the noted benefit of sodium-channel blocking agents such as lidocaine, mexiletine, phenytoin, and carbamazepine. More intriguing is the recent evidence that tricyclic antidepressants also act as sodium-channel blockers (Jacobson et al. 1995). This finding may in part explain the sometimes immediate effect (analgesia within two to three days) with these agents.

Controlled trials of lidocaine, an assumed sodium-channel blocker, in noncancer (Rowbotham et al. 1991) and cancer patients (Bruera et al. 1992) with neuropathic pain have produced different results. Lidocaine has proven effective for noncancer patients but not for those with cancer. There are no obvious reasons why neuropathic pain should respond differently in cancer and noncancer patients, unless assumed mechanisms and assessment approaches are fundamentally different. In cancer patients, tumor involvement of the nervi nervorum with "nociceptive neuropathic pain" (see below) may represent a different mechanism with variable response to therapy. These issues and controversies are under investigation. My personal experience has been that lidocaine is an effective therapy for some patients with cancer and neuropathic pain; however, responses are extremely variable and likely depend on neuropathic pain assessment approaches. The predictive value of lidocaine in determining the expected benefits of drugs such as mexiletine (Galer et al. 1996) remains important in allowing us to move more efficiently through therapeutic trials.

SYMPATHETIC DYSFUNCTION

Pain associated with sympathetic dysfunction remains an area of controversy. Recently developed animal models of neural injury may provide further insight into this clinical condition and its mechanisms (Kim and Chung 1992). It has been difficult to define such mechanisms in humans because many syndromes have been historically named based on response to therapy, for example, sympathetically maintained pain. Newer terminology (e.g., complex regional pain syndrome, types 1 and 2) will move us away from such "circular definitions" and allow us to better define the syndromes that seem to respond best to interventions involving the sympathetic nervous system.

While we continue to struggle with this terminology, it remains important to recognize that regional sympathetic block with a local anesthetic may result in pain relief through several mechanisms (Dellamijn et al. 1994). Detailed examination, including a quantitative sensory examination, may suggest that the treatment has produced a combined sympathetic and somatic nerve block from the local anesthetic. A duration of effect of three to four hours or less suggests a pharmacologic effect from the local anesthetic rather than underlying sympathetic mechanisms. Coupled interventions including (1) lidocaine infusion, (2) phentolamine infusion, and (3) epidural local anesthetic are useful in defining dominant mechanisms of action; these approaches should help in separating (1) systemic effects of regionally administered anesthetics, (2) more specific sympathetic effects, and (3) central effects of local anesthetics, respectively. All these therapies have provided relief to some of our patients with cancer and neuropathic pain; interpreting them to define mechanisms remains a concern. The further possibility of a false positive or placebo response to any of these therapies, in my opinion, remains extremely rare in patients with cancer, many of whom have failed to respond to aggressive trials of opioids.

NEUROGENIC INFLAMMATION

Neurogenic inflammation, first described by Lewis in 1936 and referred to as the triple response of Lewis, remains a prominent model for the study of pain and hyperalgesia. Recent studies of intradermal injection of capsaicin for pain and hyperalgesia have advanced our understanding of this process (LaMotte et al. 1991). Fields (1987) has best described neurogenic inflammation and the cascade of events following neural injury. Inflammatory neuropeptides (e.g., substance P) and prostaglandins (e.g., PGE_2) may be released from primary afferent nociceptors and sympathetic postganglionic neurons, respectively (Levine et al. 1993). These mechanisms may explain the clinical response of some neuropathic pain patients to topical nonsteroidal anti-inflammatory drugs (NSAIDs), lidocaine, and capsaicin. In patients with cancer, it is important to rule out a primary cause of inflammation and primary hyperalgesia before assuming the problem is inflammation and secondary hyperalgesia associated with neural dysfunction.

NERVI NERVORUM

In discussing neuropathic pain mechanisms specific to cancer patients, we must consider neural compression involving the connective tissue sheath around the nerves. Hromada (1963) first described the innervation of this sheath, termed the *nervi nervorum*. It has been hypothesized that compression and inflammation of this sheath may cause pain (Asbury and Fields 1984), but little has been written on this subject in recent decades. Nervi nervorum–related mechanisms are inferred when we see clinical resolution of neuropathic pain following tumor resection or treatment of inflammation. Pain associated with tumor compression of neural structures, sometimes referred to as *nociceptive neuropathic pain,* is clinically indistinguishable from neuropathic pain, i.e., pain without a nociceptive (somatic or visceral) cause.

The effectiveness of NSAIDs or corticosteroids in some neuropathic pain states may be due to decreased edema at the tumor site. Likewise, these agents may disrupt the inflammatory cascade associated with neurogenic inflammation and possible secondary hyperalgesia. However, these assumptions disregard the dominant membrane stabilizing effects and central analgesic effects of these therapies. Separating primary tumor-associated inflammation and involvement of the nervi nervorum from other mechanisms of neuropathic pain in cancer patients remains a clinical challenge.

As Bennett so clearly stated, "There is no reason why normal pain due to ongoing tissue injury or inflammation and neuropathic pain cannot be present simultaneously" (Bennett 1994). Such is the case in many patients with cancer, and thus observations from animal models of neuropathic pain or even human studies with focused isolated pain diagnoses have limited value. Newer animal models involving both nociceptive and neuropathic injuries (Porreca et al. 1995) may provide more insight into clinical conditions involving combined painful etiologies and mechanisms.

CENTRAL MECHANISMS

Clinical human studies of central mechanisms of pain following peripheral and central nervous system injury remain limited. Clinical assessment and insight into these mechanisms of pain associated with injury or dysfunction of the somatosensory system date back to original work by Dejerine and Roussy (1906) and have been more recently described by Boivie and Leijon (1991). Central injury to pain inhibitory systems may explain pain in some of these conditions. Endogenous analgesic systems within the central nervous system (CNS) include catecholaminergic, indolinergic, and GABAergic systems (Fields and Basbaum 1994). These systems may be directly linked to the action of opioids, endogenous or exogenous, which may turn on and off these centrally acting inhibitory pathways. Although evidence from controlled clinical trials is limited (Leijon 1989), tricyclic antidepressants appear to be the mainstay of therapy for these pain syndromes in which central lesions or central dysfunction of the nervous system is suspected. I have found that therapy with tricyclic antidepressants and opioids is an effective combination in more refractory cases.

The role of excitatory amino acids and their receptors in the mechanisms of neuropathic pain remains an important area of continued research, although clinical relevance remains speculative. Spinal neuromodulators, acting via the N-methyl-D-aspartate (NMDA) receptor, have been proposed as a mechanism to explain opioid tolerance in subjects with concurrent nerve injury (Mao et al. 1992, 1995). Up-regulation of neuromodulators, such as cholecystokinin, following neural injury may explain the relative ineffectiveness of opioids in specific neuropathic pain states (Tseng and Collins 1992). Human studies of the NMDA antagonist ketamine can be used to support such mechanisms in neuropathic pain patients (Backonja et al. 1994), although the durability of ketamine's effects and the ability to permanently reverse these conditions appear limited (Eide et al. 1995). My personal experience with ketamine has been disappointing; the primary outcome seems to be side effects with little to no report of analgesia. Future clinical trials with NMDA antagonists need to closely control for known mood-altering side effects and their possible influence on neuropathic pain assessment.

Central and peripheral changes in the nervous system have been traditionally termed "plastic": however, recent work by Woolf and colleagues (1992) suggests that new anatomic/neural connections are established in the dorsal horn following injury. Furthermore, one of the final products of excitatory amino acid pathways is nitric oxide, a recognized neurotoxin for specific neural cells. Given the seeming permanent nature of these changes, I wonder if the term "hard wired" or "fixed" might be a more appropriate term than "plastic." These findings may explain the relative treatment-refractory nature of neuropathic pain and our inability to permanently reverse these conditions in some patients. Given the possibility of such hard-wired changes, we need to place more emphasis on prophylactic therapies, i.e., therapies that prevent the barrage by primary afferent nociceptors associated with tissue injury that may lead to more CNS changes.

Given that many events associated with neural injury in cancer patients can be predicted, clinicians should always consider prophylactic therapies. Preemptive analgesia or blocking the central/afferent barrage of impulses at and around the time of neural injury remains a rational therapy, with immediate consequences on postoperative pain (Woolf and Chong 1993) coupled with possible prolonged benefits. Techniques, including epidural analgesia to prevent postamputation/phantom pain, first described by Bach in 1988, remain controversial but are the subject of continued clinical trials at M. D. Anderson Cancer Center.

CLINICAL ASSESSMENT

Clinical assessment of neuropathic pain involves taking a focused history and performing a physical examination with attention to the somatosensory system. Current assessment tools for evaluating pain involving multiple sites, as is the case in patients with cancer and neuropathic pain, are lacking. Furthermore, there is no universal agreement on terminology or standardization of the neurosensory pain examination. Focusing on specific aspects of the history (Table II) and physical examination (Table III) and clarifying these findings become important because they influence management decisions in these patients.

HISTORY

Delay in onset of pain or clinical change in the painful features is a common finding in patients with both cancer and noncancer-related nerve injury. This feature, which is common following injury to the central and peripheral nervous system, presents a diagnostic challenge in patients with cancer. Clinicians must strongly consider the possibility of tumor recurrence, and neuropathic pain becomes a diagnosis of exclusion. Until both the physician and the patient are convinced that the pain is not the direct result of cancer and likely a delayed sequela of neural injury, it may be difficult to decide on an optimal therapy.

Paroxysms of pain at rest with a tendency to disturb sleep are features consistent with neuropathic pain states. A careful history should identify patients who experience paroxysms of pain with movement and relief with rest, which is more indicative of bone pain. It is a common error to diagnose neuropathic pain based on a patient's report of "sharp," "stabbing," and "radiating" pain when, in fact, there is bone disease due to metastatic cancer of the lumbar spine and pelvis. Absence of supporting evidence, i.e., an abnormal neurological examination, should help to avoid such errors.

Patient reports of pain in an area of "numbness" or in an area that was previously numb, are highly suspicious of neural dysfunction. These reports need to be evaluated with a detailed sensory examination, as described below, with classification of features such as allodynia, hyperalgesia, and hyperpathia. Some patients with tumor progression may have a history of intermittent sensory symptoms without supporting findings on neurologic exam. Persistent absence of findings or inconsistent findings on neurological examination should raise the possibility of a visceral or myofascial etiology that mimics a neuropathic pain syndrome.

The M. D. Anderson Cancer Center Neuropathic Pain Questionnaire, a new assessment tool in development, considers our assumptions that most patients with neuropathic pain and cancer will have multiple dimensions to their pain. Dimensions specific for neuropathic pain include (1) constant pain, (2) paroxysmal pain, and (3) evoked pain or unpleasant sensations. These dimensions at times appear to be mutually exclusive features with variable but measurable responses to therapy. Additional themes built into our questionnaire include temporal dimensions of pain, beliefs about cause of pain, and expectations regarding its treatment. Patient insight and ranking of the most important features of the pain are also a critical part of our assessment (Fig. 1). Such insight relies on education and repeat assessments in each patient. This multidimensional assessment allows us to identify therapies that may be partially effective and worth continuing. It provides a rational basis for polypharmacy or polytherapy, which is frequently necessary in these patients.

EXAMINATION

A standard neurologic examination of the painful area needs to incorporate both sensory and motor findings, although the latter are frequently absent in neuropathic pain states. The distinguishing feature in patients with neuropathic pain is the presence of *positive symptoms* suggesting a hypersensitive neurologic state: (1) lowered thresholds of pain in response to stimuli (hyperalgesia), (2) pain in response to nonpainful stimuli (allodynia), or (3) elevated threshold of pain with increased pain, spread of pain, or aftersensation following repetitive stimulation (hyperpathia). The reliability of these sensory findings depends in part on examining a "normal" region

30. Of the various aspects of your pain, PLEASE RANK the pain which bothers you **most to least. RANK 1 = MOST BOTHERSOME.** Rank only those descriptions which apply to your pain.

RANK   **TYPE OF PAIN**

_____   Pain that is continuous or **constant**

_____   Pain that is **off and on,** comes and goes **on its own**

_____   Pain that is **off and on,** comes and goes with **activity**

_____   Pain or unpleasant sensations with **light touch**

_____   Pain or unpleasant sensations with applied **pressure**

_____   Pain or unpleasant sensations with **heat or cold**

_____   Pain with **itching sensation**

_____   Phantom pain

_____   Phantom sensation

_____   Other, please describe: _____

Fig. 1. Sample question (#30) from the M. D. Anderson Cancer Center Neuropathic Pain Questionnaire.

for comparison. These findings rely on the qualitative reports of each patient, somewhat independent of quantitative thresholds of pain from the applied stimuli (pinprick, cold, heat, touch, and vibration). It is important to distinguish positive features associated with most neuropathic pain states from negative features or neurologic deficits. When the examination of the painful area does not reveal supporting, _positive features,_ as described above, the clinician needs to question the cause of the pain. When bedside neurologic examination is negative or suspicious for neuropathic pain, quantitative sensory testing (QST) may permit documentation of neural dysfunction. QST, although still in its infancy, has become a recognized and sensitive means of assessing abnormal sensations (see below).

Findings of _static vs. dynamic allodynia_ are also clinically useful in separating pain due to local inflammation from neuropathic pain, i.e., pain independent of an underlying nociceptive stimuli (Koltzenburg et al. 1992; Ochoa and Yarnitsky 1993). These distinctions in type of allodynia help to define the pathophysiologic mechanisms in pain patients. Static allodynia, or pain associated with the application of a nonpainful pressure stimulus, is mediated by C fibers (nociceptors). In contrast, Aβ fibers (normally non-nociceptive) mediate dynamic allodynia, or pain associated with stroking of the skin with a moving, light touch. Patients with isolated neuropathic painful conditions often report relief of pain with pressure, which is rarely the case when a patient has regional pathology. Although pain with pressure does not rule in or out the possibility of neuropathic pain, the absence of such pain, or the report that pain is greater with light touch than with pressure, should raise the clinician's suspicion that neuropathic mechanisms are involved.

A helpful instrument in assessing neural dysfunction in association with peripheral neuropathies is the neuropathy symptom score (NSS), developed by the Neuromuscular Group at the Mayo Clinic (Dyck 1993). The NSS is a 17-point instrument that records symptoms and physical findings as present (1) or absent (0). This tool relies on physician and patient report but is not weighted toward patient response, which is the major limitation of the NSS as a measure of pain. The NSS, however, uses insightful terminology describing positive vs. negative neurologic features. This terminology is useful when applied to painful conditions with suspected neuropathic pain mechanisms. It is common for patients with cancer and nerve injury to have elevated thresholds of pain in response to sensory stimuli, i.e., negative symptoms. Many patients with cancer, pain, and recognized nerve injury may not have neuropathic pain.

QUANTITATIVE SENSORY TESTING

The past few years have brought the development of new methods to assess and quantify sensation. QST has been recommended as a means of standardizing sensory function measurements in controlled clinical trials and supplementing the standard neurologic examination (Peripheral Neuropathy Association 1993). This technology, which asks patients to identify thresholds to cold, heat, and vibratory stimuli applied by a metal probe, has yet to be standardized for most clinical pain syndromes. We need further studies that recognize that sensory function may be different in patients with cancer (Lipton et al. 1991). This technique has been largely applied to the evaluation of neural function of the extremities rather than the torso, and is a valuable tool in assessing chemotherapy-induced peripheral neuropathies. In clinical practice, we have also been applying this technology to document injury to intercostal nerves in women with breast cancer. These women with isolated injury to the intercostobrachial nerve as a consequence of breast resection or reconstruction represent a unique and ideal group in whom we might extend our understanding of neuropathic pain mechanisms through this new testing method. Studies are in progress to test the hypothesis that QST is a more sensitive and objective measure of change compared to standard neurologic sensory testing.

CONCLUSIONS

The clinical challenge that remains is to determine the dominant mechanisms of pain in a given patient based on the clinical assessment. By defining assessment approaches based on assumed neuropathology of pain and hyperalgesia, as done by Ochoa and colleagues (1993), we should gain further insight into the dominant underlying mechanisms in specific disease states. Despite the extreme heterogeneity of findings in patients with neuropathic pain, mechanisms may also be inferred based on response to selected therapies as suggested by Fields and Rowbotham (1994). The unfortunate limitation of this approach is the recognition that many therapies have multiple mechanisms of action, e.g., tricyclic antidepressants, traditionally recognized as blockers of the reuptake of norepinephrine and serotonin, have more recently been recognized as a potential sodium-channel blocker (Jacobson et al. 1995). Consequently, the therapeutic utility of these inferences based on mechanistically driven algorithms remains unproven.

At present we are unable to predict the effectiveness of a specific therapy based on our clinical assessment (Treede et al. 1992). Of some promise, in animal models of nerve injury, is the finding that response to therapy may be predicted based on the type of hyperalgesia, i.e., thermal vs. mechanical (Mao et al. 1992). This same correlation has yet to be demonstrated in human conditions, although it should become possible with refined assessment approaches including quantitative sensory testing. We hope that further advances in our basic understanding of changes and specific neurophysiologic pain pathways associated with neural injury in these models will continue to fuel hypotheses for testing in our patients.

In conclusion, I believe we need to build on the information we have gained, largely through studies performed in select neuropathic pain syndromes in patients without cancer. Unfortunately, these studies fail to capture the true clinical dimensions of our patients with cancer, including restrictions of *time* in respect to a *potentially terminal disease*. We can fully appreciate these dimensions only through clinical study of cancer populations with specific neuropathic pain syndromes. With a common language and validated instruments that clearly define these dimensions, we can then begin to assess the effectiveness of our care in these challenging patients.

REFERENCES

Asbury AK, Fields HL. Pain due to peripheral nerve damage: an hypothesis. Neurology 1984; 34:1587–1590.
Bach S, Noreng MF, Tjellden NU. Phantom limb pain in amputees during the first 12 months

following limb amputation after preoperative lumbar epidural blockade. Pain 1988; 33:297–301.

Backonja M, Arndt G, Gombar KA, Check B, Zimmermann M. Response of chronic neuropathic pain syndromes to ketamine: a preliminary study. Pain 1994; 56:51–57.

Basbaum AI, Chi SI, Levine JD. Peripheral and central contribution to persistent expression of the c-fos proto-oncogene in spinal cord after peripheral nerve injury. In: Willis WD (Ed). Hyperalgesia and Allodynia. New York: Raven Press, 1992, p 295–304.

Bennett GF. Neuropathic pain. In: Wall PD, Melzack R (Eds). Textbook of Pain, 3rd ed. Edinburgh: Churchill Livingstone, 1994, p 202.

Boivie J, Leijon G. Clinical findings in patients with central post-stroke pain. In: Casey KL (Ed). Pain and Central Nervous System Disease: The Central Pain Syndromes. New York: Raven Press, 1991, pp 65–75.

Bruera E, Ripamonti C, Brennis C, Macmillan K, Hanson J. A randomized double-blind crossover trial of intravenous lidocaine in the treatment of neuropathic pain. J Pain Symptom Manage 1992; 7(3):138–140.

Cherney NI, Thaler HT, Friedlander-Klar H, et al. Opioid responsiveness of cancer pain syndromes caused by neuropathic or nociceptive mechanisms. Neurology 1994; 44:857–861.

Dejerine J, Roussy G. Le syndrome thalamique. Rev Neurol (Paris) 1906; 14:521–532.

Dellemijn PLI, Fields HL, Allen RR, McKay WR, Rowbotham MC. The interpretation of pain relief and sensory changes following sympathetic blockade. Brain 1994; 117:1475–1487.

Devor M, Keller CH, Deerinck TJ, Ellisman MH. Sodium channel accumulation on axolemma of afferent endings in nerve ending neuromas in Apteronotus. Neurosci Lett 1989; 102:149–154.

Dyck PJ. Quantitating severity of neuropathy. In: Dyck PJ, Thomas PK, Griffin JW, Low PA, Poduslo JF (Eds). Peripheral Neuropathy. Philadelphia: W.B. Saunders, 1993, pp 686–697.

Eide PK, Stubhaug A, Oye Ivar, Breivik H. Continuous subcutaneous administration of the N-methyl-D-aspartic acid (NMDA) receptor antagonist ketamine in the treatment of postherpetic neuralgia. Pain 1995; 61:221–228.

England JD, Gamboni F, Levinson SR. Immunocytochemical localization of sodium channels form along demyelinated axons. Brain Res 1991; 548:334–337.

Fields HL. Pain. New York: McGraw-Hill, 1987, pp 13–16.

Fields HL, Basbaum AI. Central nervous system mechanisms of pain modulation. In: Wall PD, Melzack R (Eds). Textbook of Pain, 3rd ed. Edinburgh: Churchill Livingstone, 1994, pp 243–257

Fields HL, Rowbotham MC. Multiple mechanisms of neuropathic pain: a clinical perspective. In: Gebhart GF, Hammond DL, Jensen TS (Eds). Proceedings of the 7th World Congress on Pain. Progress in Pain Research and Management, Vol. 2. Seattle: IASP Press, 1994, pp 437–454.

Galer BS, Harle J, Rowbotham MC. Response to intravenous lidocaine infusion predicts subsequent response to oral mexiletine: a prospective study. J Pain Symptom Manage 1996; 12:161–167.

Hromada J. On the nerve supply of the connective tissue of some peripheral nervous system components. Acta Anatomica 1963; 55:343–351.

Inbal R, Rousso M, Ashur Haim, Wall PD, Devor M. Collateral sprouting in skin and sensory recovery after nerve injury in man. Pain 1987; 28:141–154.

Jacobson LO, Blev K, Hunter JC, Lee C. Anti-thermal hyperalgesic properties of antidepressants in a rat model of neuropathic pain [abstract 95794]. 14th Annual Scientific Meeting of the American Pain Society, Beverly Hills, CA, Nov 8–12, 1995.

Jänig W. Pathophysiology of nerve following mechanical injury in man. In: Dubner R, Gebhart GF, Bond MR (Eds). Pain Research and Clinical Management, Vol 3. Amsterdam: Elsevier, 1988; pp 89–108.

Jeanmonod D, Magnin M, Morel A. Low-threshold calcium spike bursts in the human thalamus: common physiopathology for sensory, motor and limbic positive symptoms. Brain 1996; 119:363–375.

Kim SH, Chung JM. An experimental model for peripheral neuropathy produced by segmental spinal nerve ligation in the rat. Pain 1992; 50:355–363.

Koltzenburg M, Lundberg LER, Torebjörk HE. Dynamic and static components of mechanical hyperalgesia in human hairy skin. Pain 1992; 51:207–219.

La Motte RH, Chain CN, Simone DA, Tsai EP. Neurogenic hyperalgesia. J Neurophysiol 1991; 66:190–211.

Leijon G, Boivie J. Central post-stroke pain: a controlled trial of amitriptyline and carbamazepine. Pain 1989; 36:27–36

Lenz FA. The thalamus and central pain syndromes: human and animal studies. In: Casey KL (Ed). Pain and Central Nervous System Diseases. New York: Raven Press, 1991, pp 171–182.

Levine JD, Fields HL, Basbaum AI. Peptides and the primary afferent nociceptor. J Neurosci 1993; 13:2273–2286.

Lewis T. Experiments relating to hyperalgesia. Clin Sci 1936; 2:373–421.

Lipton RB, Galer BS, Dutcher JP, et al. Large and small fiber type sensory neuropathy in patients with cancer. J Neurol Neurosurg Psychiatry 1991; 54:706–709.

Mao J, Price DD, Hayes RL, Mayer DJ. Differential roles of NMDA and non-NMDA receptor activation in induction and maintenance of thermal hyperalgesia in rats with painful peripheral mononeuropathy. Brain Res 1992; 598:271–278.

Mao J, Price DD, Mayer D. Mechanisms of hyperalgesia and morphine intolerance: a current view of their possible interactions. Pain 1995; 62:259–274.

Ochoa JL, Yarnitsky D. Mechanical hyperalgesia in neuropathic pain patients: dynamic and static subtypes. Ann Neurol 1993; 33:465–472.

Ossipov MH, Lopez Y, Nichols, ML, Bian D, Porreca F. Inhibition by spinal morphine of the tail-flick response is attenuated in rats with nerve ligation injury. Neurosci Letts 1995; 199(2):83–86.

Peripheral Neuropathy Association. Quantitative sensory testing: a consensus report from the Peripheral Neuropathy Association. Neurology 1993; 43:1050–1052.

Porreca F, et al. Loss of efficacy and potency of spinal morphine to inhibit the tail flick reflex in rats with a nerve constriction injury [abstract]. 14th Annual Scientific Meeting of the American Pain Society, Beverly Hills, CA, Nov 8–12, 1995.

Portenoy RK. Management of neuropathic pain. In: Chapman CR, Foley KM (Eds). Current and Emerging Issues in Cancer Pain, Research and Practice, Vol. 3. New York: Raven Press, 1993, pp 351–369.

Roberts WJ. A hypothesis on the physiological basis for causalgia and related pains. Pain 1986; 24:297–311.

Rowbotham MC, Reisner-Keller LA, Fields HL. Both intravenous lidocaine and morphine reduce the pain of postherpetic neuralgia. Neurology 1991; 41:1024–1028.

Torebjörk HE, Lundberg LER, LaMotte RH. Central changes in processing mechanoreceptor input. J Physiol 1992; 448:765–780.

Treede RD, Davis KD, Campbell JN, Raja SN. The plasticity of cutaneous hyperalgesia during sympathetic ganglion blockade in patients with neuropathic pain. Brain 1992; 115:607–621.

Tseng LF, Collins KA. Cholecystokinin administered intrathecally selectively antagonizes intracerebroventricular beta-endorphin-induced tail flick inhibition in the mouse. J Pharmacol Exp Ther 1992; 260:1086–1092.

Wall PD, Devor M. Sensory afferent nerve impulses originating from a dorsal root ganglia as well as from the periphery in normal and nerve injured rats. Pain 1983; 17:321–339.

Woolf CL, Chong MS. Preemptive analgesia: treating postoperative pain by preventing the establishment of central sensitization. Anesth Analg 1993; 77:362–379.

Woolf CJ, Thompson SWN. The induction and maintenance of central sensitization is dependent on N-methyl-D-aspartic acid receptor activation: implications for the treatment of post-injury pain hypersensitivity states. Pain 1991; 44:293–299.

Woolf CJ, Shortland P, Coggeshall RE. Peripheral nerve injury triggers central sprouting of myelinated afferents. Nature 1992 355:75–78.

Zeltser R, Seltzer Z. A practical guide for the use of animal models in the study of neuropathic pain. In: Boivie J, Hansson P, Lindblom U (Eds). Touch, Temperature, and Pain in Health and Disease: Mechanisms and Assessments. Progress in Pain Research and Management, Vol. 3. Seattle: IASP Press, 1994, pp 295–338.

Correspondence to: Robert R. Allen, MD, The University of Texas M. D. Anderson Cancer Center, 1515 Holcombe Blvd. Box 100, Houston, TX 77030, USA. Tel: 713-745-1736; Fax: 713-794-4999.

Assessment and Treatment of Cancer Pain,
Progress in Pain Research and Management,
Vol. 12, edited by R. Payne, R.B. Patt, and
C.S. Hill, IASP Press, Seattle, © 1998.

11

Key Issues in Anesthetic Techniques in Cancer Pain

Michael J. Cousins

Department of Anaesthesia and Pain Management, University of Sydney,
Royal North Shore Hospital, St. Leonard's, New South Wales, Australia

It is easy when dealing with cancer and postoperative pain to assume that nociception is the sole problem and consequently to focus only on its treatment. Clearly, other important factors, including psychological and environmental influences, affect cancer patients and other patients following trauma or surgery. It is essential to address all potential factors to manage any patient's pain effectively. It also is easy to base our therapies on the classic spinothalamic pathway. In fact, we not infrequently receive referrals that are totally based upon the Cartesian model of pain. The referring clinician may state: "The pain is in these dermatomes, it has been there for this amount of time; surely you can do something proximal to the painful area with alcohol or phenol and that will resolve the problem."

In the last 10 years our understanding of clinical pain has moved a long way from the Cartesian model, as is demonstrated by two diagrams of Woolf and Chong (Figs. 1 and 2). We can no longer separate innocuous sensation activating low-threshold Aβ fibers from noxious sensation activating high-threshold Aδ and C nociceptors. Such separation is all very well in the physiology laboratory where the two systems can be studied independently. Activation solely of Aδ and C fibers occurs with a *temporary* heat stimulus, for example, putting your toe near the fire or touching a hot kettle. However, in clinical pain we are dealing with low-intensity stimuli that are activating Aδ and C fibers, and also Aβ fibers, in association with sensitized nociceptors (Woolf and Chong 1993). The cancer patient often has a mass of cancer cellsthat stimulate a local reaction that is analogous to the inflammatory response. The body has only one method of mounting an injury response, basically the Lewis triple response with some nuances in different areas. Thus, cancer pain often involves peripheral sensitization and almost invariably

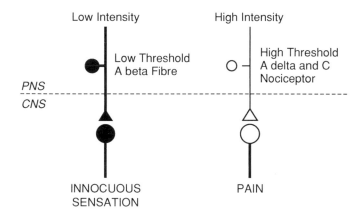

Fig. 1. Physiological pain. *PNS,* peripheral nervous system; *CNS,* central nervous system (Woolf and Chong 1993).

central sensitization, particularly if the pain generator continues, as it often does in cancer.

Activation of low-threshold mechanoreceptor Aβ fibers is new to some anesthesiologists, particularly those who work only in acute pain management, where the Cartesian model of pain often works quite well. However, when Aβ fibers are involved, and with central sensitization, "standard" treatments may not be successful. Also, we have initial experience that the Aδ and C-fiber selective drug butamben may not be ideal for pain associated with Aβ-fiber activation. In addition, if cancer or its treatment have caused nerve damage, there may be anatomical connections between normal sensory inputs and nociceptive neurons in the dorsal horn (Woolf and Chong 1993), and thus a central anatomical connection between non-noxious stimuli

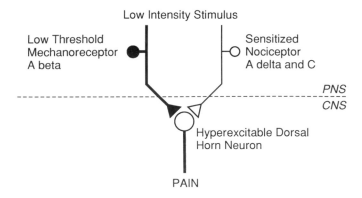

Fig. 2. Clinical pain. *PNS,* peripheral nervous system; *CNS,* central nervous system (Woolf and Chong 1993).

and continuing noxious sensations. While this concept is a rather malignant and nasty one to contemplate, it helps explain many cases of refractory chronic pain.

We have made a fundamental mistake in the past 15 years in thinking of acute post-trauma pain, postoperative pain, cancer pain, and chronic pain as totally separate entities. Regrettably, acute pain services are often run by anesthesiology departments with virtually no communication or connection with cancer pain or chronic pain services. This situation, I propose, is a fundamental error: the facilities needed for clinical care, research, and teaching are similar, the staffing can overlap to a large extent and, in my view, needs to overlap to be cost effective. It is difficult to obtain the required number of staff for each area, and integrated staffing is essential for effective delivery of care. The funding is an enormous challenge that we have addressed through a combination of government and private-sector support, and our funding increasingly comes from private-sector donations rather than patient billings.

Additionally, the pain service needs a "champion"—the pain center director—who is preferably also the head of a major hospital department such as anesthesiology or neurosurgery. Such champions are scarce and should be used to promote the full scope of activity. The clinical services need to be integrated because patients frequently progress from acute to chronic illnesses. Patients with cancer often improve, but many continue to have pain as a result of treatment or other factors, with progression from cancer pain to chronic noncancer pain and sometimes vice-versa. It makes little sense to erect discreet, isolated services that are not highly interactive. The scientific basis for the management of these three areas is a common core of knowledge as is emphasized in the *Core Curriculum for Professional Education in Pain* published by the International Association for the Study of Pain (Fields 1995). This same need to integrate information related to acute, chronic, and cancer pain also applies to undergraduate and postgraduate education.

A PAIN MANAGEMENT AND RESEARCH SERVICE

The Pain Management and Research Centre at the Royal North Shore Hospital, University of Sydney, now integrates within a single facility all activities for acute, chronic, and cancer pain programs. The Pain Centre includes consulting rooms, a large patient treatment area, an operating room, areas for patients who require physical therapy, and an area for those who require a cognitive-behavioral program (Fig. 3). There is a great deal of "cross talk," as in the example of cancer patients who enter our cognitive-

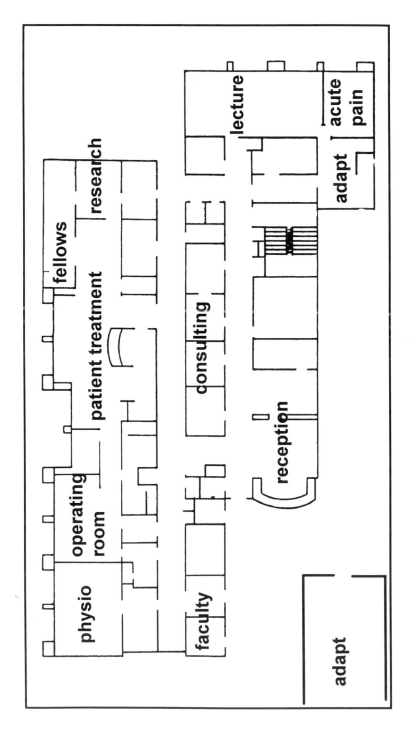

Fig. 3. Layout of the Pain Management and Research Centre at the Royal North Shore Hospital, University of Sydney.

behavioral program (active day patient treatment program, ADAPT). These patients are in remission but have complications of treatment or have become significantly deactivated and need rehabilitation to resume a "normal" life.

The Pain Centre also offers an important educational component for both undergraduate health sciences students and postgraduates. We have developed a Master of Medicine Degree in Pain Management through the University of Sydney. Thus, students from medicine, nursing, physical therapy, and a wide range of other backgrounds learn about the assessment and treatment of pain in a multidisciplinary setting. The philosophy of this masters' course is to integrate disciplines, knowledge bases, and approaches to acute, chronic, and cancer pain. Importantly, we accomplish this goal within an evidence-based context, because Australia is fully involved in the international Cochrane collaboration, which aims to base medical treatment on the best possible available evidence, as follows: the ideal standard for evidence is a randomized, prospective controlled trial, and, even better, a meta-analysis of randomized, prospective controlled trials to provide even more powerful knowledge; plotting trials on an "odds ratio" diagram enables evaluation as each trial is completed—when outcomes fall to the left of the line, a positive result is emerging, a scattering around the line indicates no clear result, and outcomes that all fall to the right of the line indicate that treatment is ineffective.

We should use methods like the Cochrane approach to assess anesthetic pain-relief techniques and evaluate the evidence not only for efficacy but also for side effects. Recently published meta-analyses of analgesic efficacy for anticonvulsants and tricyclic antidepressants evaluated "numbers needed to treat." That is, how many patients does a clinician need to treat to begin seeing an effective result for neuropathic pain? The answer in each case was about three patients. Likewise, a mean of about 3 patients also need to be treated with each drug for side effects to begin to emerge. Thus, these agents are clearly effective for neuropathic pain, but side effects appear quite frequently (McQuay et al. 1995). Unfortunately, similar data are not yet available for most neural blockade techniques, but are sorely needed if our colleagues are to confidently refer patients for neural blockade techniques, and if we are to feel comfortable about discussing such techniques with our patients.

AN ACUTE PAIN COMPONENT

An acute component of a comprehensive pain service that is responsible for organization and delivery of short-term treatments is exceptionally important for patients with cancer and AIDS. This acute pain component needs to include quality assurance, education, research, and clinical care. It also must include attention to preemption (e.g., commencing a pain-relief technique prior to a painful intervention) and prevention, which involves diagnosing and treating persisting acute pain to prevent emergence of chronic pain. A new emphasis on prevention and preemption can make an important contribution to quality of life, particularly in cancer patients who require surgery or treatments that can cause subacute or even chronic pain.

Acute rehabilitation, even in cancer patients, is also critically important. We now have data showing that many of our patients with chronic noncancer pain obtain excellent relief with anesthetic techniques, but what about their underlying problems? In patients receiving an intrathecal pump for severe arachnoiditis or excruciating generalized neuropathic pain due to multiple sclerosis, the quality of pain control is a fundamental outcome variable. But what happens to physical and other indices of function? Without the application of a program of acute rehabilitation in conjunction with pain relief, many of these patients fare poorly. We have encouraging data on rehabilitating such patients in our cognitive-behavioral program; they may indeed return to a more active life. Likewise, I believe acute rehabilitation is just as important for cancer patients once the anesthetic technique or other alternative pain relief method is effectively applied. This type of service also can manage "acute on chronic" episodes. Again, most pain management serivces underemphasize the preparation necessary to provide effective early intervention for these "acute on chronic" episodes.

Are patient-controlled analgesia pumps (PCAs) used frequently enough to manage painful medical interventions and diagnostic procedures? Are neural blockade procedures always optimally supplemented by combinations of analgesics and the wonderful new sedative drugs such as midazolam and propofol? Probably not. The routine use of midazolam and/or propofol plus an opiate revolutionizes how patients feel about painful anesthetic procedures. We should never subject patients to painful therapeutic procedures without adequate sedation and analgesia. The preventative role of anesthetic techniques is also important. Severe reflex sympathetic dystrophy (complex regional pain syndrome type I) may occur in association with cancer, but must be diagnosed early or even prevented by use of neural blockade techniques, such as in association with limb surgery.

INTEGRATION OF TECHNIQUES AND TREATMENTS

Anesthetic techniques must ultimately be considered in the context of other available treatments. One of our most exciting challenges is to optimally integrate these techniques into the other potentially applicable treatments. This goal can only be accomplished effectively through evaluation of the wider dimensions of pain. For example, psychological therapies can only be considered in conjunction with the patient's psychological profile. Optimally, the multidisciplinary team should include a psychologist or psychiatrist to conduct routine assessments so that an outside referral is not necessary. Each of our new patients is assessed for physical, psychological, and environmental factors, and the results are shared and discussed among the team members, who generate a problem list and management options. The lack of such a process, increases the likelihood that selection of an invasive technique will be based on incomplete, unidimensional data.

In the case of cancer pain, clinicians must carefully consider direct anticancer treatments that may improve the pain by modifying its cause. For example, a single session of well-planned radiotherapy may dramatically reduce pain associated with vertebral metastases. If, due to the patient's overall status, cure is impossible, then a single treatment may be just as effective as a protracted course of radiotherapy, and much less costly and inconvenient.

It is increasingly a challenge to ascertain that we are offering the best treatment recommendations and that our characterization of relative risk and benefit is realistic. We might consider, for example, the common scenario of a patient with spinal metastases and good analgesia with oral opioids and adjuvants. Inevitably, some patients will develop compression or direct invasion of a nerve root and will not obtain adequate pain relief without treatment with the more potent methods now available. My concern is that the lack of data about the efficacy and side effects of anesthetic techniques in such situations may result in their underuse even though they may be truly necessary. I suspect that this situation is common in many institutions throughout the world. Again, however, we need to look at the "total situation" for each patient, as recommended by Saunders (1987). Clinicians should explore not only the somatic source, but also seek causes of anxiety and fear (e.g., of pain, death, the hospital), feelings of loss of control, anger, depression, and so forth. If you are attentive to all the dimensions of suffering, you may, to your surprise, sometimes find that the patient's pain is not so severe as initially thought. I well remember that when I first started doing neurolytic procedures in the late 1960s, I was at times quite amazed with the poor results for a seemingly well-chosen technique for a patient who seemed to have a straightforward problem. But in those days we did not assess any of these broader dimensions; I hope that we have progressed considerably in our approach.

NEURAL BLOCKADE TECHNIQUES

Current neural blockade techniques are listed in Table I; the list does not include techniques that are termed "anesthetic" but are not strictly nerve blocks. As discussed above, we should consider infusion of opiates and nonopiate drugs such as the sedatives, and even ketamine. Such approaches are anesthetic techniques because they may require a critical care approach. Ketamine infusion is an effective way to relieve severe pain in opioid-tolerant patients, particularly when there is a neuropathic component. We also use subcutaneous lignocaine infusion for neuropathic cancer pain (Brose and Cousins 1991).

What about diagnostic local anesthetic blocks? Do they have any role in cancer pain? A chapter in the third edition of *Neural Blockade in Clinical Anesthesia and Management of Pain* should provoke significant concern about the precision of results of diagnostic local anesthetic blocks (Hogan and Abram 1998). The original concept of diagnostic nerve blocks is based upon the Cartesian model of pain. In a "hard-wired" system, a nerve blocked at a specific point will produce a certain response, and ipso facto, results will be highly reliable. If the nerve is cut at the exact site of the block, the same degree of pain relief will occur. I am aware of only one correlative study; in the mid-1960s John Loeser, a neurosurgeon, performed diagnostic spinal nerve root blocks prior to dorsal rhizotomies (Boas and Cousins 1988). The study found no correlation whatsoever between the results of those

Table I
Neural blockade and cancer pain

Diagnostic neural blockade
Local anesthetic blocks as an adjunct to physical therapy
Local anesthetic plexus infusions
Neurolytic neural blockade
  Celiac plexus block
  Lumbar sympathetic block
  Superior hypogastric plexus block
  Subarachnoid neurolytic block
  Epidural neurolytic block (rarely used)
  Pituitary ablation (rarely used)
Alternatives to neurolytic blockade
  Percutaneous cordotomy
  Dorsal root entry zone (DREZ) lesions
  Epidural butamben
  Epidural and intrathecal opioid and nonopioid (e.g., clonidine, SNX-111) drug administration
  Intrathecal "dialysis tubes" with cloned cells producing opioids and catecholamines

blocks and of rhizotomy. We now better understand the plasticity of the nervous system and other possible explanations (Hogan and Abram 1998). Nevertheless, I believe that diagnostic blocks can be useful if the physician has a reasonable understanding of neuroplasticity and controls the blocks, observes the duration of the pharmacologic effect, and considers the results in the context of other information about the patient. However, the clinician cannot simply perform a diagnostic block and accept the results in isolation. We still see inappropriate referrals for diagnostic nerve blocks: for example, a referral from a surgeon who requests an intercostal nerve block for a patient with intercostal neuralgia after thoracotomy because he is thinking of doing an intercostal neurectomy. He holds a seriously flawed concept that "positive" results would be an indication to proceed with the neurectomy.

The place of neurolytic blocks in cancer pain is more complex now that we have many alternatives. It is more difficult to discuss with patients the pros and cons of a procedure that may have serious side effects compared to other effective noninvasive alternatives (Swarm and Cousins 1993). I believe that neurolytic blocks are now appropriate for less than 5% of patients with cancer pain. Some procedures such as celiac plexus and other sympathetic blocks are associated with a relatively low incidence of complications and still offer the patient considerable relief. However, subarachnoid neurolytic techniques have nearly disappeared to the point of extinction subsequent to the emergence of exciting methods such as intrathecal and epidural opioids and new nonopioid drugs. Epidural neurolytic techniques have disappeared in our practice because of their relative unreliability, but I am aware that others are still using them. Somatic nerve blocks have also become fairly rare, although with the use of the cryoprobe they sometimes remain a valuable option. In my opinion, percutaneous cordotomy is underused. I am aware of no other technique that can provide complete pain relief in appropriately selected patients, provided they have a circumscribed life span. Dorsal root entry zone (DREZ) lesion may be valuable for appropriate patients with major plexopathies. Pituitary alcohol instillation has disappeared completely from our practice. It was a fascinating procedure that produced dramatic and early pain relief, but almost always required repetition. The risk of rendering a patient blind when good, safe alternative techniques are available is simply unacceptable in contemporary practice.

The spinal route of drug administration will continue to be the area of greatest growth and will encompass a host of techniques including implantation of tiny tubes containing cloned cells that continuously produce opioids and other neurotransmitters. Such devices act like a tiny biologic pump and may take the place of implanted machinery. While we have an exciting range of anesthetic techniques, we need to better characterize their efficacy.

CELIAC PLEXUS BLOCK

Many techniques are now available for celiac plexus block, including the classic, the transaortic, the splanchnic, and the anterior. They probably do not differ significantly in efficacy and safety, although we have little comparative data. One very nice study from Italy compared the classic approach with transaortic and splanchnic techniques and found little difference among them (Ischia et al. 1992). Blocks performed correctly under image intensifier control or computed tomography (CT) scan should give similar results, regardless of technique used.

How effective is celiac block? Numerous studies show that 75% of treated patients require minimal analgesic or none at all. For example, a follow-up study from the Seattle group reported that 85% of patients achieved good initial results and 75% experienced good pain relief through their remaining life spans (see Swarm and Cousins 1993). We continue to use alcohol celiac plexus block for upper abdominal cancer with similar results. Two meta-analyses have now been attempted. One showed similarly efficacious results to those noted above, while the other emphasized the poor quality of the nonblinded "case series" research. Unfortunately, we do not yet have a proper odds ratio diagram for celiac plexus block; neither complications nor their follow-up are well documented. One study described weakness or numbness in the T10–L2 distribution in 8% of subjects, lower chest pain in 3%, failure of ejaculation in 2% of males, urinary retention in 1% of subjects, and postural hypotension that was temporary in 20% of subjects and long lasting in 2%. We see diarrhea quite commonly, and usually regard it as a good sign because these patients were often constipated. Pneumothorax, of course, is more likely to occur with the splanchnic approach, and paraplegia is rare but possible. Paraplegia is probably due to an effect on the spinal nutrient arteries, which may be injured either by the needle or the neurolytic material.

Subarachnoid neurolysis is being performed much less frequently. Phenol injection for pain in the saddle region is suitable for very few patients, unless they have lost bladder and bowel function, in which case it can be quite useful. I often use thoracic subarachnoid alcohol in my practice. I believe patients with a mesothelioma or similar condition with unilateral chest pain, even over many spinal segments, may be suitable candidates for thoracic subarachnoid alcohol. I routinely place three needles so as to inject a very small dose at each level. Patients are treated with a propofol infusion and fentanyl, and are positioned comfortably with the affected site uppermost rather than trying to lay them on the painful side, as is required for hyperbaric phenol. In addition, the 45° semiprone position is much more comfortable than the posterior tilt that is needed with phenol. The patient is now relaxed and comfortable and the clinician can take the time to titrate the dose with good, unhurried communication. Once the needles are placed, the sedative infusion can be slowed to facilitate communication with the patient. This approach increases safety, as the injection can be halted if the patient develops distal signs in the limbs or in the sacrum. The old literature describes some appalling complication rates because earlier clinicians did not take due care to consider the relationships of the spinal cord segments to the spinous process of the vertebral bodies, to place the needles appropriately to cover the lesion, and then to titrate very, very carefully in 0.05-ml increments from a tuberculin syringe (Cousins 1988).

Although we use this technique quite frequently for patients with unilateral chest pain, what sort of data can we offer the patients? Both the literature and, unfortunately, our current results indicate that "good" relief (no analgesic or minimal amounts) occurs in only about 60% of patients. Inexplicably, pain returns 48 hours later in some patients who had excellent early results; dilution of the alcohol may explain this relapse. Careful judgment is needed regarding the speed of alcohol injection. The cord may be injuried if it is injected too quickly, and the concentration near the nerve roots may be inadequate if the drug is instilled too slowly. Regardless, if pain returns, the procedure usually can be repeated. Although the procedure carries a risk of major spinal cord injury, that has never occurred in my practice of over 25 years, but it could and no doubt will occur at some time. Some patients faced with the prospect of even a tiny risk of paraplegia or major neurologic deficit will indicate that under no circumstances do they want this technique. But again, the data are not very good. The evidence is not level I or level II; it is barely level III and more correctly level IV (the expert opinion category; see Table II).

Table II
Levels of evidence ratings

Level I	Evidence obtained from systematic review of relevant randomized controlled trials (with meta-analysis where possible).
Level II	Evidence obtained from one or more well-designed randomized controlled trials.
Level III	Evidence obtained from well-designed nonrandomized controlled trials; OR from well-designed cohort or case-control analytical studies, preferably multicenter or conducted at different times.
Level IV	The opinions respected authorities based on clinical experience, descriptive studies, or reports of expert committees.

Note: This table is an example of evidence ratings. Numerous methods are used.

AN ACCEPTABLE STUDY DESIGN

An example of an acceptable study design for spinal analgesic techniques is our randomized, prospective controlled study of different methods of epidural opioid administration in 28 patients with cancer pain. The study investigated differences between bolus injections administered through an epidural portacath and continuous epidural infusion administered via the Infusaid pump, a fully implantable volatile liquid–driven pump. In theory it should be possible to obtain more consistent dosage of drug with the infusion and produce more effective pain relief, perhaps with smaller doses and fewer complications. In addition to evaluating pain relief, patients completed several instruments intended to evaluate neuropsychological function, and we also assessed side effects and patients' treatment preference. Measurements were performed at baseline and two-week intervals. We looked at trends over time within groups and treatment differences. To our surprise, the infusion and bolus approaches to administration produced similar results for analgesic and neuropsychologic function. These results are particularly important because the pump system is quite expensive, whereas the portal system only costs several hundred dollars to implant. The increase in dose was more rapid for the infusion than for the bolus group, and again we thought the reverse would be true; in six of the 15 infusion patients, in fact, analgesia became so inadequate that we had to convert to intrathecal administration. This study produced some objective data about these two techniques and constitutes a good example of level II evidence (Gourlay et al. 1991). One implication is that the epidural port is a good option for short-term spinal bolus administration in cancer patients.

CONCLUSION

In summary, a wide range of "anesthetic techniques" are now available for control of cancer pain in addition to the venerable neurolytic neural blockade techniques. Knowledge of neuroplasticity has prompted the development of a vast array of drugs for use by the spinal route. Exciting new options are emerging, such as "pain-fiber-specific" axonal blocking drugs, N-channel calcium blockers, and others.

REFERENCES

Boas RA, Cousins MJ. Diagnostic neural blockade. In: Cousins MJ, Bridenbaugh PO (Eds). Neural Blockade in Clinical Anesthesia and Management of Pain, 2nd ed. Philadelphia: J.B. Lippincott, 1988, pp 855–898.

Brose WG, Cousins MJ. Subcutaneous lidocaine for treatment of neuropathic cancer pain. Pain 1991; 45:145–148.

Cousins MJ. Neurolytic neural blockade. In: Cousins MJ, Bridenbaugh PO (Eds). Neural Blockade in Clinical Anesthesia and Management of Pain, 2nd ed. Philadelphia: JB Lippincott, 1988, pp 1053–1084.

Fields HL (Ed). Core Curriculum for Professional Education in Pain, 2nd ed. Seattle: IASP Press, 1995.

Gourlay GK, Plummer JL, Cherry DA, et al. Comparison of intermittent bolus with continuous infusion of epidural morphine in the treatment of severe cancer pain. Pain 1991; 47:135–140.

Hogan Q, Abram S. Diagnostic and prognostic neural blockade. In: Cousins MJ, Bridenbaugh PO (Eds). Neural Blockade in Clinical Anesthesia and Pain Management, 3rd ed. Philadelphia: Lippincott-Raven, 1998, pp 837–877.

Ischia S, Ischia A, Polati E, Finco G. Three posterior block techniques: a prospective randomized study in 61 patients with pancreatic cancer pain. Anesthesiology 1992; 76:534.

McQuay H, Carroll D, Jadad AR, Wiffen P, Moore A. Anticonvulsant drugs for the management of pain: a systemic review. Br Med J 1995; 311:1047–1052.

McQuay H, Tramer M, Nye BA. A systematic review of antidepressants in neuropathic pain. Pain 1996; 68:217–227.

Saunders C. The Management of Terminal Illness. London: Edward Arnold, 1987.

Swarm RA, Cousins MJ. Anaesthetic techniques for pain control. In: Doyle D, Hanks G, MacDonald N (Eds). Oxford Text Book of Palliative Medicine. Oxford, UK: Oxford Medical Publications, 1993, pp 204–221.

Woolf CJ, Chong MS. Pre-emptive analgesia: treating postoperative pain by preventing the establishment of central sensitisation. Anesth Analg 1993; 77:362–379.

Correspondence to: Michael J. Cousins, MD, Department of Anaesthesia and Pain Management, University of Sydney, Royal North Shore Hospital, St. Leonards, NSW 2065, Australia. Tel: 61-2-9926-8423; Fax: 61-2-9906-4079.

Assessment and Treatment of Cancer Pain,
Progress in Pain Research and Management,
Vol. 12, edited by R. Payne, R.B Patt, and
C.S. Hill, IASP Press, Seattle, © 1998.

12

Methodological Issues in the Design of Clinical Trials

Perry G. Fine

*Department of Anesthesiology and Pain Management Center,
University of Utah, Salt Lake City, Utah, USA*

Sound methodology is the fulcrum upon which balance the credibility, reliability, and applicability of clinical research. All clinicians need to understand the pitfalls and constraints of past and present research methods to appreciate historical and current practical limitations. The randomized controlled trial (RCT) has become the ideal standard for clinical investigations, and for good reasons (McPeek 1987). Nevertheless, this paradigm presents real challenges and sometimes insurmountable problems that, if unquestioned, can lead to misinterpretations of results and erroneous conclusions.

Furthermore, practical and ethical barriers hinder the application of this methodological standard, especially in settings involving subjects with life-limiting illnesses and invasive (e.g., surgical) therapies. This chapter reviews the basis for the RCT as a scientific imperative and draws attention to reasons for caution in relying upon this model for "truth." Such critical evaluation is warranted because standards of care are increasingly derived from conclusions of clinical trials (i.e., evidence-based practice). Given this trend, we must have considerable confidence in the process for deriving conclusions, but also recognize potential shortcomings.

PLACEBO CONTROLS

"The strength of a trial lies principally in the strength of its control" (McPeek 1987). This statement ingenuously reflects the evolution of thought that predominates in current clinical science. Placebos formally entered the clinical science arena when Dr. James Lind (1753) evaluated the specific effects of lime juice on scurvy. Not until the middle of the twentieth century, however, did the Cornell Conference on Therapy (1946) recognize the necessary role of placebo-controlled, double-blind clinical trials. In 1955, Beecher published *The Powerful Placebo*, the seminal systematic study of patients' subjective responses to placebos.

In 1962, the Kefauver-Harris Amendment mandated that the United States Food and Drug Administration (FDA) evaluate *efficacy* as well as *safety* as a means to strengthen the regulation of purportedly therapeutic products and practices. Historically, these products have included a wide variety of interesting but unproven substances such as lizard's blood, crocodile dung, ground Egyptian mummy, and many more (Honigfeld 1964; Berg 1977, Shapiro and Morris 1978). In the long wake of specious medicinal use of nonspecifically acting substances, this federal act represented a marked shift in the culture of medicine. The demand that efficacy be demonstrated required an accepted methodology as a basis for the confident assertion of conclusions.

By 1970, the placebo control was firmly rooted in clinical trial design. In that year, the FDA published its rules for clinical evaluations and identified the placebo control as an indispensable tool (Federal Register 1970), clearly a huge step in furthering legitimate clinical science. However, the powerful momentum of this mandate and its reinforcement through the modern peer review processes for grant procurement and manuscript publication have obscured some highly relevant issues. Namely, are placebo controls always essential, possible, ethical, and interpretable? Also, can active pharmacological cues ever be adequately mimicked (controlled for) by placebos? These questions must be considered to design, carry out, and have confidence in results obtained through randomized controlled trials.

Alternatives to placebo-controlled blinded trials are all problematic. Uncontrolled trials cannot be trusted to discern nonspecific effects. Placebo effects may be potent and enduring (Fine et al. 1994). The inclusion of untreated controls does not obviate treatment effects and introduces bias because there is no blinding; studies have well demonstrated that no treatment is not the equivalent of placebo treatment (Joyce 1994). The use of nonconcurrent (i.e., historical) controls leads to ambiguity because change over time eliminates the certainty of results. Even active controls must be evaluated cautiously given that a host of cues may contaminate results and confound interpretation of differences between groups.

PROPERTIES OF PLACEBOS

The sole intent of using placebos in clinical trials is to elucidate specific effects for a postulated therapeutic intervention. This point is of utmost importance because placebos have potent salutary effects for a long list of conditions, from arthritis and angina to wound healing and varicose veins (Clark and Leaverton 1994). It is equally necessary to recognize that placebo characteristics include time-effect curves, dose-related peaks, cumulative effects, conditioning enhancement, wearing off, carryover, and side effects similar to those of "pharmacologically active" agents (Lasagna et al. 1958). The methods for using placebos and the interpretation of results thus require serious scrutiny. The characteristics of placebo effects have been far better defined than the methods for applying them and sorting out their effects in clinical studies.

Another concern is the considerable variability of subjects in time, duration, and extent of response. All of these effects can be modified by nonspecific factors, including the attributes of the intervention, doctor/researcher attitude and demeanor, and patient/subject expectations and experience (Pearce 1995). The necessity for evaluating these nonspecific determinants of response and for being attentive to the way placebos are used within protocols is underscored by the findings of Kleijnen et al (1994). In a review of 1100 studies, these investigators found only 10 RCTs that met inclusion criteria for "validity," which included accounting for nonspecific factors. We can reasonably state that a randomized, controlled, double-blinded design is not, of itself, necessarily sufficient to yield results that are clinically meaningful, let alone conclusive. For example, an RCT designed by Bergmann et al. (1994) demonstrated that the added variable of informed consent (a nonspecific factor) significantly decreased the apparent clinical efficacy of an active drug, naproxen, when compared to placebo.

Placebos may so strongly mimic active drugs that distinguishing drug-specific effects may be difficult and investigators may rightly or wrongly reach conclusions that potentially therapeutic drugs have or lack specific efficacy. For instance, it has been reported that placebo responses may increase over time; Lasagna et al. (1958) demonstrated progressive increases in appetite and energy in tuberculosis patients using placebo. However, placebo responses may diminish over time and represent a form of "tachyphylaxis" indistinguishable from the known pharmacological effects of many drugs (e.g., local anesthetics, diuretics, antihypertensives). Federle and co-workers (1989) proved this response in patients given placebos for dysmenorrhea.

Of greater practical significance, and a true confounder in clinical trials, is the potential persistence of placebo effects. Boissel reported this persistence in angina patients who sustained a 77% decrease in anginal episodes during a six-month trial using placebo alone (Boissel et al. 1986). More recent research has shown that repeated placebo dosing in patients with chronic low back pain leads to additive and sustained therapeutic effects, indistinguishable from those of a pharmacologically "active" agent (Fine and Roberts 1994). This observation strongly suggests that conventionally designed placebo-controlled trials may be inadequate to distinguish therapeutic efficacy of an "active" agent due to the influence of dosing sequence and timing. Finally, so-called hard or objective end points (e.g., oxygen delivery and consumption) may be affected equally by placebo and active pharmaceuticals, as exemplified by cardiovascular studies (Murali et al. 1988; Vayssairat et al. 1988). Recognition of these properties erects an even greater methodologic burden in efforts to elucidate specificity for subjective end points such as pain.

ETHICAL CONSIDERATIONS IN INVASIVE
THERAPEUTIC TRIALS

Designing clinical trials for the variety of available invasive therapies, especially in pain management (e.g., surgical procedures, neurolytic procedures, implanted devices, and nerve blocks), may for ethical reasons challenge and entirely frustrate efforts to randomly allocate patients into placebo control groups. Generally, the only justification for performing such invasive procedures, especially ones that are irreversible, is a reasonable expectation that they will work, coupled with a lack of reasonable alternatives. In the domain of palliative care, this situation poses a "Catch-22" dilemma: There are few clinically analogous animal models that can serve as testable bases for the requirement of "reasonable expectation" of therapeutic efficacy. Volunteer studies present obvious ethical and experimental constraints, and interventional approaches are rarely, if ever, the only choice for pain and symptom control. Direct comparisons with noninvasive therapies, which are necessary to justify the (usually) higher risk and costlier invasive interventions, do not offer patients a sufficiently similar experience upon which to make fair assessments or draw firm conclusions (Elander 1991; Clark and Leaverton 1994). Thus, provision of adequate yet ethical controls is virtually impossible.

We must openly acknowledge the tension between ethical considerations and concerns related to the potency and durability of placebo effects. This concern is heightened by the psychologically dramatic nature of invasive procedures, which may greatly amplify nonspecific effects. A reappraisal of the classic RCT paradigm is especially important in the context of such therapeutic trials. In these instances, the only reasonable alternative may be to conduct open trials with strict adherence to agreed-upon protocols with well-defined entry criteria and end points that allow data to be amassed and analyzed for comparative efficacy and safety.

The "agreed-upon protocol" portion of this process is the most important and troublesome aspect of this approach. Ideally, a credible and inclusive advocacy organization, such as the IASP, would assume a scientific jury and clearinghouse function. Interdisciplinary, nonbiased review committees need to be formed to evaluate protocols, much like an Institutional Review Board or National Institutes of Health (U.S.) Study Section. However, in this case the purpose would be to give constructive comments and generate consensus, rather than "acceptance" or "rejection."

CONCLUSIONS

It is apparent that the design of reliable and meaningful clinical trials is becoming more, rather than less, difficult. While we have moved beyond the era of accepting anecdotal reports as reproducible, we are left with the challenge of convincing ourselves that what we think we have proven with RCTs is, indeed, conclusive. Although the current models for clinical research address many shortcomings of the past, they continue to receive inappropriately high regard despite practical and ethical limitations, and despite our vastly increased knowledge of the confounding nature of placebo effects.

I conclude with two quotations that speak to the heart of these issues. The first emphasizes the complex nature of what we wish to study (Turner et al. 1994): "Symptoms, illness, and their changes over time reflect complex interactions between anatomical and neurophysiological processes, on the one hand, and cognitive behavioral and environmental factors on the other. The findings reviewed herein support the thesis that these factors are inextricably intertwined." Finally, to invite what I believe to be a necessary new chapter in the science of clinical investigations, I borrow from Pearce (1995), who states, "Nowhere in medicine is the trite conclusion: 'more experimental work needs to be done' more justifiable." To be convinced, those in doubt need only to pick up their most often-used sources of clinical science information (journals) and scrutinize the methodologies and conclusions drawn.

REFERENCES

Beecher HK. The powerful placebo. JAMA 1955; 159:1602–1606.

Berg AO. Placebos: a brief review for family physicians. J Fam Pract 1977; 5:97–100.

Bergmann JF, Chassany O, Gandiol J, et al. A randomised clinical trial of the effect of informed consent on the analgesic activity of placebo and naproxen in cancer pain. Clinical Trials and Meta-Analysis 1994; 29:41–47.

P.G. FINE

Boissel JP, Philippon AM, Gauthier E, Schbath J, Destors JM. Time course of long-term placebo therapy effects in angina pectoris. Eur Heart J 1986; 7:1030–1036.

Clark PI, Leaverton PE. Scientific and ethical issues in the use of placebo controls in clinical trials. Annu Rev Pub Health 1994; 15:19–38.

Cornell Conference on Therapy. The use of placebo in therapy. NY State J Med 1946; 46.

Elander G. Ethical conflicts in placebo treatment. J Adv Nurs 1991; 16:947–951.

Federal Register 1970; 35:7250.

Federle L, Marchini M, Acaia B, Garagiola U, Tiengo M. Dynamics and significance of placebo response in primary dysmenorrhea. Pain 1989; 36:43–47.

Fine PG, Roberts WJ, Gillette RG, Child TR. Slowly developing placebo responses obscure results of the intravenous phentolamine test in subjects with idiopathic chronic low back pain. Pain 1994; 56:235–242.

Honigfeld G. Non-specific factors in treatment: I. Review of placebo reactions and placebo reactors. Dis Nerv Syst 1964; 25:145–156.

Joyce CRB. Placebo and complementary medicine. Lancet 1994; 344:1279–1281.

Kefauver-Harris amendments of October 10, 1962, to the Food, Drugs and Cosmetic Act. Code of Federal Regulations. Washington, DC: Government Printing Office.

Kleijnen J, de Craen JM, van Everdingen J, Krol L. Placebo effect in double-blind clinical trials: a review of interactions with medications. Lancet 1994; 344:1347–1349.

Lasagna L, Laties VG, Dohan JL. Further studies on the 'pharmacology' of placebo administration. J Clin Invest 1958; 37:533–537.

Lind JA. A Treatise of the Scurvy. Edinburgh, 1753.

McPeek B. Inference, generalizability, and a major change in anesthetic practice. Anesthesiology 1987; 66:723–724.

Murali S, Uretsky BF, Kolesar JA, Valdes AM, Reddy PS. The acute effect of an oral "inotropic" placebo on the exercise capacity of patients with chronic cardiac failure. Chest 1988; 94:262–266.

Pearce JMS. The placebo enigma. Q J Med 1995; 88:215–220.

Shapiro AK, Morris LA. The placebo effect in medicine and psychological therapies. In: Bergin AI, Garfield SL (Eds). Handbook of Psychotherapy and Behavior Change: An Empirical Analysis. New York: Wiley, 1978, pp 369–410.

Turner JA, Deyo RA, Loeser JD, Von Korff M, Fordyce WE. The importance of placebo effects in pain treatment and research. JAMA 1994; 271:1609–1614.

Vayssairat M, Baudot N, Sainte-Beuve C. Why does placebo improve severe limb ischaemia? Lancet 1988; 1:356

Correspondence to: Perry G. Fine, MD, Department of Anesthesiology, University of Utah, 546 Chipeta Way, Suite 2000, Salt Lake City, UT 84108, USA. Tel: 801-585-7690; Fax: 801-585-7694; email: pfine@anesth.med.utah.edu.

Assessment and Treatment of Cancer Pain,
Progress in Pain Research and Management,
Vol. 12, edited by R. Payne, R.B. Patt, and
C.S. Hill, IASP Press, Seattle, © 1998.

13

The Current Status of Anesthetic Approaches to Cancer Pain Management

Richard B. Patt

Departments of Anesthesiology and Neuro-Oncology, and Anesthesia Pain Services, The University of Texas M. D. Anderson Cancer Center, and the Cancer, Pain and Wellness Institute International, Houston, Texas, USA

THE OUTCOME CONUNDRUM

To characterize the roles for various treatments for cancer pain, the U.S. Agency for Health Care Policy and Research (AHCPR; Jacox et al. 1994) and the American Society of Anesthesiologists (ASA; Ferrante et al. 1996) analyzed the peer reviewed literature for valid outcome data. These efforts revealed a paucity of evidence from controlled or even partially controlled trials to support specific roles for so-called "interventional" treatments. These findings, however, appear to reflect methodologic deficiencies rather than poor efficacy. Although both the AHCPR and ASA Task Force encountered voluminous support from anecdotal and expert opinion sources, they found a comparative absence of controlled investigations to support these therapies. This historic lack of adequate outcome data appears not to stem from intellectual or scientific neglect, but from factors that legitimately confound the scientific investigation of pain and interventional therapies (Sharfman and Walsh 1990; Chapman and Donaldson 1991).

Prospective research on the outcomes and indications for anesthetic therapies has been limited by logistic, scientific, and ethical constraints. Problems include accurately characterizing pain and distinguishing among subtly distinct pathologies that elicit similar complaints, variable temporal and anatomic patterns of disease in patient populations, insufficient sample sizes, variability in technique (between practitioners and even, for the same practitioner, from patient to patient), and ethical and logistical constraints on blinding, randomization, and the use of placebo. Consequently, much of what is known about neurolysis is garnered from case reports, clinical series, the observations of experienced clinicians, and extrapolations from limited basic science investigations. The relative lack of data from controlled studies on neurolysis is a major barrier to the development of scientifically supported algorithmic approaches to decision making that attempt to integrate a full range of treatment approaches. Although such schema have been proposed (Cleeland et al. 1986; Ferrer-Brechner 1988; Ferrante et al. 1996), their utility is limited by the anecdotal nature of available source documents. There is a critical need to more accurately characterize the role of neurolysis with respect to better studied pharmacologic approaches. Progress in reconciling these issues will require discrete controlled comparisons among different treatment techniques for a variety of clinical syndromes. The recent surge of interest in pain management offers promise that anesthetic approaches will not be relegated to a lost art that is merely of historical significance; this resurgent interest is expected to stimulate further basic and clinical research.

These deficiencies form the rationale for the *urgent* development of a research agenda and for political action to ensure funding for cooperative research initiatives. The success of such an effort will ultimately depend on commitment from professional organizations and governmentally funded research agencies because, in contrast to drug therapies, there is little incentive for industry-based funding. Notwithstanding the absence of data from controlled trials, we must continue providing care for patients with pain that is refractory to pharmacologic management, especially given the availability of treatments that appear to be effective. The decision-making dilemma is not uncertainty as to whether these techniques work or whether they have value, but rather, the use of acceptable scientific methods to define specific patient populations and clinical settings in which given interventions are most helpful. The provision of clinical care must thus proceed in parallel with an increased focus on the development of research initiatives. What can be surmised from available data and clinical experience and how can clinical decisions be best guided by this information?

ROLE OF ANESTHETIC / INTERVENTIONAL THERAPIES

So-called "anesthetic procedures" or "interventional" therapies include local anesthetic blocks, chemical and thermal neuroablation, the administration and maintenance of intraspinal analgesia, and electrical stimulation. Given that pharmacotherapy fails to yield adequate durable results in 10–30% of patients, these therapies continue to play an important role in the management of cancer pain. Like other interventions they should be regarded neither as a panacea nor as treatment to be instituted in isolation. Rather, they are best considered a component of a therapeutic matrix that includes antitumor therapy, various pharmacologic strategies, neurosurgical and neuroaugmentative procedures, and behavioral and psychiatric approaches, ideally implemented in a multidisciplinary setting. This matrix of complementary interventions, when individualized to each patient and applied by a compassionate, knowledgeable, and committed team of health care providers, permits extremely effective management of even complex, otherwise refractory cancer pain.

The complementary, as opposed to primary, role of anesthetic interventions is all the more apparent when viewed against the larger construct of palliative care, a philosophy of care that endeavors to control the protean symptoms of terminal illness, including pain, with quality of life as the end point (Ventafridda 1989). In general, a multimodal approach is most likely to accurately determine the cause of pain and establish a management plan that considers all its determinants. Such an approach is particularly important in considering a neurolytic block, both to establish contingency plans should treatment prove ineffective, and to provide support should a complication occur. When a multidisciplinary approach is impractical because of limited resources, the clinician at minimum needs to ensure availability of appropriate specialty consultation, when indicated. In addition, the sole practitioner must possess expertise in pharmacologic management, because careful titration of baseline opioid therapy is generally required following a block.

Patients with advanced disease are often debilitated physically and psychologically, and are emotionally overwhelmed by their prognosis and symptoms. Every intervention, no matter how "minor," must be weighed carefully against its inconvenience, recuperative time, the energy and cooperation demanded of the patient, and the potentially devastating impact of a poor outcome. Every effort should be made to select a therapeutic option with a high likelihood of success and that is not too demanding on limited resources. Patients may occasionally be too unwell to receive treatment in a traditional setting, in which case the anesthesiologist must decide whether to treat at the bedside or whether an alternative therapeutic option may be more appropriate (Patt 1989).

CLINICAL INTEGRATION OF PHARMACOTHERAPY AND NEURAL BLOCKADE

Given a historic construct that first viewed the use of opioids as undesirable, clinicians tended to correlate the outcome of nerve blocks with whether opioid use could subsequently be discontinued or dramatically curtailed. With the current emphasis on quality of life as an outcome, independent of opioid doses per se, nerve blocks are more appropriately viewed in a role that complements rather than replaces opioids. Reductions in opioid use are often still sought as a means to reduce drug side effects and as indirect evidence that the correct procedure has been properly executed. Nevertheless, efficacy is not generally judged directly in light of changes in dose requirements, but instead on clinical reports of pain and toxicity.

Most patients undergoing neurolysis receive concurrent treatment with opioids, usually chronically and often in relatively high doses. Accordingly, modification of opioid therapy after neurolysis is an important part of planning. Pain is a functional antagonist to opioid effects and reduction in nociception consequent to successful neurolysis may place patients at risk for *relative* opioid overdose. Previously well-tolerated doses may result in obtundation and even respiratory depression if nociception is suddenly and profoundly interrupted; consequently, signs of a successful procedure are an indication for early dose reduction. Abrupt discontinuation of opioids may induce physical withdrawal (abstinence syndrome). As a rule of thumb, given signs suggestive of efficacy, neurolysis may be followed by a reduction of 25–50% in basal opioids, close observation, and consideration of further upward or downward dose adjustments as needed.

Regardless of the technical success of a nerve block, most patients taking opioids chronically will require continued maintenance, albeit at lower doses. Continued opioid requirements may be due to a variety of factors including pain from other sites, incomplete neurolysis, salutary effects on anxiety and dyspnea, and rarely, psychological dependence. The likelihood that most patients will continue to use opioid analgesics even after treatment with an invasive procedure makes it imperative that the anesthesiologist pain specialist be facile in prescribing opioids.

INDICATIONS FOR ANESTHETIC INTERVENTIONS

The role of ablative techniques, the main focus of this chapter, is best considered in the context of the respective roles of other anesthetic interventions.

LOCAL ANESTHETIC BLOCKS

While therapeutic local anesthetic blocks are widely used in the management of pain of nonmalignant origin, they play a more limited role in the treatment of cancer pain (Porges 1984). The main limitation of local anes-

Table I
Indications for local anesthetic blocks for cancer pain

Diagnostic block
Prognostic block
Acute relief for pain emergencies
Secondary muscle spasm (prolonged bed rest, etc.)
Sympathetically maintained pain (e.g., Pancoast syndrome)
Premorbid chronic pain (e.g., sciatica)
Treatment-related pain (e.g., postmastectomy pain)
Herpes zoster and postherpetic neuralgia
Catheter infusions for tumor-mediated pain

thetic blockade as a therapeutic tool in patients with cancer pain that emanates from progressive tumoral activity is that pain relief tends to be transient. Indications for local anesthetic blocks are listed in Table I.

INTRASPINAL OPIOIDS

Spinal opioid therapy is a relatively new modality whose attributes resemble systemic pharmacotherapy more closely than they do those of neuroablation. The effects of both spinal and systemic analgesics are reversible, titratable, applicable to all populations, do not involve tissue destruction, and are applicable for a wide variety of pains. Thus, to the degree that these therapies are analogous, many of the same advantages apply. Intraspinal opioid therapy may provide benefits that exceed those of systemic pharmacologic therapy in select populations, to the degree that administration in proximity to centrally located drug receptors permits treatment with lower drug doses that are associated with better efficacy and fewer side effects. In addition, the administration of opioids combined with local anesthetics may be more effective than systemic therapy for movement-related pain (Du Pen et al. 1992).

In positive contrast to neuroablation, intraspinal opioid therapy more often provides effective relief of generalized pain, widely disseminated pain, and pain that is bilateral or midline, particularly when located in the trunk or lower limbs. Another feature distinguishing intraspinal opioid therapy and neuroablation is the opportunity for reliable, cost-effective screening. In negative contrast to neuroablation, spinal opioid administration requires a commitment by the clinician, patient, family, and home care system to more demanding maintenance therapy. While neuroablation is associated with significant risks, a favorable outcome requires little after-care and few resources. Thus, in rural areas and developing nations, and in some hospices, spinal opioid therapy is considerably less practical. Further, depending on a variety of factors, spinal opioids can be more costly to maintain over time than is adequate neuroablation (Hassenbusch et al., in press). However, treatment with a fully implanted system, when effective, may be much less costly than other parenteral therapies for patients with a prognosis for long-term survival.

ELECTRICAL STIMULATION

With the exception of transcutaneous electrical nerve stimulation (TENS), which is most commonly provided by a rehabilitation medicine specialist or a physical therapist, electrical stimulation does not play an important role in contemporary cancer pain management. TENS is most often used as an adjunct to other more reliably effective modalities because it rarely relieves cancer pain entirely or durably, and appears to be partially dependent on the placebo response (Ventafridda et al. 1979). It is, however, relatively innocuous and may augment patients' sense of control.

The risk:benefit ratio, cost, and durability of spinal cord stimulation (SCS) does not warrant its use in patients with cancer pain (Meglio and Cioni 1982), although stable neuropathic pain related to cancer therapies (e.g., thoracotomy, mastectomy, chemotherapy) is a relatively unexplored potential indication for SCS.

Deep brain stimulation (DBS), although intriguing, occupies a limited and controversial role in the management of intractable cancer pain (Young and Brechner 1986). Thalamic stimulation, which is associated with unilateral pain relief that corresponds topographically to the stimulated region and does not appear to be opioid-mediated, is more frequently considered for nonmalignant neuropathic pain (Turnbull et al. 1980). In contrast, DBS involves stimulation of areas of the brain with dense populations of opioid receptors (e.g., periaqueductal/periventricular gray matter) and has been advocated for cancer pain (Young and Brechner 1986). This form of stimulation may produce nonspecific, profound analgesia that appears to be mediated by the release of endogenous opioids. Interest has waned with the introduction of spinal opioid therapy and the advent of more facile use of systemic opioids. Deep brain stimulation has recently been redesignated as experimental and is available at only a few specialized centers.

NEUROABLATION

Neurolytic blocks have played an important historical role in the management of intractable cancer pain and remain a primary focus of the anesthesiologist with specialized training in pain management. As has been noted, the role of neurolytic blockade is complemented by the support offered by the multidisciplinary pain management team. Neuroablative procedures are indicated only in specific circumstances, i.e., for pain of malignant origin that is severe, expected to persist, well localized, and that is ideally somatic or visceral in origin and does not comprise a component of a syndrome characterized by multifocal aches and pains. Further, these procedures are best considered for patients with relatively short life expectancies, who are not excessively distressed, and who can both adequately and consistently characterize their pain. They may be preferable to spinal delivery systems in patients who lack access to regular medical follow-up or the means to maintain a continuous drug delivery system. Like other invasive modalities, they are generally considered only when pain persists despite thorough trials of pharmacotherapy or when drug therapy produces unwanted side effects that persist despite control efforts. Careful selection of the proper procedure and attention to technical detail will limit the incidence of side effects and unwanted neurologic deficit. The important features of patient selection are listed in Table II.

Patients with vague complaints are likely to be ill served simply because their clinical presentation renders selecting the proper procedure difficult. In addition, patients who "feel bad all over," or who volunteer that "I can't describe it, it just hurts" may be experiencing a symptom complex defined not just by nociceptive elements but by spiritual, psychological, social, and/or economic malaise, in which case no amount of opioids or nerve ablation will enhance well-being.

Most neurolytic procedures are relatively efficacious for pain that is well localized, but when extended to provide analgesic coverage for pain that is extensively distributed they are more prone to failure, or of greater concern, are associated with increased risks of undesirable neurologic deficit. There are, however, a few exceptions to this general dictum. Sympathetic blockade (stellate ganglion, celiac, lumbar sympathetic, and hypogastric block) often provides topographic analgesia that is ample for the visceral pain syndromes, most of which tend to be vague in character and relatively diffuse. Epidural neurolysis, although performed in only a few centers, can often be successfully employed to manage diffuse pain without inducing unwanted neurologic deficit, although this approach remains a risk because of the potential for unpredictable spread.

Pain that is due to somatic or visceral injury is more likely to respond beneficially to neural blockade than is neuropathic pain. Neurolytic blocks need not be summarily excluded in the management of intractable neuropathic pain, but should be preceded by careful trials of local anesthetic blocks to determine the likelihood of efficacy. Surveys of patients with

Table II
Indications for neurolysis

Pain is severe
Pain is expected to persist
Pain cannot be modified by less invasive means
Pain is well localized Although blocks are usually most effective when the topographic extent of pain is limited, sympathetic blocks may provide relief of relatively diffuse visceral pain. Epidural neurolysis has also been advocated for segmental pain distributed over several dermatomes.
Pain is well characterized and consistent Though often vague in nature, visceral pain is amenable to treatment with neural blockade.
Pain is not multifocal Pituitary destruction, although infrequently performed, may be considered for disseminated pain due to osseous metastases, especially in patients with breast or prostate cancer. Other forms of neurolysis may be cautiously considered with the goal of eliminating the most severe pain and controlling secondary pain with opioids.
Limited life expectancy Requires carefully individualized decision making. In general, problems such as deafferentation pain and transience are minimized when selection is limited to patients with predicted life expectancy of less than one year.
Pain is of somatic or visceral origin Although temporary pain relief can often be achieved with local anesthetic blocks, in general, neuropathic pain is less likely to respond favorably to neurolysis. Not an absolute contraindication.
Patient has pain otherwise amenable to spinal opioid therapy but lacks ready access to follow-up or the means to adequately maintain delivery system.

advanced cancer have determined that pain is usually present in more than one body part simultaneously (Twycross 1978). Patients may complain of one predominant source of pain only to find that when it is eliminated by a nerve block or radiotherapy other previously secondary complaints increase in severity. Nevertheless, even in patients with multiple sources of pain, a localized procedure that reduces the most severe complaint is sometimes of value and permits control of the secondary symptoms with conservative means.

HAZARDS

Nervous structures are affected indiscriminately by chemical neurolysis and great care must be exercised to relieve pain without producing unwanted motor or autonomic dysfunction. The potential for motor weakness and disturbances in autonomic function can be partly assessed in advance with local anesthetic blockade. Blockade of a purely sensory peripheral nerve will not result in motor deficit. Thorough assessment identifies patients in whom a degree of motor weakness will be well tolerated, e.g., patients already confined to bed, patients with preexisting motor deficit, and those with pain sufficiently severe to render an involved limb already useless.

The potential for damage to nontargeted tissue is of concern with any destructive procedure. Verification of needle placement and the potential for aberrant spread of the injected solution must be carefully assessed. Such localization is facilitated by careful aspiration, observation for paresthesia, manual appreciation of tissue compliance, electrical stimulation, radiographic guidance, or test doses of local anesthetic.

Neither chemical nor other means of interrupting nerve function reliably produce permanent relief of pain because of axonal regrowth, central nervous system plasticity, or the development of deafferentation pain (Ramamurthy et al. 1989). The significance of impermanence of effect is minimized by selecting patients whose life expectancy is unlikely to exceed the duration of pain relief, and by recognizing that the procedure can be repeated at the same site or more proximally if the effects are more short-lived than anticipated.

COMPARISON TO OTHER TREATMENT MODALITIES

The clinical features of neuroablation and its alternatives are compared and contrasted in Tables III–IX. Even with acceptance of the contemporary

Table III
Pharmacotherapies: favorable attributes

General Features	Wide Application
Analgesia is reversible Effects are titratable No end-organ toxicity (except meperidine) Side effects are reversible Treatment principles are easily learned Technologic, equipment requirements low Costs may be low	Topographic • diffuse pain • multiple pains • bilateral/midline pain Mechanistic • (+++) nociceptive • (+) neuropathic • (++) mixed Etiologic • tumor invasion • therapy-related • premorbid Demographic • across age groups • across cultures • across ranges of medical fitness

Table IV
Opioid pharmacotherapy: unfavorable attributes

General Considerations	Limited Efficacy
Stigma and effects on compliance	Neuropathic pain
Requirements for chronic treatment • regular drug use • regular reassessment • frequent titrations	Cutaneous pain Movement-related pain Massive nociception
Usually requires polypharmacy • multiple analgesics (atc + prn) • laxatives, antiemetics, stimulants, etc.	Debilitated patients Narrow therapeutic window Addiction as a comorbidity

construct that blocks are considered only after "failure" of more conservative pharmacologic therapies, problems arise because *vastly different criteria are applied to define "failure;"* these criteria in part depend on available resources, subtle differences in disease and personality dynamics, treatment philosophies, and which specialist dominates decision making. Features in need of more exact, consensual definition are listed in Table X.

Likewise, there is little agreement about what constitutes "unacceptable side effects." Ultimately, the patient must be regarded as the final authority on when a side effect is sufficiently disagreeable to warrant trial of an alternate modality. As with pain and delirium (Fainsinger et al. 1993), we have been slow to develop sufficiently sensitive tools to accurately characterize these effects, and their apparent incidence and seriousness will naturally differ with changes in the methods used to characterize them. Side effects, ranging from the obvious to the subtle, that accompany systemic opioid therapy may in fact be so ubiquitous that we accept their presence too uncritically. Should this premise be confirmed, early consideration of procedures with a favorable risk:benefit ratio may be warranted for patients with amenable symptoms (Table XI). Such procedures may include celiac or hypogastric plexus block for abdominopelvic pain, phenol saddle block for

Table V
Adjuvant pharmacotherapy: unfavorable attributes

Toxicity	Efficacy
NSAIDs • gastrointestinal, renal, hepatic • hematologic, cutaneous, CNS	NSAIDs • ineffective for severe pain
Other Adjuvants • CNS, GI, GU, cardiac • bone marrow, hepatic • miscellaneous	Other Adjuvants • mechanism specific • latency to effect • often ineffective • unpredictable dose-response relationship

Table VI
Attributes of neuroablation

Favorable Attributes	Unfavorable Attributes
Reduced need for follow-up	Toxicities infrequent, but may be serious and lasting
Reduced need for chronic drug therapy	New neuropathic pain
Potential cost savings	• deafferentation, regenerative neuritis
Useful in rural areas and developing nations	Unintended neurologic injury
	• sphincter or limb paresis
Targeted to painful region	• injury to nutrient vessels of spinal cord
• fewer collateral effects	Unintended non-neurologic injury (pneumothorax, etc.)
Efficacy may be superior for certain syndromes	

perineal pain in patients with urinary diversions, intercostal or thoracic sub-arachnoid neurolysis or for well-localized chest wall pain, and trials of intra-spinal opioids for movement-related pain or in patients prone to opioid side effects, such as those who are elderly or cachectic. This construct assumes relatively similar risk:benefit ratios, and is thus reasonable only with careful decision making and a high level of technical expertise. Certainly, from a strictly pharmacoeconomic perspective, the system would often be better served if a proportion of patients with chronic cancer pain and relatively long life expectancies were treated with neuroablation or implantable systems for the delivery of spinal opioids. Interestingly, preliminary data strongly suggests that relatively early in the course of treatment (3–5 months), less invasive subcutaneous and externalized epidural systems become considerably more expensive than fully implanted intrathecal systems due to charges for home care, pump leasing, nursing, and drugs (Hassenbusch et al., in press).

Table VII
Limitations of neuroablation

Applications limited in presence of long life expectancy
  • transience
  • development of new pain
  • less of an issue for sympathetic block
Applications limited for limb pain in ambulatory, continent patients
  • significant risks of paresis
Applications limited for diffuse, disseminated, or bilateral pain
May reduce but usually does not eliminate need for analgesics
Performance requires specialized training
Often requires fluoroscopy or CT guidance

Table VIII
Attributes of chronic treatment with intraspinal analgesics

General Considerations
   Potential risks and benefits more closely resemble those of systemic
     pharmacotherapy
   Targeted delivery may enhance efficacy and reduce adverse effects
   Considerations differ for alternate delivery systems
Favorable Attributes
   Reversible
   Titratable
   No tissue destruction
   Applicable for diverse patient populations
   Applicable for diverse pain syndromes
     nociceptive, neuropathic, mixed pain
     diffuse, disseminated, bilateral, and limb pain
   Screening is simple, reliable, and inexpensive
   Very cost effective in some settings
Unfavorable Attributes
   Requires (minor) surgery
   Requires committed patient, family, treatment team, and home care service
   Requires maintenance of both drug therapy and delivery system
   Practitioner requirements: specialized training, institutional support, around-the-
     clock availability

OUTCOMES

From a historical perspective and in contemporary practice, most neurodestructive techniques involve chemical neurolysis, i.e., the injection of alcohol or phenol near a nerve or nerves to destroy a portion of the targeted nerve to interrupt the transmission of impulses for a prolonged time. Cryoanalgesia is said to produce more selective destruction (Evans 1981), but is generally associated with an unacceptably short duration of action and

Table IX
Limitations of chronic spinal analgesia

Potential for device malfunction

Risk of infection

Risk of migration

Costs: system dependent
   • fully implantable: high upfront cost
   • epidural: high maintenance costs

Intrathecal analgesics
   • most pumps lack PCA capacity
   • limited efficacy for opioid-insensitive pain

Epidural analgesics
   • systemic effects at high doses

Table X
What constitutes "failure" of systemic pharmacotherapy?

Is additional antitumor therapy applicable?

Is titration to a "maximum" dose ever a criterion?

Have there been trial "rotations" of alternate analgesics?
  • How many failed rotations constitute overall failure? Two? Three?
  • Is *dramatic* failure of a single agent sufficient?

Are side effects truly refractory?
  • What constitutes sufficient trials of symptomatic management?
  • Have there been trials of multiple/combined antiemetics? Psychostimulants?
    Corticosteroids?
  • Have purported opioid "allergies" been confirmed/debunked?

For less opioid-responsive syndromes, have adjuvants received adequate trials? All
  "appropriate" classes? Multiple drugs within a class? Adequate duration of trials?

is typically reserved for patients with longer life expectancies. Radiofrequency-generated thermal lesions are an effective means of inducing therapeutic nerve injury. While results are more discrete and controllable than those achieved with chemical blockade, anesthesiologists are often unfamiliar with this technology, or it may be unavailable due to its expense; consequently, chemical techniques still predominate.

While well-controlled studies are lacking, large clinical series report significant relief of pain in an average of 50–80% of patients, with the best results obtained when studies include patients who have received multiple blocks (Perese 1958; Hay 1962; Papo and Visca 1979).

This seemingly modest outcome data is more meaningful when interpreted in the context of patient selection, because patients referred for treatment with nerve blocks by definition have pain that is refractory to other treatment modalities. Effects tend to average six months in duration, an interval that is usually sufficient for most patients. There are anecdotal reports of pain relief persisting in excess of one to two years, but alternatively, blocks frequently need to be repeated more often than expected, usually due to disease progression or the presence of tumor limiting the contact between the injected drug and the targeted nerve. Overall, significant complications are reported in less than 5% of patients (Perese 1958; Hay 1962; Papo and Visca 1979).

In patients with advanced disease, the relative risk:benefit ratio shifts considerably in favor of invasive procedures. Optimal results are ensured by the judicious use of fluoroscopic and computed tomography (CT) guidance to verify needle localization, and by the application of simple adjuncts such as careful aspiration, the use of a nerve stimulator, the administration of test doses of local anesthetic, and elicitation of paresthesias.

Table XI
Early consideration of neuroablation

Procedure	Indication
Celiac plexus neurolysis	Abdominal pain, back pain
Superior hypogastric plexus neurolysis	Pelvic pain
Phenol saddleblock	Perineal pain with urinary diversion
Thoracic subarachnoid neurolysis	Focal chest wall pain
Intercostal neurolysis	Focal chest wall pain
Lumbar subarachnoid neurolysis	Unilateral leg pain in bed-bound patient

Note: The risk:benefit ratio of these procedures in the specified settings is sufficiently favorable and well established to warrant early consideration.

CELIAC PLEXUS BLOCK

The status of celiac plexus block and related outcome data represent an excellent closing example of the problems related to the evolving role of anesthetic interventions and potential solutions. An 85–94% incidence of good to excellent relief of pain has been obtained in large series of patients receiving one or more neurolytic celiac plexus blocks for pain from pancreatic cancer, per se (Brown et al. 1987), or a variety of intra-abdominal neoplastic conditions (Jones and Gough 1977). In a series of 136 patients, analgesia was present until the time of death in 75% of cases, and in an additional 12.5% pain relief was maintained for more than 50% of survival time (Brown et al. 1987). Notwithstanding this case series retrospective data, an article was recently published that suggested that reports documenting outcomes for celiac plexus neurolysis are inadequate, even though this intervention is the single procedure with perhaps greatest consensus regarding claims for efficacy (Tables XII and XII; Sharfman and Walsh 1990). Indeed, a recent meta-analysis of 59 papers on celiac neurolysis for cancer pain found that only two involved randomization, and only one of these employed a control group (Eisenberg et al. 1995). Of note is the recent publication of a randomized double-blind, placebo-controlled study of intra-operative celiac neurolysis that demonstrated that treated patients experienced not only improved pain control, reduction in opioid use and improved function, but also statistically significant improvement in survival.

CONCLUSION

Cancer pain is comprised of a group of heterogeneous disorders characterized by variable responses to treatment. Control of pain can be achieved

Table XII
Potential limitations of pharmacologic management for abdominopelvic pain

Modality	Potential Limitation
NSAIDs	Gastropathy, renal dysfunction, bone marrow depletion, masking fever
Oral analgesics	Xerostomia, dysphagia, malabsorption, obstruction, nausea, vomiting, coma
Transdermal analgesics	Dose requirements for opioids that exceed dose limitations
Parenteral analgesics	Inadequate household or community support to manage infusions
Opioids	Ileus, partial obstruction, intractable constipation; reduced responsivity due to neuropathic component of pain; dose-limiting side effects due to asthenia and cachexia

in most patients by the application of a carefully individualized, flexible program of analgesic drugs. Anesthetic procedures comprise an important category of complementary therapeutic options that, when carefully selected and applied in the context of multimodal therapy, promote improved outcome.

The paucity of data from *controlled* studies on neuroablation is a major barrier to the development of scientifically supported algorithmic approaches to decision making that integrate a full range of treatment approaches. There is a critical need to more accurately characterize the role of neurolysis with respect to better studied pharmacologic approaches. To begin reconciling these issues, we need discrete controlled comparisons among different

Table XIII
Potential advantages of early implementation
of neural blockade for abdominopelvic cancer pain

Overall favorable risk:benefit ratio

Better efficacy before extensive perineural infiltration shelters targeted nerves

Increased ease and safety prior to development of massive organomegaly and anatomic distortion

Interventions generally better tolerated in less medically ill patients

May forestall development of chronic pain behavior

Improved performance status more likely to meaningfully increase activity and function

May improve compliance with antitumor therapy

Improved performance status may enhance candidacy for investigational therapy

Collateral effects may result in improved gastrointestinal motility

Preliminary evidence of improved survival

treatment techniques for a variety of clinical syndromes. To succeed, this effort will require multicenter collaboration, novel study designs, and new funding initiatives.

REFERENCES

Brown BL, Bulley CK, Quiel EC. Neurolytic celiac plexus block for pancreatic cancer pain. Anesth Analg 1987; 66:869–873.

Chapman CR, Donaldson GW. Issues in designing trials of nonpharmacologic treatments for pain. In: Max M, Portenoy RK, Laska EM (Eds). The Design of Analgesic Clinical Trials. Advances in Pain Research and Therapy, Vol. 18. New York: Raven Press, 1991, pp 699–711.

Cleeland CS, Rotondi A, Brechner T, et al. A model for the treatment of cancer pain. J Pain Symptom Manage 1986; 1:209–215.

Du Pen Sl, Kharasch ED, Williams A, et al. Chronic epidural bupivacaine-opioid infusion in intractable cancer pain. Pain 1992; 49:293–300.

Eisenberg E, Carr DB, Chalmers TC. Neurolytic celiac plexus block for treatment of cancer pain: a meta-analysis. Anesth Analg 1995; 80:290–295.

Evans PJD. Cryoanalgesia. Anaesthesia 1981; 36:1003–1013.

Fainsinger RL, Tapper M, Bruera E. A perspective on the management of delirium in terminally ill patients on a palliative care unit. J Palliat Care 1993; 9:4–8.

Ferrante FM, Bedder M, Caplan RA, et al. Practice guidelines for cancer pain management. A report by the American Society of Anesthesiologists Task Force on Pain Management, Cancer Pain Section. Anesthesiology 1996; 84:1243–1257.

Ferrer-Brechner T. Neurolytic blocks for cancer pain. In: Abrams S (Ed). Cancer Pain. Boston: Kluwer Academic, 1988, p 111.

Hassenbusch S, Payne R, Patt RB, Paice J, Chandler S. Modeling of patient charges for opioid therapy by different delivery routes for cancer pain management. J Pain Symptom Manage, in press.

Hay RC. Subarachnoid alcohol block in the control of intractable pain: report of results in 252 patients. Anesth Analg 1962; 41:12–16.

Jacox A, Carr DB, Payne R, et al. Management of Cancer Pain: Clinical Practice Guideline no 9. AHCPR Publication no. 94-0592. Rockville, MD: U.S. Department of Health and Human Services, Public Health Service, Agency for Health Care Policy and Research, 1994.

Jones J, Gough D. Coeliac plexus block with alcohol for relief of upper abdominal pain due to cancer. Ann R Coll Surg Engl 1977; 59:46–49.

Meglio M, Cioni B. Personal experience with spinal cord stimulation in chronic pain management. Appl Neurophysiol 1982; 45:195–200.

Papo I, Visca A. Phenol subarachnoid rhizotomy for the treatment of cancer pain: a personal account of 290 cases. In: (Eds). Advances in Pain Research and Therapy, Vol. 2, 1979, pp 339–346.

Patt RB. Interventional analgesia: epidural and subarachnoid therapy Am J Hospice Care 1989; 6:18.

Perese DM. Subarachnoid alcohol block in the management of pain of malignant disease. Arch Surg 1958; 76:347–354.

Porges P. Local anesthetics in the treatment of cancer pain. Recent Results Cancer Res 1984; 89:127.

Ramamurthy S, Walsh NE, Schoenfeld LS, et al. Evaluation of neurolytic blocks using phenol and cryogenic block in the management of chronic pain. J Pain Symptom Manage 1989; 4:72.

Sharfman WH, Walsh TD. Has the efficacy of celiac plexus block been demonstrated in pancreatic cancer pain? Pain 1990; 41:267–271.

Turnbull JM, Shulman R, Woodhurst WB. Thalamic stimulation for neuropathic pain. J Neurosurg 1980; 52:486–493.

Twycross RG. Relief of pain. In: Saunders CM (Ed). The Management of Terminal Disease. Chicago: Yearbook Publishers, 1978, p 65.

Ventafridda V. Continuing care: a major issue in cancer pain management. Pain 1989; 36:137–143.

Ventafridda V, Sganzerla EP, Fochi C, et al. Transcutaneous nerve stimulation in cancer pain. In: Bonica JJ, Ventafridda V (Eds). International Symposium on Pain in Advanced Cancer. Advances in Pain Research and Therapy, Vol. 2. New York: Raven Press, 1979, pp 509–515.

Young RF, Brechner T. Electrical stimulation of the brain for relief of intractable pain due to cancer. Cancer 1986; 57:1266–1272.

Correspondence to: Richard B. Patt, MD, Department of Anesthesiology, University of Texas M. D. Anderson Cancer Center, 1515 Holcombe Blvd., Houston, TX 77030, USA. Tel: 713-745-0091 ; Fax: 713-794-4590.

Assessment and Treatment of Cancer Pain,
Progress in Pain Research and Management,
Vol. 12, edited by R. Payne, R.B. Patt, and
C.S. Hill, IASP Press, Seattle, © 1998.

14

Neurosurgical Considerations and Options for Cancer-Related Pain

Ehud Arbit

Department of Neurosurgical Oncology, Nalitt Cancer Institute, Staten Island University Hospital, Staten Island, New York, USA

Cancer is the second leading cause of death worldwide. Of patients with cancer, 30–45% report moderate to severe pain at the time of diagnosis, and up to 90% do so at intermediate or advanced disease stages (Daut and Cleeland 1982; Bonica 1985; Levin et al. 1985). Up to 25% of patients die with pain that is inadequately controlled (World Health Organization 1990).

The last two decades have seen significant progress in the management of cancer pain. These strides have largely resulted from clarifications of the pathophysiology and pharmacology of nociception, the systematic identification of distinct cancer-related pain syndromes, and advent of the analgesic ladder approach to therapy (Yaksh and Rudy 1976; Foley 1979; Yaksh and Hammond 1982; Bonica 1985; Breitbart 1989; Elliot and Foley 1989; Cleeland 1990; Inturrisi et al. 1990; Portenoy 1990). Effective pharmacological management of pain has led to a significant decrease in the number of patients requiring invasive interventions. It is estimated that a neurosurgical intervention to relieve pain is required in only 1–2% of patients with cancer-related pain (Gildenberg 1976).

To overcome problems that result from the infrequent use of neurosurgical pain intervention, and to simultaneously make neurosurgical approaches universally available, a simple "book of recipes" similar to the analgesic ladder concept needs to be developed for surgical interventions. The following generic and procedure-specific guidelines may be helpful in developing such an approach to pain procedures.

GENERIC GUIDELINES

A. The basic treatment approach must initially address the neoplastic process and concurrently use pharmacological means directed at the pain and its psychological and physical sequelae.

B. Failure of medical management must be recognized at the point when pain relief cannot be attainable without side effects that interfere with the patient's quality of life (e.g., encephalopathy) or are unacceptable to the patient (e.g., intractable nausea, vomiting, and constipation).

C. Of the procedures to alleviate pain, those that are reversible (e.g., augmentative modalities) should generally have priority over procedures that cause irreversible neurological sequelae (ablative modalities).

D. Cancer is a dynamic, evolving process, and end-stage pain may be multifocal or diffuse and is likely to emanate from a mix of somatic-visceral and neuropathic mechanisms. Augmentative modalities are anticipatory in the sense that they may correlate with changes in the disease stage, pain level, and pain sites.

E. In certain clear situations the use of an ablative modality as a "onetime" procedure can be less invasive and demanding of the patient than continued aggressive medical management or augmentative modalities that require ongoing care.

PROCEDURE-SPECIFIC GUIDELINES

A. The procedure most likely to be effective in alleviating the pain should obviously be performed, but if there is a choice, the one associated with fewer and less serious risks is preferred. For example, bilateral cordotomy, midline myelotomy, and spinal opioid infusion are all viable options to alleviate abdominopelvic pain. As spinal opioid infusion is reversible and least likely to cause serious and permanent sequelae, it is the preferred first choice.

B. Applicable for both ablative and augmentative modalities, the lowest or most peripheral point relative to the location of pain is the more appropriate site for intervention. For example, if pain is located in the torso or lower extremities, spinal opioid infusion is more appropriate, initially, than ventricular opioid infusion. Also, if ablation is indicated, for example for trigeminal nerve territory pain, rhizotomy or ganglionectomy of the trigeminal nerve is more appropriate than a trigeminal tractotomy or thalamotomy.

C. The pattern and temporal evolution of the pain syndrome, and the likelihood of the development of multifocal or diffuse pain (e.g., breast cancer and multiple bone metastases) should prompt consideration of an anticipatory procedure, such as spinal or ventricular opioid infusion.

Choosing the most appropriate procedure for an individual patient involves two considerations apart from the site of pain: the pathophysiological mechanism underlying the pain and the patient's functional and disease status. From the pathophysiologic perspective, nociceptive pain implies pain commensurate with tissue damage associated with an identifiable somatic or visceral process activating well-localized nociceptors in skin, bone, or deep tissues. Nociceptive pain often responds well to opioid drugs, and is also the most amenable and responsive to ablative treatment modalities. While most cancer-related pain is predominantly nociceptive, at least initially, many patients also develop an underlying component of neuropathic pain. This pain results from damage by compression, encasement, or infiltration by tumor of peripheral nerves, plexus, or spinal cord elements. Neuropathic pain superimposed on the primary somatic-nociceptive pain is often overlooked, which leads to the less than optimal results achieved by procedures strictly aimed at nociceptive pain.

Neuropathic pain is a consequence of damage to the peripheral or central nervous system, and given that ongoing nociception is not a prerequisite for occurrence of this pain, the removal of a nociceptive lesion may not produce relief. Neuropathic pain is regarded as less opioid responsive than is nociceptive pain and is not as well served by ablation of peripheral nerves or pain tracts. The treatment of neuropathic pain is primarily with adjuvant drugs, including antidepressants and anticonvulsants. Surgical treatments include spinal and central nervous system (CNS) stimulation procedures, and procedures aimed at modulating pain perception at spinal cord level, such as dorsal root entry zone lesions (DREZ-otomies).

Visceral pain, the result of activation of visceral nociceptors by stretch or distention, is conducted afferently through the sympathetic nerves to corresponding segmental ganglia. In the spinal cord, visceral pain is conducted by crossed and uncrossed ascending fibers. Ablative procedures aimed at visceral pain need be directed at segmental ganglia, and in the spinal cord must be carried out bilaterally and more rostrally than for pure somatic-nociceptive pain.

The functional and disease status of patients is an important determinant of the most appropriate procedure. At present, most patients considered for surgical interventions have advanced, often end-stage disease with weeks to a few months expected longevity. In these patients, the procedure most likely to alleviate the pain is the most appropriate whether it is ablative or augmentative. In cancer patients with potential protracted longevity whose focal or systemic disease may be eradicable or controllable for many months or years by antineoplastic therapy, the procedure must be chosen more carefully. Functionality and quality of life are of paramount concerns, so procedures that are reversible and least destructive to the nervous system or associated with the least risk of complication are preferred.

NEUROSURGICAL PROCEDURES

Numerous neurosurgical procedures alleviate pain, including cancer-related pain. The four most common procedures in this author's practice are percutaneous cordotomy, midline myelotomy, and spinal or ventricular opioid infusions. On rare occasions, other procedures tailored for a specific pain syndrome are considered. Nonablative procedures that use stereotactic radio-surgery (gamma knife) directed at the pituitary gland or cerebral-thalamic and subthalamic nuclei represent a new and promising modality. Stereotactic ablations, such as cingulotomy or thalamotomy, should be considered for specific situations, as is the case with dorsal rhizotomies (Hassenbusch and Pillay 1993).

CORDOTOMY

During cordotomy, the anterolateral spinothalamic tract is interrupted to produce contralateral loss of pain and temperature sensibility (Rosomoff et al. 1965; Arbit 1990). Patients with severe unilateral pain arising in the torso or lower extremity are most likely to benefit from this procedure (Ischia et al. 1984; Sanders and Zuurmond 1995). Impressive results have also been observed in patients with chest wall pain (Stuart and Cramond 1993; Sanders and Zuurmond 1995). The percutaneous technique is generally preferred (Arbit 1990). Surgical cordotomy, which is rarely used, is reserved for patients who are unable to undergo a percutaneous procedure, or patients who require lesioning on the side of the only functional lung (Arbit 1990). Significant pain relief is achieved in more than 90% of patients during the period immediately following cordotomy (Rosomoff et al. 1965; Ischia et al. 1984; Tasker et al. 1988; Arbit 1990; Stuart and Cramond 1993; Sanders and Zuurmond 1995). Fifty percent of surviving patients have recurrent pain after one year, and repeat cordotomy can sometimes be effective. The neurologic complications of the procedure include paresis, ataxia, bladder dysfunction, and "mirror-image" pain (Tasker et al. 1988; Sanders and Zuurmond

1995). These complications are usually transient, but may be protracted and disabling in up to 5% of cases. Rarely, patients with long survival develop a delayed-onset dysesthetic pain. The most serious potential complication is respiratory dysfunction, which manifests as phrenic nerve paralysis or sleep-induced apnea (in patients who undergo bilateral high cordotomy) (Polatty and Cooper 1986). This risk explains the contraindication for performing bilateral high cervical cordotomies in one sitting or a unilateral cervical cordotomy ipsilateral to the site of the only functioning lung.

A small but an important group of patients, namely those with bilateral lower extremity pain, midline spinal, or abdominopelvic pain may derive great benefit from a bilateral thoracic surgical cordotomy. Many patients with this kind of pain from spinal or abdominopelvic malignancies have lost their ability to ambulate and have bowel and bladder diversions. The bilateral thoracic cordotomy carries a minimal risk of further neurologic compromise in these patients and is likely to result in excellent and lasting pain relief.

MIDLINE C1–C2 MYELOTOMY

C1 commissural myelotomy is a percutaneous technique in which a radiofrequency lesion is produced in the central cord. Until recently the procedure was performed under stereotactic guidance using a designated spinal frame, which limited its wide acceptance. Recently, a freehanded CT-guided technique has led to a resurgence of interest in the procedure (Kanpolat et al. 1988, 1990). Intraoperative stimulation to ensure appropriate placement of the radiofrequency probe is essential. Data suggests that this approach may relieve bilateral arm, leg, and pelvic pain without altering proprioceptive or motor function (Hitchcock 1974; Schvarc 1976; Papo 1979). Transient gait disturbance is common, but usually resolves within 48 hours. Experience with this approach is limited, and relief is sometimes incomplete and short lived (Papo and Luongo 1976; Papo 1979).

The exact mechanism by which myelotomy is effective is not entirely clear, but it is postulated that interruption of a nonspecific polysynaptic pain pathway in the central cord is responsible for the wide analgesia produced (Jones 1993). High cervical myelotomy is effective for bilateral upper or lower extremity pain, abdominopelvic pain, and axial pain.

SPINAL (EPIDURAL OR INTRATHECAL) OPIOID INFUSION

Perhaps the greatest advance in the last two decades in the management of cancer-related pain has been the introduction and evolution of spinal and ventricular opioid therapy (Yaksh 1981; Yaksh and Reddy 1981). The concept of direct instillation of opioids into the cerebrospinal fluid is the logical consequence of the discovery of opioid receptors in the spinal cord and brain. These modalities are now used routinely to manage acute and chronic pain (Campbell 1987; Ross and Hughes 1987; Arner et al. 1988; Cousins et al. 1988; Hardy and Wells 1990; Tobias et al. 1990; Cousins and Plummer 1991; Plummer et al. 1991; Sjöberg et al. 1994). The delivery of low doses of opioids near their sites of action in the spinal cord may decrease supraspinally mediated adverse effects. In the absence of randomized trials that compare the various intraspinal techniques with other analgesic approaches, the indications for the spinal route remain empiric (Krames 1993) but are based on an evaluation of a relative therapeutic index (Devulder et al. 1994). A recent survey reported that only 16 of 1205 cancer patients with pain required intraspinal therapy (Hogan et al. 1991). Compared with neuroablative therapies, spinal opioids have the advantage of preserving sensation, strength, and sympathetic function. Contraindications include bleeding diathesis, profound leukopenia, and sepsis. A temporary trial of spinal opioid therapy should be performed to assess the potential benefits of this approach before implantation of a permanent catheter.

Opioid selection for intraspinal delivery is influenced by several factors. Hydrophilic drugs, such as morphine and hydromorphone, have a prolonged half-life in cerebrospinal fluid and significant rostral redistribution (Max et al. 1985; Moulin et al. 1986; Brose et al. 1991). Lipophilic opioids, such as fentanyl and sufentanil, have less rostral redistribution (Chrubasik et al. 1988) and may be preferable for segmental analgesia at the level of spinal infusion. The addition of a low concentration of a local anesthetic, such as 0.125% to 0.25% bupivacaine, to an epidural (Nitescu et al. 1990; Hogan et al. 1991; Sjöberg et al. 1991; DuPen and Williams 1992) or intrathecal opioid (Goucke 1993; van Dongen et al. 1993; Crul et al. 1994; Sjöberg et al. 1994) increases analgesic effect without increasing toxicity. Other agents have also been coadministered with intraspinal opioids, including clonidine, somatostatin, and calcitonin (Chrubasik 1980; Coombs et al. 1985; Coombs et al. 1986; Bonnet et al. 1988; Mok et al. 1988; Eisenach et al. 1989; Poli et al. 1993), but additional studies are required to assess their potential utility and safety.

There are no trials comparing the intrathecal and epidural routes in cancer pain. A combined analysis of adverse effects observed in numerous trials of epidural or intrathecal administration suggests that the risks associated with these techniques are similar (DeCastro et al. 1991). The potential morbidity for these procedures indicates the need for a well-trained clinician and long-term monitoring.

INTRAVENTRICULAR OPIOID INFUSION

Until recently, ventricular opioid infusions were reserved for patients with cervicofacial pain syndromes and brachial plexopathies. The indications for this treatment method have recently been expanded to include other pain syndromes. The appeal of a ventricular route of administration is in the simplicity of placing a ventricular cannula and the adequacy of using an Ommaya reservoir as a port of drug instillation. The pain relief obtained with this technique is in the range of 70–90%, which is attainable in over 90% of patients so treated. The main complication of repeated ventricular drug instillation is infection. Other complications are drug-related, and are similar to those of spinal opioid infusions. Data suggest that the administration of an opioid into the cerebral ventricles can provide long-term analgesia in selected patients (Leavens et al. 1982; Nurchi 1984; Roquefeil et al. 1984; Lobato et al. 1987; Obbens et al. 1987; Dennis and DeWitty 1990; Lee et al. 1990; Crammond and Stuart 1993). This technique has been used for patients with craniofacial pain, upper body pain including brachial plexopathies, abdominoperineal pain, pelvic pain, and severe diffuse pain. Schedules have included both intermittent injection via an Ommaya reservoir (Lobato et al. 1987; Obbens et al. 1987; Crammond and Stuart 1993; Lazorthes et al. 1995) and continual infusion using an implanted pump (Dennis and DeWitty 1990).

CONCLUSION

Most patients with cancer-related pain will respond adequately to pharmacological therapy. Only a small percentage of patients will need neurosurgical modes of therapy. A variety of interventions have been described, but the four most common procedures are percutaneous cordotomy, myelotomy, and spinal and ventricular opioid infusions. The selection of the most appropriate procedure depends on the site of pain, its underlying mechanism, the patient's functional status, life expectancy, and general condition.

REFERENCES

Arbit E. Neurosurgical management of cancer pain. In: Foley KM, Bonica JJ, Ventafridda V (Eds). Second International Congress on Cancer Pain. Advances in Pain Research and Therapy, Vol. 16. New York: Raven Press, 1990, pp 289–300.

Arner S, Rawal N, Gustafsson LL. Clinical experience of long-term treatment with epidural and intrathecal opioids: a nationwide survey. Anaesthesiol Scand 1988; 32:253–259.

Bonica JJ. Treatment of cancer pain: current status and future needs. In: Fields HL, Dubner R, Cervero F (Eds.). Proceedings of the Fourth World Congress on Pain. Advances in Pain

Research and Therapy, Vol. 9. New York: Raven Press, 1985, pp 589.

Bonnet F, Boico O, Rostaing S, et al. Clonidine for postoperative analgesia: Epidural vs. I.M. study. Anesthesiology 1988; 69:A395.

Breitbart W. Psychiatric management of cancer pain. Cancer 1989; 60:2336–2342.

Brose WG, Tanalian DL, Brodsky JB, et al. CSF and blood pharmacokinetics of hydromorphone and morphine following lumbar epidural administration. Pain 1991; 45:11–17.

Campbell C. Epidural opioids: the preferred route of administration [editorial]. Anesth Analg 1987; 68:869–873.

Chrubasik J. Somatostatin, a potent analgesic. Lancet 1980; 2:1208.

Chrubasik J, Wust H, Schulte MJ, et al. Relative analgesic potency of epidural fentanyl, alfentanil, and morphine in treatment of postoperative pain. Anesthesiology 1988; 68:929–933.

Cleeland CS. Assessment of pain in cancer: measurement issues. In: Foley KM, Bonica JJ, Ventafridda V (Eds). Proceedings of the Second International Congress on Cancer Pain. New York: Raven Press, 1990, pp 47–56.

Coombs DW, Saunders RL, LaChance D, et al. Intrathecal morphine tolerance: use of intrathecal clonidine, DADLE, and intraventricular morphine. Anesthesiology 1985; 62:357–363.

Coombs DW, Saunders RL, Fratkin JD, et al. Continuous intrathecal hydromorphone and clonidine for intractable cancer pain. Neurosurgery 1986; 64:890–894.

Cousins MJ, Plummer J. Spinal opioids in acute and chronic. In: Max MB, Portenoy RK, Laska E (Eds). The Design of Analgesic Clinical Trials. Advances in Pain Research and Therapy, Vol 18. New York: Raven Press, 1991, pp 457–480.

Cousins MJ, Cherry DA, Gourlay GK. Acute and chronic pain: use of spinal opioids. In: Cousins MJ, Bridenbaugh PO (Eds). Neural Blockade in Clinical Anesthesia and Management of Pain. Philadelphia: JB Lippincott, 1988, pp 955–1029.

Crammond T, Stuart G. Intraventricular morphine for intractable pain of advanced cancer. J Pain Symptom Manage 1993; 8:465–473.

Crul BJ, van Dongen RT, Snijdelaar DG, et al. Long-term continuous intrathecal administration of morphine and bupivacaine at the upper cervical level: access by a lateral C1-C2 approach. Anesth Analg 1994; 79:594–597.

Daut RL, Cleeland CS. The prevalence and severity of pain in cancer. Cancer 1982; 50:1913–1918.

DeCastro MD, Meynadier MD, Zenz MD. Regional opioid analgesia. In: Portenoy RK, Laska E (Eds). Developments in Critical Care Medicine and Anesthesiology, Vol. 20. Dordrecht: Kluwer Academic, 1991.

Dennis GC, DeWitty RL. Long-term intraventricular infusion of morphine for intractable pain in cancer of the head and neck. Neurosurgery 1990; 26:404–407.

Devulder J, Ghys L, Dhondt W, et al. Spinal analgesia in terminal care: risk vs. benefit. J Pain Symptom Manage 1994; 9:75–81.

DuPen S, Williams AR. Management of patients receiving combined epidural morphine and bupivacaine for the treatment of cancer pain. J Pain Symptom Manage 1992; 7:125–127.

Eisenach JC, Rauck RL, Buanell C, et al. Epidural clonidine analgesia for intractable cancer pain: Phase I. Anesthesiology 1989; 71:647–652.

Elliot K, Foley KM. Neurological pain syndromes in patients with cancer. In: Portenoy RK (Ed). Neurologic Clinics: Pain: Mechanisms and Syndromes. Philadelphia: Saunders, 1989, pp 333–360.

Foley KM. Pain syndromes in patients with cancer. In: Bonica JJ, Ventafridda V (Eds). International Symposium on Pain in Advanced Cancer. Advances in Pain Research and Therapy, Vol. 2. New York: Raven Press, 1979; pp 59–75.

Gildenberg, PL. Considerations in the selection of patients for surgical treatment caused by malignancy. In: Arbit E (Ed). Management of Cancer-Related Pain. Mt. Kisco, NY: Futura, 1993, pp 221–230.

Goucke R. Continuous intrathecal analgesia with opioid/local anaesthetic mixture for cancer pain. Anaesth Intensive Care 1993; 21:222–223.

Hardy PAI, Wells JCD. Patient controlled intrathecal morphine for cancer pain. Clin J Pain 1990; 6:57–59.

Hassenbusch SJ, Pillay PK. Cingulotomy for treatment of cancer-related pain. In: Arbit E (Ed). Advances in Surgical Management of Cancer-Related Pain. Mt. Kisco, NY: Futura, 1993, pp 297–312.

Hitchcock E. Stereotactic myelotomy. Proc R Soc Med 1974; 67:771–772.

Hogan Q, Haddox JD, Abram S, et al. Epidural opiates and local anesthetics for the management of cancer pain. Pain 1991; 46:271–279.

Inturrisi CE, Portenoy RK, Max MB, et al. Pharmacokinetic pharmacodynamic (PK-PD) relationships of methadone infusions in patients with cancer pain. Clin Pharmacol Ther 1990; 47:565–577.

Ischia S, Luzzani A, et al. Subarachnoid neurolytic block (L5-S1) and unilateral percutaneous cervical cordotomy in the treatment of pain secondary to pelvic malignant disease. Pain 1984; 20:139–149.

Jones MW. Commisural myelotomy for relief of intractable pain. In: Arbit E (Ed). The Management of Cancer Pain. Mount Kisco, NY: Futura, 1993, pp 313–319.

Kanpolat Y, Atalag M, Deda H, et al. CT-guided extralemniscal myelotomy. Acta Neurochir 1988; 91:151–152.

Kanpolat Y, Atalag M, Deda H, et al. CT-guided pain procedures. Neurochirurgie 1990; 36:394–398.

Krames ES. Intrathecal infusional therapies for intractable pain: patient management guidelines. J Pain Symptom Manage 1993; 8:36–46.

Lazorthes YR, Sallerin, BA-M, Verdie JP. Intracerebro-ventricular administration of morphine for control of irreducible cancer pain. Neurosurgery 1995; 37:422–429.

Leavens ES, Hill CS, Cech DA, et al. Intrathecal and intraventricular morphine for pain in cancer patients. J Neurosurg 1982; 56:241–245.

Lee TL, Kumar A, Baratham G. Intraventricular morphine for intractable craniofacial pain. Singapore Med J 1990; 31:273–276.

Levin DN, Cleeland CS, Dar R. Public attitudes toward cancer pain. Cancer 1985; 56:2337.

Lobato RD, et al. Intraventricular morphine for intractable cancer pain: rationale, methods, clinical results. Acta Anaesthesiol Scand 1987; 31(Suppl):68–74.

Max MB, Inturrisi CE, Kaiko RF, et al. Epidural and intrathecal opiates: cerebrospinal fluid and plasma profiles in patients with chronic cancer pain. Clin Pharmacol Ther 1985; 38:631–641.

Mok MS, Wang JJ, Chan JH, et al. Analgesic effect of epidural clonidine and nalbuphine in combined use. Anesthesiology 1988; 69:A398.

Moulin DE, Inturrisi CE, Foley KM. Epidural and intrathecal opioids: cerebrospinal fluid and plasma pharmacokinetics in cancer pain patients. In: Foley KM, Inturrisi CE (Eds). Opioid Analgesics in the Management of Clinical Pain. Advances in Pain Research and Therapy, Vol 8. New York: Raven Press, 1986, pp 369–384.

Nitescu P, Appelgran L, Einarsson S, et al. Epidural versus intrathecal morphine-bupivacaine: assessment of consecutive treatment in advanced cancer pain. J Pain Symptom Manage 1990; 5:18–26.

Nurchi G. Use of intraventricular and intrathecal morphine in intractable pain associated with cancer. Neurosurgery 1984; 15:801–804.

Obbens EAMT, Hill CS, Leavens MD, et al. Intraventricular morphine administration for control of chronic cancer pain. Pain 1987; 28:61–68.

Papo I. Spinal posterior rhizotomy and commisural myelotomy in the treatment of cancer pain. In: Bonicca JJ, Ventafridda V (Eds). Advances in Pain Research and Therapy, Vol. 2, New York: Raven Press, 1979, pp 325–327.

Papo I, Luongo A. High cervical commisural myelotomy in the treatment of pain. J Neurol Neurosurg Psychiatry 1976; 39:705–710.

Plummer JL, Cherry DA, Cousins MJ, et al. Long-term spinal administration of morphine in cancer and non-cancer pain: a retrospective study. Pain 1991; 44:212–220.

222   E. ARBIT

Polatty RC, Cooper KR. Respiratory failure after percutaneous cordotomy. South Med J 1986; 79:367–379.
Poli P, Sabbia E, Venturi L, et al. Intrathecal octreotide for cancer pain: our experience. In: Abstracts: 7th World Congress on Pain. Seattle: IASP Publications, 1993.
Portenoy RK. Pain and quality of life: clinical issues and implications for research. Oncology 1990; 4:172–178.
Roquefeil B, Blanchet P, et al. Intraventricular administration of morphine in patients with neoplastic intractable pain. Surg Neurol 1984; 21:155–158.
Rosomoff HL, Carroll F, Brown J. Percutaneous radiofrequency cervical cordotomy: technique. J Neurosurg 1965; 23:639–644.
Ross BK, Hughes SC. Epidural and spinal narcotic analgesia. Clin Obstet Gynecol 1987; 30:552–565.
Sanders M, Zuurmond W. Safety of unilateral and bilateral percutaneous cervical cordotomy in 80 terminally ill cancer patients. J Clin Oncol 1995; 13:1509–1512.
Schvarc JR. Stereotactic extralemniscal myelotomy. J Neurol Neurosurg Psychiatry 1976; 39:53–57.
Sjöberg M, Appelgren L, Einarsson S, et al. Long-term intrathecal morphine and bupivacaine in "refractory" cancer pain: results from the first series of 52 patients. Acta Anaesthesiol Scand 1991; 35:30–43.
Sjöberg M, Nitescu P, Appelgren L, et al. Long-term intrathecal morphine and bupivacaine in patients with refractory cancer pain: results from a morphine:bupivacaine dose regimen of 0.5:4.75 mg/ml. Anesthesiology 1994; 80:284–297.
Stuart G, Cramond T. Role of percutaneous cervical cordotomy for pain of malignant origin. Med J Aust 1993; 158:667–670.
Tasker RR, Tsuda T, Howrylyshn P. Percutaneous cordotomy: the lateral high cervical technique. In: Schmidek HH, Sweet WH (Eds). Operative Neurological Technique Indications, Methods and Results. New York: Grune and Stratton, 1988, pp 1191–1205.
Tobias JD, Deshpande JK, Wetzel RC, et al. Post-operative analgesia: use of intrathecal morphine in children. Clin Pediatr (Phila) 1990; 29:44–48.
van Dongen RT, Crul BJ, DeBock M. Long-term intrathecal infusion of morphine and morphine/bupivacaine mixtures in the treatment of cancer pain: a retrospective analysis of 51 cases. Pain 1993; 55:119–123.
World Health Organization. Cancer Pain Relief and Palliative Care. Geneva: World Health Organization, 1990.
Yaksh TL. Spinal opiate analgesics: characteristics and principal action. Pain 1981; 11:293–346.
Yaksh TL, Hammond DL. Peripheral and central substrates in the rostral transmission of nociceptive information. Pain 1982; 13:1–85.
Yaksh TL, Reddy SVR. Studies in the primate on the analgesic effects associated with intrathecal actions of opiates, alpha adrenergic agonists and baclofen. Anesthesiology 1981; 54:451–467.
Yaksh TL, Rudy, TA. Analgesia mediated by a direct spinal action of narcotics. Science 1976; 192:1357–1358.

Correspondence to: Ehud Arbit, MD, Director, Neurosurgical Oncology, Nalitt Cancer Institute, Staten Island University Hospital, Staten Island, New York 10305, USA.

Assessment and Treatment of Cancer Pain,
Progress in Pain Research and Management,
Vol. 12, edited by R. Payne, R.B. Patt, and
C.S. Hill, IASP Press, Seattle, © 1998.

15

Intrathecal Opioid Therapy
and Implantable Devices

Sannichie Quaicoe[a], Russell McLaughlin[a],
and Samuel Hassenbusch[b]

*Departments of [a]Anesthesiology and [b]Neurosurgery,
The University of Texas M. D. Anderson Cancer Center, Houston, Texas, USA*

BASIC SCIENCE

ANATOMY

Noxious (mechanical, thermal, or chemical) stimuli affect the perception of pain by activating the pain receptors (nociceptors) at the free nerve endings of afferent fibers. These nociceptive afferents are the finely myelinated Aδ fibers and unmyelinated C fibers. The exact mechanism by which noxious stimuli are transduced into electrical nociceptive impulses is not known. Certain substances such as bradykinin, acetylcholine, and potassium activate the nociceptor afferents and produce pain when applied locally. Others, such as the prostaglandins, do not produce pain directly. Instead, they sensitize the nociceptors and thereby facilitate the pain evoked by chemicals that activate the nociceptive afferents. Mediators such as substance P produce local extravasation. At the dorsal horn of the spinal cord the nociceptive afferents contact second-order neurons in the dorsal horn. The C polymodal nociceptive afferents synapse exclusively in laminae I, II, and V of the dorsal horn, while the Aδ nociceptors terminate in laminae I and II, and can also penetrate deeper into laminae V and X (Fig. 1) (Raj 1996).

A high degree of complex sensory processing occurs in the various laminae of the dorsal horn. Such processing includes local abstraction, integration, selection, and appropriate dispersion of sensory impulses. This highly complex circuit is activated through central convergence and central summation and through excitatory and inhibitory influences coming from the periphery, from local interneurons, and from the brain stem and cortex.

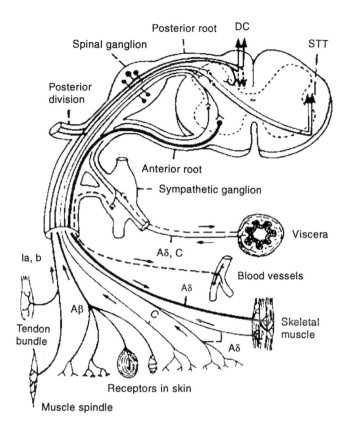

Fig. 1. A graphic illustration of a mixed spinal nerve connecting receptors from the periphery to the spinal cord (Bonica 1990).

Most afferent impulses enter the spinal cord through the dorsal root, but the ventral roots also carry afferent input. The afferents of the ventral root consist mostly of unmyelinated nociceptive afferents, which explains the incomplete relief of pain after a dorsal rhizotomy (Portenoy and Kanner 1995).

After processing in the dorsal horn of the spinal cord, some nociceptive impulses pass directly through the interneurons to the anterior and antero-lateral horn cells where they stimulate other neurons. The anterolateral neurons provoke autonomic segmental nociceptive reflex responses. The other nociceptive impulses are transmitted to neurons that project to supraspinal centers via their ascending systems (Fig. 2) (Wall and Melzack 1994; Portenoy and Kanner 1995; Raj 1996).

The ascending tracts are found in the ventrolateral quadrant and consti-tute the spinothalamic tract (STT), the spinoreticular tract (SRT), and the

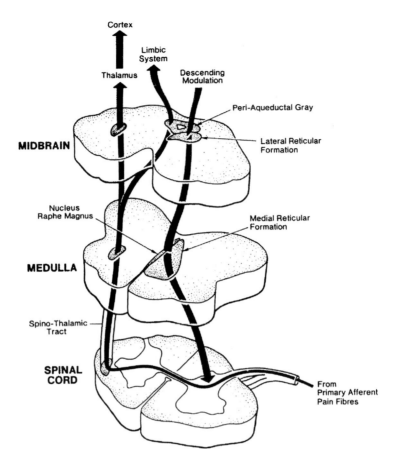

Fig. 2. A simplified schema of modulation of pain at the spinal cord, medulla, and midbrain (Cousins and Phillips 1986).

spinomesencephalic tract (SMT). These are the primary pathways for transmission of nociceptive information from the periphery to the brain. Almost all spinothalamic tract neurons send myelinated axons to the contralateral thalamus via the anterolateral quadrant of the spinal cord. It is hypothesized that the spinothalamic tract ascends for several segments before decussating. This theory is based on the observation that the analgesia produced by cordotomy begins several segments below the level of the lesion. Axons from the spinothalamic tract cells terminate in both the medial and lateral thalamus. Some of the STT fibers branch and synapse in both regions and some send collaterals to the brain stem structures en route. These collaterals have been identified in both the periaqueductal gray and the medullary reticular formation (Portenoy and Kanner 1995).

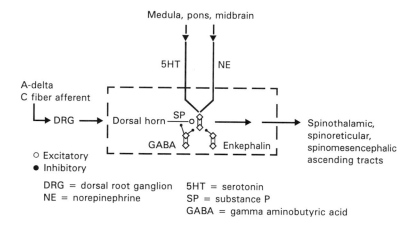

Fig. 3. Schematic diagram of input modulation at the dorsal horn of the spinal cord (Faust 1991).

The descending pain control system includes serotonergic and adrenergic fibers that originate from cortical and diencephalic systems, the periaqueductal gray (PAG) and periventricular gray areas of the mesencephalic system, and the nucleus raphe magnus and adjacent nuclei of the rostroventral medulla. The nucleus raphe magnum receives excitatory input from the PAG and sends serotonergic and noradrenergic fibers via the dorsolateral funiculus in the medullary dorsal horn. There the spinal and medullary dorsal horn receives terminal axons from the nucleus raphe magnum and adjacent nuclei. These descending pain control fibers terminate in the dorsal horn of the spinal cord and influence modulation of nociception via inhibitory impulses (Raj 1996). The dorsal horn of the spinal cord is a station where both relay and processing of nociceptive impulses from the periphery occur (Fig. 3).

CYTOARCHITECTURE

The dorsal horn is divided into the marginal zone, also known as Rexed's lamina I (Fig. 4), the superficial layer composed of large neurons oriented transversely across the cap of the dorsal gray matter. Some of these cells project to the thalamus via the contralateral pathways; others project intra- and intersegmentally along the dorsal and dorsolateral white matter. Lamina I neurons are activated by Aδ and C fibers that respond to mechanical stimulation and by Aδ fibers that respond to innocuous skin cooling; and a small percentage are activated by polymodal C fibers afferents. Lying deeper and ventral to the marginal zone is the substantia gelatinosa, which is a clear band of neural tissue. The substantia gelatinosa is composed of Rexed's

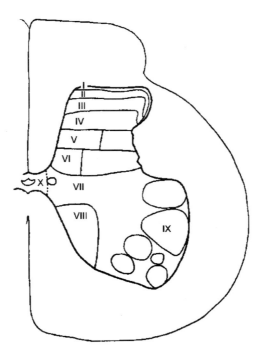

Fig. 4. Schematic drawing of the Rexed laminae of the 7th lumbar spinal cord segment in the full-grown cat (adapted from Rexed 1952).

laminae II and III, with lamina II superficial to lamina III.

Lamina II is further divided into an outer and inner layer and is characterized by small densely packed cells. The principal type is the stalk cell whose dendrites course through lamina II into lamina III and whose axons branch into lamina I. Terminals of Aδ afferents project into lamina II. Lamina III lies beneath lamina II and is composed predominantly of the islet cells. Lamina IV is composed of a broad layer of relatively large neurons. Its dendrites spread transversely and dorsally to laminae II and III. Lamina V is located along the neck of the dorsal horn and like lamina IV is composed mostly of larger neurons (Rexed 1952; Yaksh 1988).

Neurons from lamina V project to the ventrobasal thalamus and mesencephalon and the lateral cervical nucleus. Lamina IV and V compose the nucleus proprius. Lamina X, the central canal, is a parvicellular region. Neurons from this lamina project both ipsilaterally and contralaterally in the ventrolateral tract into the bulbar reticular formation (Portenoy and Kanner 1995).

Multiple discoveries in the 1970s led to a better understanding and applica-tion of intrathecal opioid analgesia. Significantly, these discoveries included endogenous peptides with opioid-like activities, opioid receptors in the dorsal horn of the spinal cord, and production of segmental analgesia by direct intrathecal injection of opioid (Dichiro 1966; Pert and Snyder 1973; Atweh and Kuhar 1977; Yaksh 1988; Bonica 1990).

Opioid receptors exist on both presynaptic and postsynaptic sites in the dorsal horn. The opioid receptors involved in the modulation of nociception at the level of the spinal cord are densely packed in the substantia gelatinosa. Opioid receptors are subcategorized as mu, kappa, delta, and sigma (μ, κ, δ, and σ). The μ, κ, and δ receptors occur in the spinal cord. The μ receptors respond to the natural ligands met-enkephalin and leu-enkephalin, which are derived from proenkephalin A. The natural ligand for the δ receptor is an enkephalin derived from proenkephalin B. The κ receptor's natural ligand is dynorphin, which is derived from prodynorphin B. These receptors produce analgesic effects of approximately 40% for μ, 10% for δ, and 50% for κ (Yaksh 1988; Portenoy and Kanner 1995; Raj 1996).

Activation of the μ and δ receptor subtypes alters potassium conductance. Mu and δ receptor activation is thought to result in hyperpolarization of membranes and a reduction in neuronal responses to excitatory transmitters. Kappa receptor activation blocks calcium ion influx in axon terminals and thus inhibits transmitter release. Inhibition of adenyl cyclase activity occurs during this process. Opioid binding to the opioid receptors on the presynaptic neurons inhibits release of transmitters such as substance P. Binding to opiate receptors on the postsynaptic neuron inhibits neurons in the pain pathway. Presence of the opioid in the ionized state appears to be necessary for strong binding at the anionic opioid receptor sites. Also, only the levorotatory form of the opioid exhibits agonist activity. The affinity of most opioid agonists for the receptor correlates well with their analgesic potency. It is assumed that increasing opioid receptor binding results in a parallel increase in opioid effects.

PHARMACOKINETICS

The documented practice of oral administration of opioids dates back to the Sumarian era of around 5000 B.C. Opioids have been administered parenterally since the invention of the hypodermic needle and syringe over a century ago. Knowledge gained from the discovery of opioid receptors in the dorsal horn and analgesic effects of direct intraspinal administration of opioid about two decades ago has greatly influenced the management of certain types of chronic pain (Layfield et al. 1981; Penn 1984; Murphy et al. 1987; Jacobson et al. 1990; Plummer et al. 1991; Portenoy and Kanner 1995).

It is well known that constant administration of systemic opioid in a subject with intact hepatic and renal function results in a steady-state serum concentration of the opioid. Accompanying this steady serum concentration is a concomitant but far lower steady-state concentration of opioid in the cerebrospinal fluid (CSF) (Fig. 5). The serum concentration required to achieve a CSF opioid concentration for satisfactory analgesia is sometimes not attained before undesirable side effects occur. However, a constant intrathecal infusion of opioid results in a steady serum opioid concentration that is much lower than the CSF opioid concentration (Fig. 6) and is less likely to result in an undesirable opioid side effect.

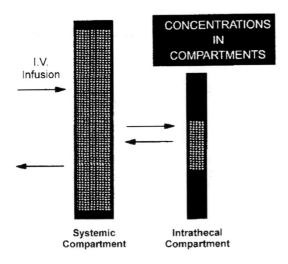

Fig. 5. Systemic infusion of opioid results in a higher systemic concentration.

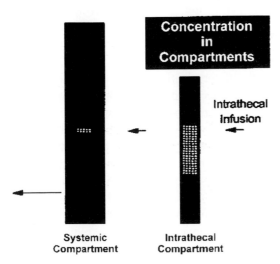

Fig. 6. Intrathecal administration results in a lower systemic concentration, and fewer side effects are likely.

The relative impermeability of the blood-brain barrier to systemically administered drugs is well known. Among the determinants of transport of molecular particles across the blood-brain barrier are molecular weight, concentration gradient, lipid solubility, and the ionic to nonionic ratio (a function of their dissociation constants). When an opioid is directly injected into the CSF the blood-brain barrier is no longer a factor, and an easily created reservoir of drug diffuses passively into the dorsal horn of the spinal cord where it binds with the opioid receptors.

Opioid receptors of the dorsal horn are confined not only to the superficial layer (lamina I) but also to the lipid-rich substantia gelatinosa (lamina II), which is thought to have a large population of opioid receptors, and in lamina V. This implies that the opioid molecules have to diffuse into the deeper layers of the dorsal horn. Similar to diffusion across the blood-brain barrier, this diffusion also depends on molecular weight, concentration gradient, ionic to nonionic ratio, and the lipid solubility of the respective opioid. Clinical observations suggest that the rate of diffusion into the lipid-rich tissues correlates well with lipid solubility. For example, lipophilic opioids such as fentanyl and meperidine have a rapid onset of action as a result of faster transfer from CSF phase to tissue-rich phase. Other observations are that: (1) a higher lipid solubility is also associated with faster clearance of the drug from the intrathecal space and thus shorter duration of action and higher blood concentration of the opioid; (2) a higher lipid solubility is associated with small areas of distribution of the drug along the length of the spinal cord and thus a limited area of analgesia (Portenoy and Kanner 1995); (3) hydrophilic opioids such as morphine exhibit slower onset of action and prolonged duration of action due to slower clearance. The hydrophilic nature of morphine allows it to remain longer in the CSF, so rostral spread may occur with potentially significant respiratory depression. This possibility is a major impediment to the more liberal use of intraspinal opioids in acute care settings such as for labor and postsurgical pain.

The exact role of metabolism in the termination of opioid action at the level of the spinal cord following intrathecal administration has yet to be established. However, given the high concentration of drug still present after loss of clinical effect, it is unlikely that metabolism is a major contributor. Rather, loss of analgesia following intrathecal administration results from clearance of opioids from the receptor. Stronger receptor binding with polar agents such as morphine retards clearance compared to that of more lipophilic agents. Intrathecally administered opioids are predominantly removed by vascular absorption, which is most significant for the lipophilic agent. Opioid that has spread rostrally is also removed by the intracranial arachnoid granulations (Bonica 1990).

Repeated intrathecal administration of opioid has not produced neurologic injury. However, antioxidant preservatives such as sodium bisulfate possess neurotoxic properties (Bonica 1990). Consequently, opioids prepared for intrathecal injection come in preservative-free glass ampules (i.e., Astromorph and Duramorph). The pH range of solutions of the commonly used intrathecal opioids (e.g., morphine and fentanyl) in normal saline ranges from 4.52 to 6.85, but when they are mixed with CSF they all lower the pH of the CSF by 0.3 or less, and the mixture remains clear. Addition of heroine solution to CSF produces a turbid mixture that implies protein precipitation (Yaksh 1988).

CLINICAL APPLICATIONS

While most cancer patients obtain adequate analgesia with systemic medications, a small but significant number (10–20%) will require alternative therapies because of inadequate analgesia or intolerable side effects (Malone et al. 1985). Compared to systemic administration, intraspinal administration results in a lower drug dosage with resultant decreases in cost and incidence of side effects, and the possibility of a totally implanted system (Table I). While neuroablative and neurosurgical procedures are often used, intraspinal opioid therapy is increasingly offered because it is reversible, generally will not lead to centrally mediated pain, and is more likely to be effective for multiple painful sites including bilateral disease. Most

Table I
Properties of opiods for intraspinal use

Drug	Lipid Sol.	Average Effective Dose* (mg/70kg body weight)			Onset (min)	Peak (min)	Duration (hr)
		IV	EPI	IT			
Morphine	1.42	10	5–10	0.1–0.5	20–35	30–60	8–22
Diamorphine	1.7	5–10	5–10	1	5–10	30–60	6–12
Meperidine	38.8	100	25–50	35–70	15–20	20	7–10
Methadone	116	10	4–5	—	10–15	20–30	7–9
Alfentanil	131	0.5–1	0.5–1	—	5	15	1.5
Hydromorphone	—	1–2	1–1.5	—	10–20	20–30	6–19
Fentanyl	813	0.1	0.1	—	4–6	10–20	2–3
Sufentanyl	1778	0.02	0.05	—	5	10	4–6
Buprenorphine	—	0.3	0.1–0.3	—	5–10	30–60	4–10

Source: Adapted from Patt 1993.
*IV = intravenous, EPI = epidural, IT = intrathecal.

patients with symptomatic cancer have or will develop pain in multiple sites (Twycross and Lack 1986). Furthermore, the ability to provide "test doses" helps ensure efficacy prior to a longer term implantation for spinal or epidural delivery.

Not all painful syndromes respond favorably to opioid therapy. It has been observed that acute, sharp, "incidental" breakthrough or surgical pain (so-called "first pain," usually associated with rapid transmission along the myelinated Aδ fibers) is relieved less readily by intraspinal opioids. In contrast, dull constant pain (so-called "slow" or "second" pain, associated with C-fiber transmission in the neospinothalamic tract) is more amenable to opioid therapy. In decreasing order of favorable response to intraspinal opioids are the following types of pain: (1) continuous somatic, (2) continuous visceral, (3) intermittent somatic, (4) intermittent visceral, (5) neurogenic, and (6) cutaneous, ulcer, or fistula-related pain (Artner and Arner 1985).

PATIENT SELECTION

The cornerstone of a successful intrathecal opioid therapy is appropriate patient selection. Spinal opioid therapy is used most commonly in the management of cancer-related pain (Ventafridda et al. 1987). It also may be used for carefully selected noncancer pain conditions such as severe inoperable peripheral vascular disease (Layfield et al. 1981; Portenoy and Kanner 1995), vertebral crush fractures, inoperable myocardial ischemia (Murphy et al. 1987; Plummer et al. 1991; Portenoy and Kanner 1995), postherpetic neuralgia, phantom-limb pain, sympathetic dystrophy, and inoperable spinal stenosis (Layfield et al. 1981; Penn et al. 1984; Murphy et al. 1987; Jacobson et al. 1990; Plummer et al. 1991; Portenoy and Kanner 1995). The general indication for spinal opioid therapy is pain that cannot be controlled with systemic opioids because of dose-limiting side effects.

Several criteria must be met before beginning spinal opioid therapy. The general indications for intraspinal opioid therapy follow:

Failure of more conservative therapies. Note that multiple routes of administration (oral, transdermal, subcutaneous, transbuccal, transrectal, intravenous, and subcutaneous), multiple opioids (morphine, oxycodone, fentanyl, hydromorphone, etc.), multiple adjuvant medications (nonsteroidals, anticonvulsants, beta-blockers, alpha-blockers, alpha-2 agonists, antidepressants, benzodiazepines, etc.), and multiple nonpharmacologic treatments (radiation, braces, corsets, physical therapy, biofeedback, relaxation training, etc.) are available and the clinician should consider whether continued trials are likely to be beneficial before instigating more invasive modalities. This is not to say that all permutations should be tried as clearly this would result in an excessive delay, but merely that consideration is necessary.

Absence of more beneficial procedures. For example, it is impractical to insert a intrathecal pump when the pain is secondary to a mass that is amenable to simple resection, or to a pathologic humeral fracture that may be surgically stabilized. Furthermore, a neurolytic procedure often is indicated.

Adequate resources. Inability or unwillingness by the designated personnel to care for the intraspinal opioid delivery system has significant implications for selecting the appropriate system. Cancer patients who are able to self-inject their drug delivery device in the early stages of the disease may be unable to do so later in its course (Du Pen and Williams 1996).

Life expectancy. The patient must have an adequate life expectancy for the required device. Although prediction of a cancer patient's life expectancy can be difficult, an estimate in terms of days, weeks, months, or years is essential to guide the selection of the most appropriate implantable drug delivery system. Often the patient's general condition will improve when adequate analgesia is provided, a possibility that must be addressed. Some authors recommend a life expectancy of at least three months for consideration of an intrathecal pump. The expensive start-up costs for implantable infusion technology decreases the overall costs of therapy only if the patient survives at least three months (Bedder et al. 1991; Lanning and Hrushesky 1990).

Successful trial. A trial of intraspinal opioids should have been successful.

There are several contraindications to intrathecal pump placement:

Local alteration of skin. Infection, inflammation, and an alteration in the integrity of the skin at the entry site of the subarachnoid catheter are absolute contraindications.

Coagulopathy. Abnormal bleeding is an absolute contraindication. The cause of any coagulation abnormality must be sought and corrected before implantation of a drug delivery device.

Altered mental status. Physiologically abnormal states such as electrolyte abnormalities and drug-induced organic brain syndrome may affect the patient's judgment and result in the inability to adequately assess symptom relief. Correction of these disturbances prior to the preimplantation trial is warranted. The patient and physician might incorrectly attribute the confusion secondary to these physiologic abnormalities to uncontrolled pain. Many clinicians refer every patient for a psychiatric evaluation prior to implantation to rule out psychiatric contraindications (Maeyaert and Kupers 1996).

Allergy. The patient cannot be allergic to pump device components. Although uncommon, such allergy is possible. For example, the clinician should investigate any information regarding allergy to metals.

Noncompliance. The patient cannot be noncompliant. Such patients may be lost to follow-up and refills of the implantable system, and therefore also lost to adequate management of the painful condition (Yaksh 1981; Wisenfield and Gustafsson 1982).

TEST DOSE

Given correct diagnosis, a well-defined disease state, optimized oncologic and pain therapy, and absence of contraindications, it is appropriate to embark on a trial of spinal opioid (morphine challenge). A spinal opioid trial can be done in many ways, but should be convenient and closely simulate the final device. For example, the clinician should consider intrathecal vs. epidural injection and bolus vs. continuous infusion. One common test-dose procedure prior to placement of an intrathecal infusion device involves injecting 1.0 mg of preservative-free opioid into the intrathecal space through a spinal needle. The patient is then observed for six hours to guard against rare complications, respiratory or otherwise. If the patient reports a 50% reduction in pain during follow-up, device placement may proceed. The patient must have moderate to severe pain prior to the test dose because reductions in mild pain are difficult to assess. Opioid intake may need to be reduced by 50% prior to the test dose, which is considered successful if pain scores decline by 50% and the patient tolerates the medication well. If the test dose does not result in a 50% reduction in the pain scores, the injection may be repeated on a later day with an escalated opioid dose. Escalation schedules may involve 1, 1.5, and then 2 mg morphine, or rarely, faster escalation in patients with substantial opioid tolerance or very high pain levels. Some clinicians also use a single blinded placebo dose to further assess patient response.

Clinicians should attempt placement of a temporary epidural catheter and test dosage prior to placing a permanent system. With intraventricular systems, lumbar or cisternal test doses usually precede implantation (Waldman et al. 1993).

IMPLANTABLE DEVICE SELECTION

After determining that an intrathecal delivery system would be beneficial, that contraindications are lacking, and that the patient has an adequate personnel support system, the clinician needs to select the type of device. In addition to oral, intravenous, transdermal, transrectal, transbuccal, and subcutaneous routes, this chapter reviews three more invasive methods for administration of opioids to the central nervous system: intrathecal, epidural, and intracerebroventricular. Evidence is lacking for important distinctions in

Table II
Decision-making for the use of neuroaxial opioids for cancer pain

1. Selection of drug
   Morphine vs. a more lipophilic opioid
   Opioid alone vs. opioid + local anesthetic

2. Selection of route
   Epidural vs. intrathecal vs. intraventricular

3. Selection of catheter
   Percutaneous/externalized vs. tunneled catheter
   If a tunneled catheter is selected:
   Externalized hub vs. subcutaneous port vs. totally implanted subcutaneous
   pump

4. Selection of schedule/means of administration
   Intermittent bolus versus continuous infusion ± patient-administered boluses
   Self-administration vs. external portable pump vs. totally implanted pump

Source: Patt 1993.

the efficacy of these routes, but clinicians must consider important clinical distinctions and numerous other factors (Table II). Ultimately, the route selection, hardware, drug, dosage, and administration regimen must be individualized to each patient's unique circumstances.

The decision between epidural and intrathecal administration relies on consideration of several factors. Clinical experience is greater for epidural administration, which has several advantages, including a lower incidence of postspinal headache. If infection occurs, an epidural abscess is more likely than meningitis because the dura acts as a barrier to leptomeningeal infection. Also, a wider selection of agents can conveniently be given epidurally for chronic pain management because adjuvant medications are available in limited concentrations. For example, the highest concentration of bupivacaine commercially available is 0.75%, and for clonidine 100 µg/ml. These concentrations require too frequent refilling for administration via an intrathecal infusion with an implanted reservoir (typically 18–50 cc). While Nitescu and colleagues (1991) reported on long-term experience with patients receiving subarachnoid infusions via externalized catheters, the safety of this approach is questionable as the data on infectious complications are not convincing. Furthermore, the availability of preservative-free medications for intrathecal administration is limited.

While less commonly used, intrathecal administration has several important advantages. The intrathecal space is technically easier to locate than the epidural space. In one study involving guinea pigs, indwelling epidural catheter tips rapidly became encased in a fibrous sheath that limited drug spread (Edwards et al. 1986), which should not be a problem with intrathecal catheters. Injection into the epidural space typically requires a much

Table III
A classification of implantable drug delivery systems

Type I	Percutaneous subarachnoid or epidural catheter
Type II	Percutaneous subarachnoid or epidural catheter with subcutaneous tunneling
Type III	Totally implanted subarachnoid or epidural catheter with subcutaneous injection port (see Fig. 7)
Type IV	Totally implanted subarachnoid catheter with implanted manually activated pump (see Fig. 8)
Type V	Totally implanted subarachnoid catheter with implanted infusion pump (see Fig. 9)
Type VI	Totally implanted subarachnoid catheter with implanted programmable infusion pump (see Fig. 9)

Source: Modified from Waldman and Coombs 1989.

larger injectate volume, and if the epidural space is or becomes less compliant secondary to epidural disease, spinal cord compression with irreversible neurologic deficits can result (S. Reddy, personal communication, 1996). This risk of this complication is greatly lessened with intrathecal administration, which also is more rarely associated with pain on injection. Catheter migration from the epidural to subarachnoid space has been documented (Barnes 1990) and is hazardous because it typically results in a large intrathecal overdose. This risk of overdosage is negated by intentional subarachnoid placement, as catheter migration to other spaces typically results only in a decrease in analgesia.

There are several types of implantable drug delivery systems. The classification scheme of Waldman and Coombs (1989) is commonly used (Table III). An understanding of the benefits of each system is necessary before making a decision on which type to install.

Type I: Percutaneous subarachnoid or epidural catheter. These catheters have gained widespread acceptance for short-term use, usually for cancer patients during the perioperative period and for the administration of test doses prior to placement of a more long-term solution (see above). Preterminal patients (less than three weeks life expectancy) who are unable to tolerate even minor surgery are also candidates for this type of device (Patt 1989). Regardless of the indication, consideration should be given to the wire-reinforced catheter, which has greater durability and radiopacity, but higher cost. Type I systems have the disadvantage of increased risk of catheter migration and central nervous system (CNS) infection (Wang et al. 1979). Although the chronic use of the type I catheter is reliable and safe (Edwards et al. 1988), the type II systems are generally thought to be safer for long-term use (greater than 2–3 days).

Type II: Percutaneous catheter with subcutaneous tunneling. Decreased risk of migration and infection and ease of placement make this delivery system ideal for patients with life expectancy of weeks to months. A bedside tunneling technique using a second epidural catheter to tunnel the catheter 4–8 cm laterally is easily performed and appropriate for up to three weeks of therapy. To ensure superior infection control beyond this time frame, a surgeon should tunnel a catheter to the anterior abdominal wall of the patient. Over time, catheters intended for short-term use can become stiff and migrate into the subarachnoid space (Barnes 1990). Also, catheters for short-term use have a connector for injection that frequently becomes detached, which necessitates further intervention (Ali et al. 1989). The most commonly used long-term catheter approved for epidural use by the U.S. Food and Drug Administration (FDA) is likely the Du Pen catheter (R Bard Inc., Salt Lake City, UT), which remains flexible because of its silastic composition and also has a superior clamp-on connector.

Type III: Totally implanted catheter with subcutaneous reservoir. This type of system has a subcutaneous stainless steel reservoir with a silicone injection port (Fig. 7). The silicone dome reseals after puncture with an atraumatic Huber needle and is designed to withstand more than 1000 punctures without leakage (Waldman et al. 1996). Injections to the port can be easily taught, and the port can be attached to an infusion device. This type of device usually lacks externalized components and bulky subcutaneous components, and does not require large incisions so it is less cosmetically disfiguring than other long-term systems. It is ideal for patients with life expectancies of months to years. The most commonly used type III system is likely the Port-a-Cath epidural port system (Pharmacia-Deltec, Inc., St. Paul, MN), which is FDA approved.

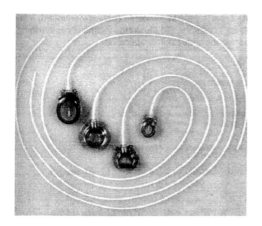

Fig. 7. An assortment of type III devices consisting of implantable ports with silastic catheters (Patt 1993).

Fig. 8. A type IV fully implantable patient-controlled infusion device. Pushing the left button loads the right dome with drug. Then, pushing the right dome delivers a bolus through the silastic catheter to the intrathecal space. In the center is a self-sealing access port to load the reservoir (Patt 1993).

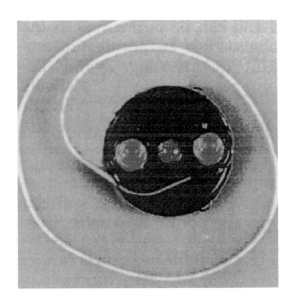

Type IV: Totally implanted mechanically activated pump. Poletti and colleagues devised one of the earliest totally implanted patient-activated reservoirs consisting of a spinal catheter, a hydrocephalus shunt valve, and an implantable blood bag attached in series (Poletti et al. 1981). Several other devices have been constructed, but none have received FDA approved to date (Fig. 8). The AlgoMed (Medtronic, Minneapolis, MN) patient-activated reservoir device is available in Australia and Europe, and FDA approval is likely by 1998. These devices lack of electrical components and all have the advantage of easy patient self-administration.

Type V: Totally implanted constant infusion system. The prototype of this system is Shiley's Infusaid pump (Norwood, MA), which was initially developed for transarterial hepatic chemotherapy (Fig. 9). The pump is about the size of a hockey puck. It is implanted subcutaneously and connected to a silastic catheter to the intrathecal space. The pump contains two chambers separated by a diaphragm, one containing Freon and the other a 47-cc drug reservoir. As the drug reservoir is filled, the drug pushes on the diaphragm to compress the Freon. After filling is complete, the pressurized Freon expands at a consistent, predictable rate to push the drug out of the reservoir. The flow rate is determined at the factory by varying the resistance to reservoir outflow and is not adjustable after assembly. Patient dosage can be altered by varying the concentration of drug in the reservoir. Unfortunately, this procedure requires percutaneous access, drainage, and refilling of the drug reservoir each time the infusion is to be altered. The difficulty with infusion titration and pump cost are its main disadvantages.

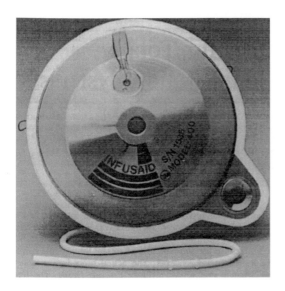

Fig. 9. Type V fully implantable intraspinal infusion device (Infusaid model 400 by Shiley) with silastic catheter and sideport. With filling of the drug reservoir, a Freon system becomes pressurized and supplies the force to gradually push the drug out of the reservoir. A set rate of infusion is determined at the factory. This pump is attractive because of its large 30-cc reservoir and absence of a battery (Patt 1993).

Type VI: Totally implanted programmable infusion pump. These pumps (Fig. 10) are similar to the type V devices (Fig. 9) in appearance, placement procedure, and high cost. However, they have the advantage of easy reprogramming with a transmitter, which does require additional investment in a specialized laptop computer assembly (Fig. 11). Reprogramming is accomplished by entering the data into the computer and placing a hand-held wand on the skin overlying the pump. The computer provides a printout of the infusion data that can be attached to the patient's chart. The programs can be sophisticated, with a different day and nighttime infusion rate, for example. It is important to remember that the reservoir volume is a calculated entry and possibly may not represent actual reservoir contents. The battery must be surgically replaced every few years; a faint audible alarm signals impending battery failure. Perhaps the most commonly used type VI device is the Medtronic series (Medtronic Inc., Minneapolis, MN), which is FDA approved for subarachnoid infusions of both morphine and baclofen.

Intracerebroventricular devices. Increasing experience with small doses of morphine administered intraventricularly suggests that this is a safe and effective method of relieving pain in appropriate patients (Waldman et al. 1996). In one study, cancer patients exposed to both modalities consistently rated intraventricular administration as more effective than subarachnoid administration (Roquefeuil et al. 1984). This technique is typically used for cervicofacial pain after more conservative measures fail (Patt 1985), but it should be considered for midline, bilateral, or any other pain refractory to more conservative therapies. The optimum life expectancy is about six months.

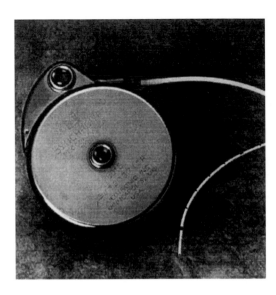

Fig. 10. The SynchroMed model 8611 programmable pump. Note the centrally located refill port and the peripherally located access port. Injection into the access port bypasses pump components and goes directly to the catheter and intrathecal space (from Medtronic, Inc., Minneapolis, MN, with permission).

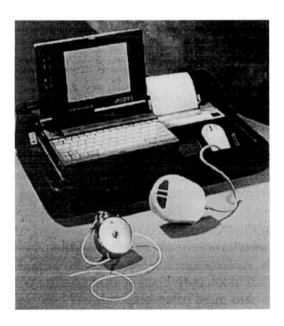

Fig. 11. The Medtronic Programmable SynchroMed Drug Delivery System includes the pump, a portable computer with necessary software, and a telemetry wand in addition to the implantable device (from Medtronic, Inc., Minneapolis, MN, with permission).

In imminently terminal patients, known to have a high incidence of both confusion and opioid tolerance, new onset of confusion can be difficult to interpret. Access to the cerebral ventricles is through a coronal bur hole usually made under local anesthesia, and an Ommaya reservoir is typically placed. An alternative technique involves passage of a percutaneous catheter through a 14-g Touhy needle into the cisterna magna (Schoffler et al. 1987). Most practitioners suggest that a family member or home health care agency personnel administer the medication. Doses of morphine between 0.2 and 4 mg are given, with a duration of analgesia of about 24 hours per dose. When needed, dosage is escalated by about 20% per day. A bag of premixed syringes and Betadine wipes are the only supplies required for home management. Minor side effects are similar to those with intrathecal and epidural administration. Published reports of dose-related respiratory depression and infection are extremely rare (Black 1985; Lenzi et al. 1985).

SELECTION OF INFUSATE

A wide variety of opioids have been injected intraspinally to obtain analgesia, but morphine is the most common (Waldman et al. 1996). As a rule, peak analgesic effects are obtained within 30–60 minutes of administration, and an analgesic duration of 6–24 hours is obtained from a single dose. The opioid-naive patient may be given intrathecal doses of 0.1–0.5 mg, or alternatively, epidural doses of 2.5–5.0 mg. The opioid-tolerant patient may require substantially higher doses regardless of the route of administration. Tolerance occurs in a variable percentage of patients and appears to be related primarily to the dose of systemic opioids given prior to the start of intraspinal therapy rather than to the specific intraspinal regimen (Ventafridda et al. 1987).

The hydrophilicity of the intraspinal opioid should be considered. Morphine is the prototypical hydrophilic opioid, and the synthetic opioids fentanyl and sufentanil are the prototypical lipophilic agents. Because of their high lipophilicity, analgesia is more regional and segmental, so more attention should be given to accurate catheter placement at the dermatome of pain origin. Also, fentanyl and sufentanil have a negligible incidence of delayed side effects (Lam et al. 1983), which is attributed to rostral spread of hydrophilic opioids in CSF.

The clinician should also consider the addition of nonopioid substances including dextrose, epinephrine, preservatives, and adjuvant medications. When dextrose 7% was added to morphine to increase the baricity for intrathecal administration, rostral redistribution was reduced and the duration of analgesia increased (Caute et al. 1988). The addition of epinephrine to epidural sufentanil intensifies the segmental nature of the analgesia and its duration (Klepper et al. 1987). Preservatives should be withheld from intrathecal injections, but low concentrations of chlorobutanol in common morphine preparations is safe for epidural administration (Du Pen et al. 1987). Adjuvant medications are discussed elsewhere in this chapter.

ADMINISTRATION BY CONTINUOUS INFUSION VERSUS INTERMITTENT BOLUS

Both techniques have their advantages, but continuous infusion is generally regarded as more favorable when available, primarily because it produces relatively stable CSF concentrations of opioid with fewer toxic peaks, less cephalad diffusion, and fewer painful troughs (Oyama et al. 1987). If the catheter migrated from the epidural to subarachnoid space, a continuous infusion would result in a safer, more gradual onset of sequelae than would occur with intermittent boluses. Finally, constant infusions can be used in patients unable to request or self-administer medication, as is common in preterminal cancer patients.

However, continuous infusion typically requires an expensive infusion device, al though less expensive disposable balloon-type infusion devices are available (Travenol Infusor, Travenol Inc., Deerfield, IL). In developing nations, any type of constant infusion device may be unobtainable or unaffordable. Patients often welcome the control given to them with intermittent boluses, as they often have little control over much of the rest of their cancer care. Intermittent boluses also give some protection against medication-induced sedation and confusion, as patients become less able to administer medication under these conditions.

There is some debate as to which method, continuous infusion or intermittent boluses, leads to a more rapid development of tolerance and dose escalation. Gourlay and others examined bolus versus continuous infusion in 29 cancer patients treated with epidural analgesia (Gourlay et al. 1991) and found no difference in analgesic efficacy or patient satisfaction. However, a significant degree of dose escalation occurred in the continuous infusion group, which indicated a more rapid development of tolerance. Other clinicians suggest that continuous infusion of intraspinal opioids may result in a delayed development of tolerance (Waldman et al. 1996).

A decision to use intermittent boluses requires that precise directions be given. In general, the drug concentration, the background infusion rate, the bolus dose, and the lockout interval are determined. The lockout interval refers to the minimum time between doses in which the system is refractory to additional patient requests. Some clinicians might also include a schedule for upward or downward titrations in doses. A typical order might be "preservative-free morphine 5 mg in 10 ml given epidurally every 8 hours as needed" or "fentanyl 50 µg/cc with 2 cc/hour basal rate per epidural catheter and 2 cc every 15 min as needed."

OPERATIVE TECHNIQUE FOR PLACEMENT OF PERMANENT INTRASPINAL OPIOID DELIVERY DEVICES

The first step is to determine the location for the intrathecal device pocket; abdominal, thoracic, and gluteal pockets have all been used. The abdominal pocket is most common, and care must be taken to ensure that it is not located at the patient's belt line, as this would surely decrease comfort and pose some risk to the device components. Also, anecdotal evidence supports placement away from possible sources of infection such as colostomies. Low thoracic pockets are used so that ribs can provide a firm support for the access port of type III devices and the patient-activated buttons of type IV devices. Subclavian sites are usually reserved for possible pacemakers and central venous access.

The pump position is outlined with the patient awake, and then general anesthesia is usually administered. Although analgesia and sedation may be adequate in selected patients, it typically is extremely uncomfortable for cancer patients to remain still in one position for the duration of the procedure. While general anesthesia is being administered, the surgeon should examine pump components, verify completeness of the kit, and perform all necessary preimplantation procedures. These procedures vary from one device to the next, but typically involve loading the reservoir and checking device functionality.

Next, the patient is definitively positioned for the procedure. Some authors recommend the left lateral decubitus position if the surgeon is right handed and the right lateral decubitus position if the surgeon is left handed (Waldman and Coombs 1989). Often, desired pump placement location dictates patient positioning because it is impossible to make a left abdominal pocket if the patient is in the left lateral decubitus position. Rarely, the prone position is used and a gluteal pocket is formed. The neck and hips should be flexed to assist in intrathecal space access. Furthermore, all pressure points should be well padded and an axillary roll should be placed.

After cleansing of the skin, drapes are applied. An area should remain exposed that extends from the sacrum to the lower thoracic spine, and horizontally from approximately 4 cm lateral to the midline to approximately 2 cm lateral of the umbilicus. An iodine-impregnated adhesive sheet then covers this area. Biplanar fluoroscopy is helpful, and the fluoroscope is aseptically draped and brought into the field.

A paramedian lumbar incision of approximately 2 cm is made. Because the spinal catheters available for this application are rather fragile and prone to obstruction or fracture, the sharp angles produced by a midline approach through the interspinous ligament may potentially lead to catheter failure at the site of entrance or exit from the supraspinous ligament. The paramedian approach is also favored over the midline approach because the former allows more layers to be closed over the catheter to further protect it as it exits the fascia. This incision is carried down to the level of the lumbodorsal fascia. The interspinous ligament is identified. There is no fixed level at which the catheter must be inserted. We routinely use the L2–3, L3–4, or L4–5 interspace. A Tuohy needle is then used to perform a dural puncture. The Tuohy needle is advanced through the incision at a shallow angle, superiorly and toward the midline to puncture the dura at the next higher interspace.

Once the stylette is removed and CSF has been obtained, the catheter is advanced through the needle under direct fluoroscopic visualization. While the catheter may pass without apparent obstruction, only with fluoroscopic visualization can kinking or looping of the catheter or migration of the catheter tip into a dural root sleeve be definitely recognized. While initially allowing adequate CSF flow, these suboptimal catheter positions may ultimately lead to failure of the system and require subsequent revision.

Some investigators suggest that the catheter be advanced routinely to about the L1 level because mixing of the drug in the CSF results in wide distributed. This practice is reasonable, especially if only hydrophilic compounds are employed. In our practice, the catheter is typically advanced to the T10 to T12 level. For pain involving the upper extremities, we attempt a placement at the T6 level, which we believe allows for somewhat greater efficacy, especially when infusing hydrophobic agents.

CSF flow is confirmed at each step of the procedure. Occasionally, positive contrast myelography using nonionic contrast may be necessary to confirm catheter position. When adequate catheter placement has been obtained, the catheter guide wire is withdrawn. A 2-0 silk purse string suture is placed around the needle (Fig. 12) and the catheter is stabilized while the Tuohy needle is removed. Gentle rotation of the needle during its withdrawal may minimize comigration of the catheter. The pursestring suture is then tightened and secured; this helps to limit catheter migration and prevent CSF leakage. A silastic fixation device is then placed around the catheter and secured to the lumbodorsal fascia with a nonabsorbable suture such as 3-0 silk (Fig. 13). This fixator should be placed as close as possible to the site where the catheter exits the fascia. Care should be taken to secure the sutures tightly enough to prevent catheter migration, but not so tightly as to obstruct CSF flow.

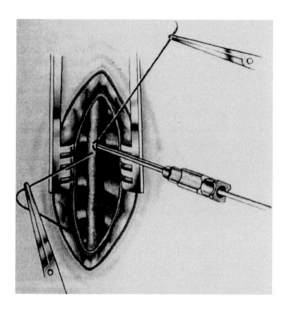

Fig. 12. A pursestring suture is placed around the catheter with the protecting needle still in place (from Medtronic, Inc., Minneapolis, MN, 1996, with permission).

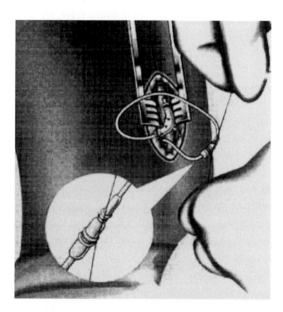

Fig 13. A silastic cover is secured over the connector connecting the access port catheter to the subarachnoid catheter with 3-0 silk. At our institution, this connection typically lies 10–15 cm laterally from the incision (from Medtronic, Inc., Minneapolis, MN, 1996, with permission).

For a subcutaneous reservoir (type III device), the thoracic wall incision is 2 cm lower and a small pocket is bluntly dissected. Blunt dissection is most safely accomplished with fingers alone. A tunneling device is then used to draw the access port catheter from the anterior incision to the lumbar incision. This step is particularly painful; the awake patient may require additional sedation and analgesia to remain comfortable. After trimming the lumbar catheter to the necessary length, the surgeon connects the two catheters with a straight connector that should lie near the paramedian incision when the lumbar catheter is correctly trimmed. A silastic sleeve and non-absorbable sutures can be used to secure this connection (Fig. 13). After again ensuring free flow of CSF, the surgeon attaches the proximal end of the catheter to the access port and secures it with nonabsorbable suture. The reservoir itself is then secured to the chest wall to prevent migration or rotation and to provide stability for access.

For implantation of a continuous pump, the preparation of the patient and initial procedures are exactly the same as for the implanted reservoir, except that optimal pump position is between the inferior costal margin and the anterior superior iliac crest. Improper placement can result in significant discomfort if the pump hits against either of these bony structures. Generally, placement below the level of the umbilicus is best. A transverse incision of roughly 8 cm is made at the superior margin of the ideal pump position. A subcutaneous pocket is then dissected; it must be at least 0.7 cm deep to the skin but no deeper than 2.5 cm from the skin. Deeper placement will make access for refilling and programming the pump difficult, while shallower placement may result in loss of skin integrity and contamination of the hardware. This pocket should be bluntly dissected, initially with fingers and by spreading the surgical scissor tips. An occasional fibrous band may need to be severed, which is best done with electrocautery to maintain hemostasis. The pump should be placed within this pocket to confirm its adequacy. Care should be taken to ensure hemostasis within this pocket. A flexible tunneling device is then used to draw the catheter between the lumbar and abdominal incisions. This part of the procedure is particularly painful and often requires liberal use of sedatives and analgesics. The pump catheter is then secured to the lumbar catheter by a straight connector, with nonabsorbable sutures and/or a silastic sleeve used to secure the connector. The proximal end of the catheter is attached to the pump and secured with a nonabsorbable suture, and the pump is placed into the subcutaneous pocket (Fig. 14). In the abdominal pocket, the pump should be secured to the rectus fascia by nonabsorbable sutures to prevent inferior migration of the pump over time and the potential for the pump to flip over and obscure the access port.

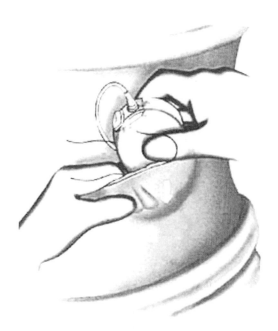

Fig. 14. After the catheter is connected, the intrathecal infusion device is placed into the subcutaneous pocket (from Medtronic, Inc., Minneapolis, MN, 1996, with permission).

Before closing the wounds, the surgeon should ensure that the lumbar catheter lies loosely in the subcutaneous space without kinking. This positioning often requires dissecting a small plane above the fascia. A loop of catheter in this space will allow for movement and prevent tension of the catheter.

The wounds are then well irrigated with solution containing antibiotic and are closed. The anterior incision requires a two-layer closure, while the posterior incision requires a three-layer closure. The wounds are covered with antibiotic ointment and sterile dressings (North and Levy 1997). Neurological responses are documented when the patient awakens, and the patient is monitored in the recovery room until alert and then checked for neurological symptoms.

PERIOPERATIVE COMPLICATIONS

Intraoperative bleeding. Intraoperative bleeding is usually a simple problem because the areas involved with device placement are not highly vascular. Bleeding is best avoided by identifying and correcting bleeding problems preoperatively, infiltrating the skin before incision with a 1:200,000 solution of epinephrine, using electrocautery for extending the scalpel incision to deeper layers, and using blunt dissection whenever possible. When curved scissors are used for blunt dissection, the tips should be concave anteriorly to prevent digging into deeper structures and so they can be visualized at all times. If bleeding occurs, simple pressure with dry gauze and electrocautery are usually all that is needed. Occasionally, a vessel will need ligation with absorbable suture or a clip.

Subarachnoid and epidural bleeding is more worrisome because of the risk of neurological morbidity. Deep bleeding is best avoided by identifying and correcting bleeding disorders preoperatively and by accurately placing the Tuohy needle with as few attempts as possible. Placement of the Tuohy can be assisted with correct patient position, use of fluoroscopy, and use of a 22-gauge finder needle if necessary. Occasionally, frank bleeding from the epidural or subarachnoid space occurs if entry was difficult. Although this problem is not usually associated with morbidity, it does require increased observation. The needle should be irrigated with saline until clearing is seen. Persistent bleeding requires intraoperative consultation from a neurosurgeon. Postoperatively, patients should be assessed frequently for new back pain and cauda equina syndrome.

Postoperative bleeding. New back pain and progressive neurological dysfunction should raise suspicion of a subarachnoid or epidural hematoma. An accurate preoperative examination is a prerequisite for recognition of new neurological deficits. Postoperatively, subjective complaints and objective incontinence, weakness, and sensory loss indicate a significant bleed. Typically, neurological deficits are progressive over hours, and emergent imaging studies and neurosurgical consultation must be obtained to avoid permanent sequelae. The appropriate imaging study may be a magnetic resonance imaging (MRI), computed tomography (CT) scan, myelogram, or combination depending on the clinical situation. Previously, it was thought that MRI was contraindicated after pump placement, but now most agree that MRI can be performed safely given that the rotors are the only ferrous portions on a SynchroMed pump. However, the device should be turned off, and increased artifact will probably result. Spinal cord stimulators, while not previously mentioned in this chapter, must be removed prior to MRI.

Hematomas, seromas, and hygromas. A hematoma is a collection of blood, a seroma is a collection of serum, and a hygroma may represent either lymph or cerebrospinal fluid. Typically, a postoperative bulge is common, and reassurance is needed but not intervention, which would increase the risk of infection (Hahn 1992). These collections typically resolve spontaneously. Rarely, a large or chronic subcutaneous pocket may require sterile percutaneous drainage with a needle. Care must be taken to avoid the underlying apparatus and tubing.

Peripheral infection. Local infection is typically diagnosed by fever, leukocytosis, and characteristic skin changes (erythema, edema, tenderness, and drainage). Treatment is controversial. While some would treat conservatively with intravenous antibiotics and wound care, others believe all hardware should be removed (the usual recommendation if an infectious disease consultation is obtained). Additionally, consider evidence of infection near the subarachnoid catheter, which may progress into the central nervous system.

Meningitis. Early diagnosis is necessary as meningitis is rapidly progressive. Meningitis is usually heralded by fever, malaise, headache, vomiting, stiff neck, and back or neck pain. Two commonly used signs of meningeal irritation are Kernig's sign and Brudzinski's sign. Kernig's sign is pain or resistance while straightening the patient's leg at the hip and the knee from the flexed position. Brudzinski's sign is spontaneous flexion of the patient's knees and hips after flexing the neck. Patients may appear ill and have neurological findings, including seizures. Laboratory examination of blood and cerebrospinal fluid is warranted. The opening pressure on lumbar puncture may also be abnormally elevated. An infectious disease or neurological consultation should be obtained, and all hardware should probably be removed. Early antibiotic coverage is essential. Ceftriaxone is often initially administered for meningitis because of its broad spectrum and excellent penetration across the blood-brain barrier, and more tailored therapy is begun when cultures return.

Post–dural puncture headache. Post–dural puncture headache is classically recognized by symmetrical headache pain (usually occipital or frontal) that is postural—it resolves with lying down. Tinnitus and photophobia occasionally occur. Post–dural puncture headaches are thought to be due to leakage of cerebrospinal fluid resulting in stretch on the dural vessels of the brain. While blood patches are about 90% effective, conservative therapy is often best after pump placement to avoid damage to device components. Conservative therapy consists of bed rest, analgesics, hydration, caffeine, and possibly abdominal binder. Caffeine can be given orally or intravenously (caffeine sodium benzoate 500 mg diluted in a liter of 5% dextrose Ringer's Lactate and administered at 200 cc/hour). Persistent headaches may be treated with a blood patch of 10–20 ml of autologous blood placed sterilely in the epidural space near the presumed interspace of cerebrospinal fluid loss.

Reservoir refilling errors. The many types of refilling errors include accidental subcutaneous administration, accidental intrathecal administration, inaccurate programming, and loading the wrong drug. Potentially devastating errors can be avoided with vigilance and proper technique. When refilling, the clinician must be aware of the pump model, use the proper template, and correctly following the instructions provided in the pump manual. The procedure usually involves inserting a Huber needle sterilely into the center hole of the template; a definite resistance should be felt as the needle hits the posterior wall of the pump. Resuscitative equipment including naloxone for opiate refills and physostigmine for baclofen refills should be immediately available. Accidental bolus injection into accessory ports is a serious problem that has proved fatal in two of four reported cases (Patt et al. 1993). If confusion exists as to which port is accessed, an aspirate should be tested for glucose (which would not be present if the reservoir were correctly accessed). Emptying the reservoir completely before refilling may provide additional protection. Risk factors for problems during refilling include obesity, the presence of a "deep" implant, and, as is common after recent implantation, local edema (Patt and Hassenbusch 1996).

TOLERANCE

The decrease in effectiveness over time with a given dose of opioid is not a common observation in clinical practice. When it does occur, it is often due to tolerance (a constant dose resulting in decreased effect over time due to cellular adjustments). Rapid development of tolerance similar to that seen in animals has been reported in cancer patients who receive 1 mg/day of intrathecal morphine (Bonica 1990). Tolerance should not be confused with situations where the decrease in drug effect is due to a progressive disease state.

The exact mechanism of tolerance to opioids is not known. Tolerance is a pharmacodynamic event thought to be related to receptor down-regulation, that is, an uncoupling or inactivation of some receptors resulting in a decease in receptor reserve. Down-regulation is characterized by continued agonist stimulation of receptors resulting in a state of desensitization to opioid. Research at a variety of institutions suggests that tolerance is to some extent time dependent, concentration dependent, and receptor selective (Rogers et al. 1986; Stevens 1989).

Tolerance to some nonanalgesic effects of opioids commonly occurs and is often desirable. After the initiation of dosing, patients often report somnolence, mental clouding, and nausea, all of which diminish with days or weeks. Opioid-induced respiratory depression is a worrisome side effect that is much less common with patients on chronic opioid therapy compared with opioid-naive patients treated for acute postsurgical pain (Portenoy and Kanner 1995). However, constipation is a static problem that usually does not improve with time.

Treatment strategies for tolerance to the analgesic effects of opioids initially involve upward titration of the opioid dose. Maximum daily doses reported in the literature are 150 mg of intrathecal morphine daily (Ventafridda et al. 1987) and 480 mg of epidural morphine daily (Arner et al. 1988). When upward titration is no longer practical, another strategy involves using nonopioid analgesic to recruit receptors and provide a "drug holiday." However, no substances besides morphine and baclofen are approved for administration via an implanted Medtronic infusion device. Compounds that have been beneficial either intrathecally or epidurally include droperidol (Lanning and Hrushesky 1990), clonidine (Coombs et al. 1985), local anesthetics, somatostatin (Chrubasik et al. 1984; Meynadier et al. 1985), and calcitonin (Fiorcde et al. 1983). Additionally, use of a different opioid will allow a degree of receptor rest, as cross-tolerance between opioids is incomplete (Yaksh 1987). In addition, it has been proposed that use of sufentanil results in a less rapid receptor down-regulation, which may result in some additional protection against tolerance to analgesic effects (Patt 1993). In addition, it is thought that continuous infusion of opioids results in less susceptibility to tolerance than do intermittent boluses, although this observation has not been proven convincingly (Bonica 1990).

SIDE EFFECTS AND THEIR MANAGEMENT

Respiratory depression. Respiratory depression is one side effect of opioids that generates the most clinical concern because of its potentially fatal consequence. The temporal feature of respiratory depression may be associated with the lipophilic properties of the opioid. Lipophilic opioids such as fentanyl and sufentanil display early respiratory depression, which may be caused by systemic absorption of the opioid and its effect on the respiratory center. However, hydrophilic opioids exhibit a biphasic pattern of respiratory depression. The early peak in incidence occurs less than two hours after administration and results from systemic absorption and intravenous transport of opioid to the respiratory center. A second delayed or late peak occurs four to 24 hours after administration and is thought to result from subarachnoid diffusion of opioid to the respiratory center. Activity at both the μ and δ receptors is associated with both types of respiratory depression. Kappa receptor activation may not be associated with significant respiratory depression (Sosnowski and Yaksh 1990; Patt 1993). Factors that predispose to respiratory depression include accidental overdose, an absence of severe pain, advanced age or debility, coexisting pulmonary disease, sleep apnea, the coadministration of opioid analgesic by alternative routes, and opioid naiveté (Patt 1993). Opioid respiratory depression is characterized by reduced respiratory rate resulting in hypercarbia and a CNS depressive effect. Respiratory depression can be reversed by titration of the μ antagonist naloxone (40 μg intravenously at a time) or the κ agonist/μ antagonist nalbuphine. The effects of respiratory depression can be combated by vigorously encouraging the patient to breath deeply or by assisted ventilation via endotracheal intubation and mechanical ventilation (Patt 1993).

Gastrointestinal dysfunction. Constipation is particularly common in cancer patients on systemic opioids; intrathecal opioids decrease peristalsis to a lesser extent. Constipation in the cancer patient may be multifactorial, and the clinician should consider other causes such as obstruction secondary to mass effect, tricyclic antidepressant side effects, or dehydration. The mainstay of the management of constipation is an aggressive regimen of generous fluid intake, laxatives, and enemas. It is much easier to prevent constipation than to treat it.

As with constipation, nausea and vomiting in a cancer patient on intrathecal opioids is often multifactorial and all reversible causes must be sought. The incidence of nausea and vomiting in patients with intrathecal opioid therapy may range from 25–30% in opioid-naive patients, but it is infrequent in patients with chronic exposure to opioids. Nausea and vomiting are thought to be due to activity at the chemoreceptor trigger zone (the area postrema) and the vomiting center, and also to involvement of the vestibular system. Changing to a more lipophilic opioid may resolve the problem. Nausea and vomiting can be managed symptomatically by standard medications such as the phenothiazine metoclopramide, a butyrophenone, a hydroxyzine, an anticholinergic such as scopolamine, or the antiserotoninergic ondansetron. Nausea and vomiting may also be relieved by partial opioid reversal with small doses of naloxone or nalbuphine.

Urinary retention. Urinary retention in a patient on intrathecal opioids is mediated via the μ and δ receptors but not the κ receptor. The incidence is 20–40% and occurs most frequently in opioid-naive male patients. Hesitancy is caused by decreased detrusor muscle tone and dyssynergy of the detrusor-urethral sphincter. Management of severe urinary retention involves bladder catheterization. If tolerance does not rapidly develop, other approaches may include conversion to a more lipophilic opioid or a trial of small doses of μ antagonists (Patt 1993).

Pruritus. This side effect is uncommon in cancer patients on intrathecal opioid infusion, but is common in opioid-naive patients and can be quite disturbing and upsetting. Treatment with diphenhydramine and other antihistamines, opioid antagonists, and droperidol have been recommended, but all such interventions have yielded mixed results.

Mental status and other effects. Dysphoria is an uncommon side effect of intrathecal opioid. However, it is more common with parenteral administration. A low incidence of sedation has been reported in cancer patient treated with intrathecal opioid after prior treatment with oral opioids

(Cousins and Bridenbaugh 1988). Hyperesthesia has been reported after high doses of spinal morphine in patients with cancer pain (Portenoy and Kanner 1995). It seems that this symptom results from an action of morphine on receptors other than those involved in nociception, because the hyperesthesia is not antagonized by naloxone.

TROUBLESHOOTING

Even with careful patient selection and flawless implantation techniques, a patient with initial satisfactory pain relief from the intrathecal opioid delivery system may later begin to complain of returning pain. The exact cause is determined by obtaining a careful history and physical examination. Possible explanations include prescription error, development of tolerance, progression of the underlying disease, and mechanical difficulties. Possible mechanical reasons for intrathecal pump failure include incorrect loading, pump malfunction, and catheter compromise (including disconnection, perforation, breakage, obstruction, or tip migration). In addition to data obtained from the patient and the physical examination, communication with patient's family, primary care physician, oncologist, nurses, and the pharmacy personnel will often yield invaluable information that can help in diagnosing and resolving the problem.

A simple, methodical approach for evaluating possible device failure is to work from the periphery to the catheter tip. This process involves: (1) determination that the current drug and drug delivery rate is appropriate; (2) examination of the infusion device and verification that the program is correct, the battery is functioning, and that the volume in the reservoir is appropriate; (3) examination of external portions of the system for kinking, and to confirm that the drug is exiting the pump; (4) examination of the tunneled portion of the catheter to detect kinks or rents in the tubing or evidence of infection or subcutaneous drug deposition; and (5) plain X-ray studies to determine the presence and location of the catheter in the intrathecal space. In the absence of demonstrable defects in the integrity of the delivery system, a local anesthetic test dose or radiopaque contrast medium should be injected (Hirsch et al. 1985; Patt 1993).

FUTURE HORIZONS

Since the 1970s, when intrathecal opioid administration was shown to produce segmental analgesia, remarkable progress has occurred in using intrathecal opioid to manage of pain, especially in the cancer patient population. However, several areas need to be addressed with respect to efficacy, especially in patients with noncancer pain. Properly controlled, large-scale trials are lacking in this patient population and should be performed.

There is a strong need for better defined and validated patient selection criteria. The psychosocial evaluation of potential candidates for implantable opioid delivery system is invaluable to predict success or failure of the system. Pain states that may respond to this intervention need to be better elucidated. Given the cost and invasiveness of this modality of pain control, great attention should be paid to refining the patient selection criteria to ensure a good chance of successful pain relief.

Unlike systemic analgesic therapy, which includes dozens of pharmacologic agents, intrathecal analgesia until recently was restricted only to opioids. With better understanding of the neurochemistry of pain transmission, newer and more specific agents designed for intrathecal use will become available. New, nonopioid agents such as adrenergic agonists (clonidine), neuronal-specific calcium-channel blockers (SNX-111), and N-methyl-D-aspartate (NMDA) antagonists (dextrorphan) are now being examined in clinical or animal studies. The technology of pumps and catheters is progressing at a rapid rate with an ever-increasing variety of equipment. Improved intrathecal drugs and drug administration, when used appropriately, can in fact be employed more often to help limit the suffering of patients with otherwise intractable pain.

REFERENCES

Ali N, Hanna N, Joffman J. Percutaneous epidural catheterization for intractable pain in terminal cancer patients. Gynecol Oncol 1989; 32:22–25.

Artner S, Arner B. Differential effects of epidural morphine in treatment of cancer related pain. Acta Anaesthesiol Scand 1985; 29:32.

Arner S, Rawal N, Gustafsson LL. Clinical experience of long-term treatment with epidural and intrathecal opioids: a national survey. Acta Anaesthesiol Scand 1988; 32:253.

Atweh SF, Kuhar MJ. Autoradiographic localization of opiate receptors in rat brain, spinal cord and lower medulla. Brain Res 1977; 124:53.

Barnes RK. Delayed subarachnoid migration of an epidural catheter. Anaesth Intensive Care 1990; 18:564–566.

Bedder MD, Burchiel JK, Larson A. Cost analysis of two implantable narcotic delivery systems. J Pain Symptom Manage 1991; 6:368.

Black P. Neurosurgical management of cancer pain. Semin Oncol 1985; 12:438.

Bonica J.J. The Management of Pain, 2nd ed. Philadelphia, PA: Lea and Febiger, 1990, pp 1967–1997.

Caute B, Monsarrat B, Gouardes C, et al. CSF morphine levels after lumbar intrathecal administration of isobaric and hyperbaric solutions for cancer pain. Pain 1988; 32:141.

Chrubasik J, Meynadier J, Blond S, et al. Somatostatin, a potent analgesic. Lancet 1984; 2:1208.

Coombs DW, Saunders RL, LaChance D, et al. Intrathecal morphine tolerance: use of intrathecal clonidine, DADL, and intravenous morphine. Anesthesiology 1985; 62:358.

Cousins MJ, Bridenbaugh PO. Neurologic mechanisms of pain. In: Cousins MJ, Bridenbaugh

PO (Eds). Neural Blockade in Clinical Anesthesia and Management of Pain, 2nd ed. Philadelphia: Lippincott, 1988.

Cousins MJ, Phillips GD (Eds). Acute Pain Management. London: Churchill Livingstone, 1986.

Du Pen SL, Peterson DG, Bogosian AC, et al. A new permanent exteriorized catheter for narcotic self-administration to control cancer pain. Cancer 1987; 59:986.

Dichiro G. Observation on the circulation of cerebral spinal fluid. Acta Radiol 1966; 5:988.

Downing JE, Busch EH, Stedman PM. Epidural morphine delivered by a percutaneous epidural catheter for outpatient treatment of cancer pain. Anesth Analg 1988; 67:1159.

Edwards WT, DeGirolami U, Burney RG, et al. Histopathologic changes in the epidural space of the guinea pig during long-term morphine infusion. Reg Anesth 1986; 11:14.

Faust RJ. Anesthesiology Review. New York: Churchill Livingstone, 1991, p 250.

Fiorcde CE, Castorina F, Malatino LS, et al. Analgesic activity of calcitonin: effectiveness of the epidural and subarachnoid routes in man. Int J Clin Pharmacol Res 1983; 3:257.

Gourlay G, Plummer J, Cherry D, et al. Comparison of intermittent bolus with continuous infusion of epidural morphine in the treatment of severe cancer pain. Pain 1991; 37:135–140.

Hahn M. Faculty Handbook. Minneapolis, MN: Medtronic, Inc., 1992.

Hirsch LF, Manki A, Nowak T. Sudden loss of pain control with morphine pump due to catheter migration. Neurosurgery 1985; 17:965.

Jacobson L, Chabal C, Brody MC, et al. A comparison of the effects of intrathecal fentanyl and lidocaine on established post amputation stump pain. Pain 1990; 40:137–141.

Klepper ID, Sherrill DL, Boetger CL, et al. Analgesic and respiratory effects of epidural sufentanil in volunteers and the influence of adrenaline as an adjuvant. Br J Anaesth 1987; 59:1147.

Lam AM, Knill RL, Thompson WR, et al. Epidural fentanyl does not cause delayed respiratory depression. Canadian Anaesthesia Society Journal 1983; 30(Suppl):S78.

Lanning RM, Hrushesky WJM. Cost comparison of wearable and implantable drug delivery systems. Proc Am Soc Clin Oncol 1990; 9:322.

Layfield DJ, Lensberger RJ, Hopinson BR, et al. Epidural morphine for ischemic rest pain. Br Med J 1981; 282:697–698.

Lenzi A, Galli G, Gandolfini M, et al. Intraventricular morphine in paraneoplastic painful syndrome of the cervicofacial region: experience in 38 cases. Neurosurgery 1985; 17:6.

Malone BT, Beye R, Walker J. Management of pain in the terminally ill by administration of epidural narcotics. Cancer 1985; 55:438.

Meynadier J, Chrubasik J, Dubar M, Wunsch E. Intrathecal somatostatin in terminally ill patients: a case report of two patients. Pain 1985; 23:9.

Murphy TM, Hind S, Cherry DA. Intraspinal narcotics for non-malignant pain. Acta Anaesthesiol Scand 1987; 31(85):75–76.

Nitescu P, Appelgren L, Jultman E, et al. Long term, open catheterization of the spinal subarachnoid space for continuous infusion of narcotic and bupivacaine in patients with refractory cancer pain. Clin J Pain 1991; 7:143–161.

North RB, Levy RM. Neurosurgical Management of Pain. Berlin: Springer, 1997, pp 302–324.

Oyama T, Murkawa T, Baba S, et al. Continuous vs. bolus epidural morphine. Acta Anaesthesiol Scand 1987; 21(Suppl 85):77.

Patt RB. Neurosurgical management of cancer pain. Semin Oncol 1985; 12:438.

Patt RB. Letter to the editor. American Journal of Hospice Care 1989; 6:18.

Patt RB. Cancer Pain. Philadelphia: J.B. Lippincott, 1993, pp 287–316.

Patt RB, Hassenbusch SJ. Implantable technology for pain control: identification and management of problems and complications. In: Waldman SD, Winnie AP (Eds). Interventional Pain Management. Philadelphia: W.B. Saunders, 1996, pp 483–500.

Patt RB, Wu C, Bressi J, Catania J. Accidental intraspinal overdose revisited. Anesth Analg 1993; 76:202.

Penn RD, Parce JA, Gottochalk W, et al. Cancer pain relief using chronic morphine infusions: early experience with programmable implanted drug pumps. J Neurosurg 1984; 61:302.

Pert CB, Synder SH. Opiate receptor: demonstration in the nervous tissue. Science 1973; 179:1011.

Plummer JL, Cherry DA, Cousins MJ, et al. Long term spinal administration of morphine in cancer and noncancer pain: a retrospective study. Pain 1991; 44:215–220.

Poletti CB, Cohen AL, Todd DP, et al. Cancer pain relieved by long-term epidural morphine with a permanent indwelling system for self-administration. J Neurosurg 1981; 56:581.

Portenoy RK, Kanner RM. Pain Management, Theory and Practice (Contemporary Neurology Series). Philadelphia: FA Davis, 1995.

Raj PP. Pain Medicine, A Comprehensive Review. St. Louis: Mosby–Year Book, 1996, pp 15–23, 279–282.

Rexed B. The cytoarchitectonic organization of the spinal cord in the cat. J Comp Neurol 1952; 96:415–495.

Rogers NF, El Fakahany EE. Morphine induced opioid receptor down regulation detected intact adult rat brain cells. Eur J Pharmacol 1986; Bol. 124, p 221.

Roquefeuil B, Benezech J, Blanchet P, et al. Intraventricular administration of morphine in patients with neoplastic intractable pain. Surg Neurol 1984; 21:155.

Schoeffler PF, Haberer JP, Monteillard CM, et al. Morphine injections in the cisterna magna for intractable pain in cancer patients. Anesthesiology 1987; 67(Suppl):A246.

Sosnowski M, Yaksh TL. Spinal administration of receptor-selective drugs as analgesics: new horizons. J Pain Symptom Manage 1990, 5:204.

Stevens CW, Yaksh TL. Potency of spinal antinociceptive agents is inversely related to magnitude of tolerance after continuous infusion. J Pharmacol Exp Ther 1989; 250:1.

Twycross RG, Lack SA. Therapeutics in Terminal Cancer. Edinburgh: Churchill Livingstone, 1986, p 9.

Ventafridda V, Spoldi E, Caraceni A, et al. Intraspinal morphine for cancer pain. Acta Anaesthesiol Scand 1987; 47(suppl 85).

Waldman SD, Coombs DW. Selection of implantable narcotic delivery systems. Anest Analg 1989; 68:377–384.

Waldman SD, Winnie AP (Eds). Interventional Pain Management. Philadelphia: WB Saunders, 1996.

Waldman SD, Leak DW, Kennedy LD, Patt RB. Intraspinal opioid therapy. In: Patt RB (Ed). Cancer Pain, 1st ed. Philadelphia:J.B. Lippincott, 1993, pp 287–316.

Waldman SD, Leak DW, Kennedy LD, Patt RB. Intraspinal opioid therapy. In: Patt RB (Ed). Cancer Pain, 2nd ed. Philadelphia: J.B. Lippincott, 1996, pp 285–328.

Wall PD, Melzack R. Textbook of Pain, 3rd ed. Edinburgh: Churchill Livingstone, 1994, pp 13–51, 103–113.

Wang JK. Intrathecal morphine for intractable pain secondary to cancer of the pelvic organs. Pain 1985; 21:99.

Wang JK, Nauss LA, Thomas JE. Pain relief by intrathecally applied morphine in man. Anesthesiology 1979; 50:149.

Wisenfeld, Gustafsson LL. Continuous intrathecal administration of morphine via osmotic minipump in the rat. Brain Res 1982; 247:195.

Wu C, Patt RB. Accidental overdose of systemic morphine during intended refill of intrathecal infusion device. Anesth Analg 1992; 75:130–132.

Yaksh TL. Spinal opiate analgesia: characteristics and principles of action. Pain 1981; 11:293.

Yaksh TL. Spinal opiates: a review of their effect on spinal function with an emphasis on pain processing. Acta Anaesthesiol Scand 1987; 85(Suppl):25.

Correspondence to: Samuel Hassenbusch, MD, PhD, Department of Neurosurgery, University of Texas M. D. Anderson Cancer Center, 1515 Holcombe Blvd., Houston, TX 77023. Tel: 713-792-2400; Fax: 713-794-4950.

Assessment and Treatment of Cancer Pain,
Progress in Pain Research and Management,
Vol. 12, edited by R. Payne, R.B. Patt, and
C.S. Hill, IASP Press, Seattle, © 1998.

16

Mechanisms of Bone Metastasis

Randy N. Rosier[a], David G. Hicks[a,b], Lisa A. Teot[a,b], J. Edward Puzas[a], and Regis J. O'Keefe[a]

Departments of [a]Orthopaedics and [b]Pathology,
The University of Rochester, Rochester, New York, USA

METASTASIS

Metastasis remains the dominant problem in the clinical care of the cancer patient. Many of the most common malignancies have a strong propensity to metastasize to bone, including breast, prostate, lung, kidney, and thyroid carcinomas. In particular the incidence of bony involvement can exceed 90% in metastatic breast and prostate carcinomas. Thus, given the high and rising incidence of these cancers, chronic bone pain, pathologic fractures, and other complications such as hypercalcemia are all too common problems. Pathologic fractures secondary to metastatic carcinomas are one of the most frequent tumor-related problems for the orthopaedic surgeon. Chronic bone pain due to metastatic carcinoma also represents one of the most difficult treatment challenges and greatest impediments to quality of life in cancer patients. Recent scientific developments have enhanced our understanding of mechanisms of cancer metastasis and suggest new opportunities for both suppression and prevention of metastatic disease. In addition, advances in knowledge of the molecular mechanisms that govern bone resorption and cancer cell adhesion in bone present further opportunities for novel therapeutic strategies. Clinical applications for such new approaches could ultimately contribute to a badly needed paradigm shift in the prevention and therapy of cancer metastasis.

Metastasis involves an intricate and complex sequence of events and is fundamental to the definition of malignancy. Thus, an extremely diverse spectrum of neoplastic diseases share this one feature of metastatic capability. The long-standing "seed and soil" concept suggests that metastasis results from both biological properties of the malignant cell and conducive

All MMPs have two highly conserved zinc binding domains—a catalytic site and a structural site. In addition there are two conserved calcium binding domains. Thus, molecules with chelating properties can potentially interfere with these metal binding sites and inhibit activity, providing one obvious therapeutic approach. The enzymes are all secreted in a proenzyme form; the propeptide is folded in a way that blocks the catalytic zinc site and is maintained in this inactive conformation by a so-called cysteine switch. Upon cleavage of the propeptide, the MMP becomes activated and can degrade substrate molecules. MMPs can cleave the proenzyme forms of each other and thus become activated in a cascade-type fashion. MMP expression is also regulated at the transcriptional level by growth factors, cytokines, and intracellular signaling molecules, including TGF-β, TNF-α, and cAMP (Overall 1994; Mann et al. 1995; Tanaka et al. 1995; Callaghan et al. 1996).

Manipulation of these regulatory pathways affords another possible approach to metastatic suppression. All cells that secrete MMPs also secrete endogenous inhibitor proteins of these enzymes, called tissue inhibitors of metalloproteinases (TIMPs). These molecules bind stoichiometrically to MMPs to maintain them in an inactive state. Thus, the balance between TIMP and MMP expression ultimately controls the amount of matrix degradative activity. Overexpression of TIMP experimentally by transfection of malignant cell lines leads to inhibition of metastasis in animal models, while underexpression enhances metastasis (Montgomery et al. 1994; Watanabe et al. 1996). Three forms of TIMP have been identified; TIMP1 and TIMP2 are the most prevalent, while TIMP3, a matrix-bound form, is less well characterized (Apte et al. 1995). Some studies have reported that MMP expression correlates with metastasis and prognosis in patients with several different cancers, as does underexpression of TIMP (Baker et al. 1994; Naylor et al. 1994; Onisto et al. 1995).

One of the most promising areas of anticancer research is the pharmacologic manipulation of MMP activity. An appealing aspect of this approach is that several agents have significant MMP inhibiting activity but have minimal toxicity. Examples include tetracyclines and hydroxamates, which function by chelating the active metal-binding domains of the MMPs. Tetracyclines have demonstrated beneficial clinical effects in periodontal disease and arthritis, putatively through suppression of MMPs involved in these pathologic conditions (Greenwald et al. 1992; Rifkin et al. 1993). In addition, tetracyclines have suppressed metastasis in animal models (Masumori et al. 1994). Batimastat (BB-94), a synthetic hydroxamate MMP inhibitor, has shown a dramatic effect on ovarian and colon carcinomas in animal models and has also been used with some apparent benefit in a human clinical trial with this tumor (Wang et al. 1994). Several new MMP inhibitors with varying specificity are under development and will exploit the critical nature of the catalytic metal-binding site. In addition, retinoids and cAMP analogs have down-regulated MMPs at a transcriptional level, while prostaglandins may up-regulate these genes in some cells. Thus, the use of phosphodiesterase inhibitors, retinoids, or prostaglandin inhibitors could provide additional pharmacologic methods of inhibition of MMP expression in malignant tumors, although considerable further study of these approaches is needed.

Besides MMPs, several other metastatic markers or predictors have been identified. A protein called nm23 (nonmetastatic 23), which is negatively associated with metastasis, is a nucleotide diphosphate kinase and is also homologous to a transcription factor called PuF. While controversial, the expression of this marker and its inverse correlation with poor prognosis and metastasis has been demonstrated in a number of studies. However, some studies have not demonstrated a correlation, and the significance of nm23 expression as a predictor remains uncertain. Other markers predictive of metastasis that have been identified include maspins, metastasin, and several proto-oncogenes. Identification of novel metastatic markers may lead to an understanding of their functional role in the metastatic process and thereby to new therapeutic or preventive strategies.

BONE METASTASIS

Metastasis to bone requires both progressive displacement of marrow elements and resorption of bone to allow local tumor progression. Bone resorption and intraosseous tumor growth lead to bone pain, possibly due to necrosis, inflammation, and elevation of intraosseous pressure. In addition, loss of mechanical strength due to structural damage leads to pathologic fractures, an unfortunately common problem with metastatic carcinomas. Extensive bone resorption, or osteolysis, by metastatic tumors can lead to systemic hypercalcemia, an additional cause of morbidity and mortality. Metastatic bone deposits initially tend to displace marrow elements preferentially and seem to take the path of least resistance. For this reason, radiographs frequently appear normal, even with extensive metastatic involvement of bone. Up to 50% loss of the trabecular bone mass may be required before radiographic evidence of bone lysis is readily apparent. Radionuclide bone scans, which detect subtle bony reaction to the advancing lesion, are a much more sensitive method of detection in most tumors, in part due to the local coupling of bone resorption and formation that occurs between osteoblasts (bone forming cells) and osteoclasts (bone resorbing cells). Whenever osteoclasts resorb bone, they release so-called coupling factors locally from the bone matrix that putatively stimulate osteoblast progenitors to differentiate into osteoblasts in that area and form new bone (Fig 1). Thus, even when tumors cause osteolysis and a net loss of bone locally, some reactive bone formation also generally occurs, which accounts for radionuclide uptake on nuclear bone scans.

The spectrum of cytokines and growth factors secreted by tumor cells within bone is also a determinant of the type of local bony reaction to the lesion. Metastatic carcinomas can have a predominantly lytic radiographic appearance (commonly seen with lung, renal, and thyroid), a purely blastic appearance (prostate), or a mixed pattern of bone lysis and blastic areas (breast). Understanding of the factors that account for these differences is still limited, but several molecules have been identified that may be involved in determining the type of bony reaction to the lesion. Blastic prostatic tumors contain acid phosphatase, which is a glycosylated enzyme containing mannose-6-phosphate. This substance may activate the mannose-6-phosphate/IGF-II receptor of osteoblasts, which causes an anabolic effect and stimulates local bone formation (Ishibe et al. 1991a,b). In addition, calcitonin gene-related peptide (CGRP) has been reported in prostatic tumors and may have osteoclastic inhibitory properties similar to calcitonin. FGF (fibroblast growth factor) and BMPs (bone morphogenetic proteins) also have been expressed in prostate carcinoma and could contribute to the abnormal bone formation observed (Nakamoto et al. 1992; Harris et al. 1994). Although patients with blastic lesions may have serious problems with bone pain, they tend not to have fractures due to the sclerotic nature of the reactive bone within and around the metastatic lesions.

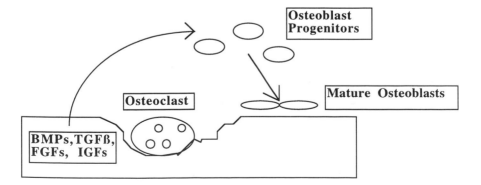

Fig. 1. Coupling of bone resorption and formation through bone matrix growth factors.

There are two theories for the mechanism of progression of lytic lesions in bone: direct osteolysis of bone by tumor cells and stimulation of host osteoclastic bone resorption by the tumor cells. Recent evidence suggests that both methods may be operant. In our laboratory, histologic study of tissue from lytic bony metastases and primary round cell tumors such as Ewing's sarcoma and lymphoma with bone destruction has consistently demonstrated bone resporbtion by large numbers of osteoclasts. This phenomenon is not observed in predominantly blastic tumors. In addition, three cytokines have been identified as important mediators of osteoclastic bone resorption: interleukin-1 (IL-1), interleukin-6 (IL-6), and TNF-α. Pathologic bone resorption has been associated with local expression of these bone resorptive cytokines in a variety of pathologic conditions, including rheumatoid arthritis, osteomyelitis, wear debris–induced periprosthetic osteolysis, bone cysts, and multiple myeloma. TNF-α is particularly important in malignancy, because its secretion may be responsible for local normal cellular cytotoxicity, and it contributes to many of the severe systemic effects of disseminated malignancy, including constitutional symptoms such as fever, malaise, weight loss, and cachexia. In addition, TNF-α is secreted in a membrane-bound form that requires cleavage by an extracellular MMP to be released and activated (Gearing et al. 1994). Thus, antimetastatic therapy targeted to MMPs may have additional beneficial effects as treatment for systemic symptoms and metastatic bone resorption.

Immunohistochemical analysis of lymphoma of bone has demonstrated these cytokines in the tumor cells in areas of bone lysis and osteoclastic stimulation (Hicks et al. 1995). Similarly, in lytic metastatic carcinomas and Ewing's sarcoma, we have observed expression of one or more of these three cytokines in all cases; they possibly represent a significant component of the mechanism of bone destruction. Direct tumor-mediated osteolysis remains a possibility, but efficient bone resorption is a fairly complex process that requires cell attachment, acidification of the space between the cell and the bone by means of a proton pump to dissolve mineral, and then secretion of acid-stable lysosomal enzymes to dissolve matrix. Thus, it is unclear to what extent tumor cells are able to duplicate the complex activities of the highly specialized osteoclast, although clearly they can lyse bone readily simply by locally stimulating these host cells.

Tumors that are predisposed to metastasize to bone may do so via expression of cell surface receptors such as integrins or CD44, which may target bone matrix components for cell attachment. Integrins are heterodimeric cell surface receptors composed of α and β subunits that transduce signals through cytoskeletally associated kinases, and are expressed at high levels in most cells of mesenchymal origin. Cells of epithelial origin such as carcinomas normally express relatively low levels of these receptors, although upregulation may occur in malignancy. Integrins bind to matrix components containing a common RGD (arginine-glycine-aspartate) sequence. Bone contains numerous matrix proteins with RGD sequences, including collagens, fibronectin, and osteopontin. Synthetic or natural peptides containing the integrin binding motif (RGD) can block tumor attachment to bone in vitro and in animal models. These molecules can also block osteoclastic bone resorption because osteoclasts must attach to bone surfaces by an integrin known as the vitronectin receptor. CD44 is a hyaluronan receptor expressed in malignant cells that also may have a role in cell attachment to bone matrix (Miyasaka 1995). Thus, blockade of tumor attachment factors provides another potential route to therapeutic suppression of bony metastases or their progression.

Many carcinomas secrete PTHrP (parathyroid hormone-related peptide); it can cause hypercalcemia of malignancy due to stimulation of osteoclastic bone resorption. PTHrP is thought to act through the same receptor as PTH; it stimulates osteoblasts to release IL-6, which then secondarily induces osteoclasts to resorb bone. This mechanism is thought to drive the response of bone to PTH in regulating calcium homeostasis under normal physiological conditions, but is pathologically stimulated in cases of tumor secretion of PTHrP. In addition, evidence suggests that PTHrP expression may in fact be a determinant of the propensity of a tumor to metastasize to bone. In a series of patients with metastatic breast carcinoma, Kitazawa recently found that the only patients who did not have bony metastases were those whose tumors did not express PTHrP (Kitazawa and Maeda 1995). It is possible that PTHrP expression, by inducing local osteoclastic bone resorption, results in exposure of integrin ligands or other adhesion molecules in the bone matrix and facilitates malignant tumor cell attachment in this organ.

EXPERIMENTAL THERAPEUTICS

Can this new information on mechanisms of metastasis be used clinically to prevent or retard metastatic disease in patients? Preliminary data from several laboratory groups suggests that some relatively nontoxic agents that interfere with various aspects of metastasis may be efficacious adjunctive treatments. We have recently studied a malignant murine lung carcinoma cell line called line 1, which is readily transplantable in syngeneic mice due to low expression of HLA-DR antigens. When injected intramuscularly in mice, these highly malignant cells rapidly develop into a primary tumor and predictably spread selectively to the surface of the lungs within a few weeks. The surface metastases can be readily quantified. Initial in vitro studies demonstrated production of MMP9 and a stromelysin by the line 1 cells by zymography. Two agents with theoretical MMP inhibitory activities—minocycline and 9-cis-retinoic acid—were chosen after screening studies. Both these agents potently suppressed (> 90%) the MMP activity of the line 1 cells at pharmacologically relevant clinical dose levels. Next, the cells were studied using an in vitro metastasis model of invasion assay, i.e., rate of tumor migration through a synthetic basement membrane-like material called Matrigel. Again, both retinoic acid and minocycline suppressed in vitro invasion by these cells by more than 90%, although the combination showed no additive effect.

Subsequently, mice were inoculated intramuscularly with the line 1 cells in control (saline), minocycline, retinoic acid, or minocycline + retinoic acid groups treated daily by IP injection. At sacrifice, while we observed no effect of any of the treatments on primary tumor size or necrosis, the treatment groups demonstrated a 93% decrease in lung tumor burden in the retinoic acid group, 74% decrease in the minocycline treated group, and 57% decrease in the combination group as compared with control (Pearson et al. 1996). Further experiments clarified the lack of synergistic or additive effects of the MMP inhibitors and demonstrated that the effect of retinoic acid was mediated by a seven-fold stimulation of TIMP expression, which was abrogated by minocycline through a mechanism not yet defined. Thus, in vitro experimental observations in this particular model correlated quite well with in vivo effects. Both these agents are relatively nontoxic and could be used as adjunctive clinical therapies to retard metastatic disease. Continued research may uncover other combinations of MMP inhibitors or agents that inhibit other phases of the metastatic process and that could be combined with MMP blockade to achieve additive or synergistic effects in the suppression of metastasis. Hydroxamates are under intensive development as other possible nontoxic MMP inhibitors for use in antimetastatic therapy.

Finally, another therapeutic target of enormous potential clinical benefit is the osteoclastic bone resorption of lytic bony metastases. Besides the theoretical use of bone antiresorptive cytokine therapy mentioned earlier, other pharmacologic agents can be used clinically to prevent bone resorption. Some of the earlier bone antiresorptive agents, such as etidronate and calcitonin, have not demonstrated clear clinical efficacy in malignancy except in cases of treatment of hypercalcemia. However, these agents have not reliably acheived the goals of reducing bone pain and preventing pathologic fractures. Bisphosphonates are thought to act by adsorbing to the hydroxyapatite surfaces of bone and interfering with osteoclast function through an as yet incompletely understood mechanism. The first bisphosphonate, etidronate, also caused significant inhibition of mineralization. However, the recent development of a new generation of far more potent bisphosphonate antiresorptive agents with minimal or no inhibitory effects on bone formation offer exciting opportunities to ameliorate the morbidity of bone metastases. Clinical trials using pamidronate, clodronate, and ibandronate have been reported, and these agents are now becoming well established for their efficacy in treatment of hypercalcemia in patients with metastatic cancer. However, several clinical trials have also reported average decreases in rates of pathologic fractures of 50%, significant decreases in bone pain, and even increases in mean survival with intermittent i.v. pamidronate therapy (Conte et al. 1994; Houston and Rubens 1995). Current availability of orally active bisphosphonates, such as alendronate, could make therapy even more practical for cancer patients. In addition, some recent in vitro work indicates that bisphosphonates may have a protective effect against tumor cell attachment to bone, which suggests possible uses in the prevention of metastases. Our group recently began using oral alendronate therapy to treat patients with extensive lytic bone disease; several patients showed dramatic radiographic changes of lesions from lytic to blastic and some experienced a decrease in bone pain and cessation of recurrent pathologic fractures. The rapid change from a lytic to a blastic radiographic appearance is not surprising given the recent advances toward elucidation of bone formation and resorption coupling mechanisms. In the context of an aggressive lytic malignancy in bone, enormous amounts of bone matrix are being dissolved by osteoclastic activity, releasing a large amount of anabolic growth factors into the local area. The catabolic, cytokine-mediated osteolytic effect of the tumor obviously dominates; however, initiation of bisphosphonate therapy causes sudden cessation of the profuse resorptive activity, and the released growth factors that normally couple formation to resorption then can trigger rapid bone formation in and around the lesion. Although much larger numbers of patients and controlled clinical trials are needed to confirm the efficacy of this treatment, the preliminary evidence suggests a highly beneficial effect for this otherwise relatively harmless therapy.

CONCLUSIONS

Recent insights into the mechanisms of metastasis, factors facilitating bony localization, and mechanisms of tumor-mediated bone resorption have revealed several novel and exciting potential approaches to the prevention or suppression of metastatic cancer. Clearly, the failure of current treatment methods to control metastasis and bone involvement underscore the need for a paradigm shift in our treatment of cancer. The use of nontoxic adjuvant antimetastatic therapies is in its infancy, but shows tremendous promise. At present, the most practical approaches for clinical application include the bisphosphonates and MMP inhibitors such as tetracyclines and hydroxamates. Early clinical results already suggest efficacy for hydroxamate MMP inhibitors and bisphosphonates in suppressing metastasis and bony progression. This approach in combination with other more traditional methods of systemic treatment might achieve even greater efficacy. Other work in angiogenesis inhibition, cell adhesion prevention, and immunotherapy provides further options for the development of novel programs of therapy that may ultimately improve cancer care and prognosis.

REFERENCES

Apte SS, Olsen BR, Murphy G. The gene structure of tissue inhibitor of metalloproteinases (TIMP)-3 and its inhibitory activities define the distinct TIMP gene family. J Biol Chem 1995; 270:14313–14318.

Baker T, Tickle S, Wasan H, et al. Serum metalloproteinases and their inhibitors: markers for malignant potential. Br J Cancer 1994; 70:506–512.

Callaghan MM, Lovis RM, Rammohan C, Lu Y, Pope RM. Autocrine regulation of collagenase gene expression by TNF-alpha in U937. J Leukoc Biol 1996; 59:125–132.

Conte PF, Giannessi PG, Latreille J, et al. Delayed progression of bone metastases with pamidronate therapy in breast cancer patients: a randomized, multicenter phase III trial. Ann Oncol 1994; 5(Suppl)7:S41–44.

Gearing AJ, Beckett P, Christodoulou M, et al. Processing of tumour necrosis factor-alpha precursor by metalloproteinases. Nature 1994; 370(6490):555–557.

Greenwald RA, Moak SA, Ramamurthy NS, Golub LM. Tetracyclines suppress matrix metalloproteinaseactivity in adjuvant arthritis and in combination with flurbiprofen, ameliorate bone damage. J Rheumatol 1992; 19(6):927–938.

Harris SE, Harris MA, Mahy P, et al. Expression of bone morphogenetic protein messenger RNAs by normal rat and human prostate and prostate cancer cells. Prostate 1994; 24:204–211.

Hicks DG, Gokan T, O'Keefe RJ, et al. Primary lymphoma of bone: correlation of magnetic resonance image features with cytokine production by tumor cells. Cancer 1995; 75:973–980.

Houston SJ, Rubens RD. The systemic treatment of bone metastases.Clin Orthop 1995; 312:95–104.

Ishibe M, Rosier RN, Puzas JE. Activation of osteoblast insulin-like growth factor-II/cation-independent mannose-6-phosphate receptors by specific phosphorylated sugars and antibodies induce insulin-like growth factor-II effects. Endocr Res 1991a; 17:357–366.

Ishibe M, Rosier RN, Puzas JE. Human prostatic acid phosphatase directly stimulates collagen synthesis and alkaline phosphatase content of isolated bone cells. J Clin Endocrinol Metab 1991b; 73:785–792.

Kitazawa S, Maeda S. Development of skeletal metastases. Clin Orthop 1995; 312:45–50.

Kuratsu S, Uchida A, Araki N. Mechanism of organ selectivity in the determination of metastatic patterns of Dunn osteosarcoma. Trans Ortho Res Soc 1992; 17:196.

Mann EA, Hibbs MS, Spiro JD, et al. Cytokine regulation of gelatinase production by head and neck squamous cell carcinoma: the role of tumor necrosis factor-alpha. Ann Otol Rhinol Laryngol 1995; 104:203–209.

Masumori N, Tsukamoto T, Miyao N, et al. Inhibitory effect of minocycline on in vitro invasion and experimental metastasis of mouse renal adenocarcinoma. J Urology 1994; 151:1400–1404.

Miyasaka M. Cancer metastasis and adhesion molecules. Clin Orthop 1995; 312:10–18.

Montgomery AM, Mueller BM, Reisfeld RA, Taylor SM, DeClerck YA. Effect of tissue inhibitor of the matrix metalloproteinases-2 expression on the growth and spontaneous metastasis of a human melanoma cell line. Cancer Res 1994; 54:5467–5473.

Nakamoto T, Chang CS, Li AK, Chodak GW. Basic fibroblast growth factor in human prostate cancer cells. Cancer Res 1992; 52:571–577.

Naylor MS, Stamp GW, Davies BD, Balkwill FR. Expression and activity of MMPS and their regulators in ovarian cancer. Int J Cancer 1994; 58:50–56.

Onisto M, Riccio MP, Scannapieco P, et al. Gelatinase A/TIMP-2 imbalance in lymph-node-positive breast carcinomas, as measured by RT-PCR. Int J Cancer 1995; 63(5):621–626.

Overall CM. Regulation of tissue inhibitor of matrix metalloproteinase expression. Ann N Y Acad Sci 1994; 732:51–64.

Pearson W, Batley J, O'Keefe RJ, et al. Suppression of metastatic potential by inhibition of matrix metalloproteinases. Trans Ortho Res Soc 1996; 21:184.

Rifkin BR, Vernillo AT, Golub LM. Blocking periodontal disease progression by inhibiting tissue-destructive enzymes: a potential therapeutic role for tetracyclines and their chemically-modified analogs. J Periodontol 1993; 64(8 Suppl):819–827.

Tanaka K, Iwamoto Y, Ito Y, et al. Cyclic AMP-regulated synthesis of the tissue inhibitors of metalloproteinases suppresses the invasive potential of the human fibrosarcoma cell line HT1080. Cancer Res 1995; 55:2927–2935

Wang X, Fu X, Brown PD, Crimmin MJ, Hoffman RM. Matrix metalloproteinase inhibitor BB-94 (batimastat) inhibits human colon tumor growth and spread in a patient-like orthotopic model in nude mice. Cancer Res 1994; 54:4726–4728.

Watanabe M, Takahashi Y, Ohta T, et al. Inhibition of metastasis in human gastric cancer cells transfected with tissue inhibitor of metalloproteinase 1 gene in nude mice. Cancer 1996; 77(8 Suppl):1676–1680.

Correspondence to: Randy Rosier, MD, PhD, University of Rochester Medical Center, 601 Elmwood Ave., Rochester, NY 14642, USA. Tel: 716-275-3100; Fax: 716-461-9299.

Assessment and Treatment of Cancer Pain,
Progress in Pain Research and Management,
Vol. 12, edited by R. Payne, R.B. Patt, and
C.S. Hill, IASP Press, Seattle, © 1998.

17

Management of Metastatic Bone Pain

Richard Payne[a] and Nora Janjan[b]

*[a]Pain and Symptom Management Section, Department of Neuro-Oncology,
and [b]Department of Radiation Oncology, The University of Texas
M. D. Anderson Cancer Center, Houston, Texas, USA*

Bone metastasis is the most common cause of pain for patients with advanced cancer (Foley 1996). Rosier (Chapter 16) has reviewed the mechanisms of bone metastasis. The many options for the management of metastatic bone pain provide an opportunity for individualizing therapy to achieve an optimal outcome for each patient, but also create opportunity for confusion. Fig. 1 illustrates a flowchart generally used to assess and manage metastatic bone pain at The University of Texas M. D. Anderson Cancer Center Bone Metastasis Clinic.

Patients reporting pain should be treated with analgesics according to established guidelines (Jacox et al. 1994, also see Chapter 2). Nonsteroidal anti-inflammatory analgesics may be particularly effective in metastatic bone pain (Levick et al. 1988; Eisenberg et al. 1994) because prostaglandin-mediated mechanisms are important in the establishment of bone metastasis (Glasko 1976), and the potent antiprostaglandin effects of nonsteroidal anti-inflammatory drugs (NSAIDs) are essential for analgesic response (Vane 1971). Opioids are necessary when pain intensity increases beyond the ceiling dose of NSAIDs (see Chapters 18 and 19).

Radiotherapy is a nearly universal treatment option for patients with metastatic bone pain (Tong et al. 1982; Bates 1992; Jacox et al. 1994). Conventionally, external beam radiotherapy is given in 10 fractions for a total dose of 30 Gray (Gy) to the symptomatic site or sites. In aggregate, pain relief has been reported in 75–80% of patients completing radiotherapy (Kagan 1987), although the dose of radiotherapy, the site of bone metastasis, and the primary histology all influence response. The role of reduced radiotherapy fractions, and even the delivery of a single large fraction (6–10 Gy), is an area of intense interest and controversy (Price et al. 1986; Barak et al. 1987; Cole 1989) and is being actively studied in several institutions,

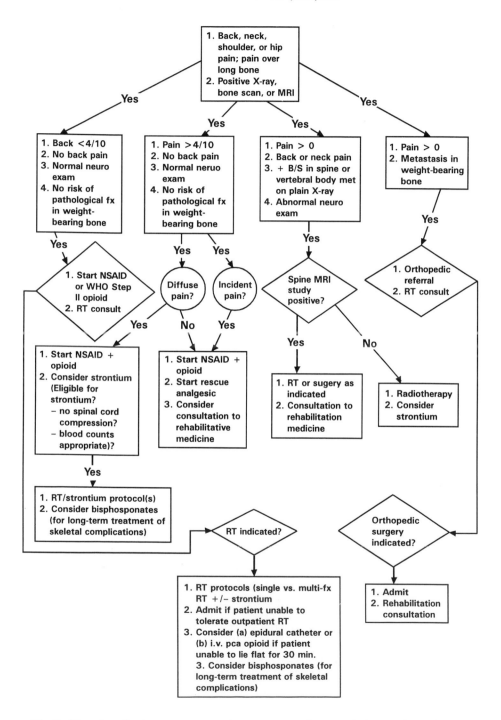

Fig. 1. Flowchart for the assessment and management of metastatic bone pain used at the M.D. Anderson Bone Metastasis Clinic. *B/S*, bone scan; *fx*, effects; *pca*, patient-controlled analgesia; *RT*, radiation therapy.

including at the M. D. Anderson Cancer Center (Fig. 1). Evaluation of the rates of fracture or refracture and the effects on pain relief, analgesic requirements, and general quality of life must be evaluated to justify the administration of single or reduced radiotherapy fractions, but the available studies report that single-fraction radiotherapy may be efficacious in 70% of patients, with the obvious additional benefits of decreased costs and increased convenience to the patient.

Radiopharmaceuticals such as strontium-89 and samarium may be used to manage diffuse or metastatic bone disease with pain, or to treat single sites of disease and pain that have recurred or progressed after treatment with external beam radiotherapy. Samarium has only recently been approved by the U.S. Food and Drug Administration (FDA). Clinical experience with samarium is not as extensive as with strontium-89, which has been available for several years. Strontium-89 is taken up into sites of active bone turnover (similar to calcium) and delivers local radiotherapy to the bone. A large randomized controlled trial that evaluated strontium-89 as an adjuvant to external beam radiotherapy indicated that a significantly greater proportion of patients treated with single intravenous doses of strontium-89 reported improved pain relief, cessation of analgesic drug use, increase in physical activity, and general improvement in quality of life, as compared to a placebo-control group (Porter et al. 1993). In addition, the strontium-89 treated patients reported a significant delay in the appearance of new painful sites, and at three months, nearly 59% of patients were free of pain. Pain relief is usually delayed for two to three weeks following treatment and may not peak until six weeks, so this radiopharmaceutical is not indicated for management of acute severe bone pain, and analgesic therapy must be continued while awaiting the therapeutic response. Suppression of blood counts is the most frequent toxicity, and patients must be followed carefully, especially if chemotherapy or other bone marrow suppressant drugs are being administered.

Bisphosphonate compounds that inhibit osteoclast resorption of bone are indicated for the treatment of hypercalcemia and pain associated with bone metastasis. Recent studies have shown that pamidronate, a commonly used bisphosphonate, reduces the morbidity of skeletal complications associated with breast cancer (Hortobagyi et al. 1996) and myeloma (Berenson et al. 1996). Pamidronate is given as an intravenous infusion of 90 mg over two hours, once a month. The drug is generally well tolerated, with the most commonly reported side effects being weakness and fatigue. Symptomatic hypocalcemia may occur and, rarely, bone pain may increase during the infusion (Hortobagyi 1996).

The use of adjuvant analgesic drugs is generally delayed until after the application of these primary analgesic therapies and specific antineoplastic therapies such as radiotherapy and osteoclast inhibition with bisphosphonates. Corticosteroids may be used to manage acute metastatic bone pain and are essential components of therapy when spinal metastasis are complicated by epidural spinal cord compression (See Chapter 19). Although declining in frequency of use given newer and effective oral bisphosphonate and intravenous radiopharmaceutical therapies, the administration of adjuvant analgesic drugs such as calcitonin (Ambrus et al. 1992) and levo-dopamine are more specific for bone pain than for soft tissue, visceral, or neuropathic pain because of their particular actions on osteoclasts. Calcitonin may have more general analgesic effects related to pharmacological effects in the central nervous system, but also appears to have direct effects on bone in disorders such as osteoporosis (Ambrus et al. 1992) and Paget's disease.

Recently, mitoxantrone, a chemotherapeutic agent that inhibits DNA synthesis, has provided palliative benefit for patients with bone pain complicating hormone-refractory prostate cancer (Tannock et al. 1996). The onset of pain relief may occur within days of mitoxantrone administration, and thus may have an advantage over strontium-89 in this regard. However, comparative studies evaluating the palliative effects of strontium-89 relative to mitoxantrone in prostate cancer have not been done.

Orthopedic consultation and treatment is important, particularly for patients with spinal instability and metastasis to weight-bearing bones of the extremities. Early consultation often allows prophylactic management of pathological fractures and provides the best opportunity to maintain function, especially mobility. Consultation with rehabilitation medicine specialists is often critical to assess a patient's functional status and needs, and it is important to work with radiotherapists, orthopedic surgeons, and pain management physicians to coordinate treatment.

As indicated from the flowchart and text above, the optimal management of patients with metastatic bone pain requires interdisciplinary assessment and expertise in specific bone pain syndromes and treatment options. Specialized bone metastasis clinics that offer interdisciplinary consultation and dialogue and allow the convenience of "one-stop shopping" for the patient are attractive and are the model used at the M. D. Anderson Cancer Center (Janjan et al. 1994).

REFERENCES

Ambrus JL, Hoffman M, Abrus CM, et al. Prevention and treatment of osteoporosis. One of the most frequent disorders in American women: a review. J Med 1992; 23:369–388.
Barak F, Werner A, Walach N, Horn Y. The palliative efficacy of a single high dose of radiation

in treatment of symptomatic osseous metastases. Int J Radiat Oncol Biol Phys 1987; 13:1233–1235.

Bates T. A review of local radiotherapy in the treatment of bone metastases and cord compression. Int J Radiat Oncol Biol Phys 1992; 23:217–221.

Berenson JR, Lichtenstein A, Porter L, et al. Efficacy of pamidronate in reducing skeletal events in patients with advanced multiple myeloma. N Engl J Med 1996; 334:488–493.

Cole DJ. A randomized trial of a single treatment versus conventional fractionation in the palliative radiotherapy of painful bone metastasis. Clin Oncol 1989; 1:56–62.

Eisenberg LE, Barkey CS, Carr DB, Mosteller F, Chalmers TC. Efficacy and safety of nonsteroidal anti-inflammatory drugs for cancer pain: a meta-analysis. J Clin Oncol 1994; 12:2756–2765.

Foley KM. Pain syndromes in patients with cancer. In: Portenoy RK, Kanner RM (Eds). Pain Management: Theory and Practice. Philadelphia: F.A. Davis, 1996, pp 191–216.

Glasko CSB. Mechanisms of bone destruction in the development of skeletal metastasis. Nature 1976; 263:507–510.

Hortobagyi GN, Theriault RL, Porter L, et al. Efficacy of pamidronate in reducing skeletal complication in patients with breast cancer and lytic bone metastases. N Engl J Med 1996; 335:1785–1791.

Jacox A, Carr DB, Payne R. Management of Cancer Pain. Clinical Practice Guideline no. 9. AHCPR Publication no. 94-0592. Rockville, MD: U.S. Department of Health and Human Services, Public Health Service, Agency for Health Care Policy and Research, 1994.

Janjan NA, Payne R. Podoloff D, Libshitz HI, et al. Outcomes in a multidisciplinary clinic for bone metastasis. Proceedings of the 77th Annual Meeting of the American Radium Society, April 29–May 3, 1995, Paris, France.

Kagan AR. Radiotherapeutic management of the patient for palliation. In: Perez CA, Brady LW (Eds). Principles and Practice of Radiation Oncology. Philadelphia: J.B. Lippincott, 1987, pp 1271–1282.

Levick S, Jacobs C, Loukas D, et al. Naproxen sodium in treatment of bone pain due to metastatic cancer. Pain 1988; 35:253–258.

Porter AT, McEwan AJ, Powe JE, et al. Results of a randomized phase-III trial to evaluate the efficacy of strontium-89 adjuvant to local field external beam irradiation in the management of endocrine resistant metastatic prostate cancer. Int J Rad Oncol Biol Phys 1993; 25:805–813.

Price P, Hoskin PJ, Easton D, et al. Prospective randomized trial of single and multifraction radiotherapy schedules in the treatment of painful bone metastases. Radiother Oncol 1986; 6:247–255.

Tannock IF, et al. Chemotherapy with mitoxantrone plus prednisone or prednisone alone for symptomatic hormone-resistant prostate cancer: a Canadian randomized trial with palliative end point. J Clin Oncol 1996; 14:1754–1764.

Tong D, Gillick L, Hendrickson FR. The palliation of symptomatic osseous metastases: final results of the study by the Radiation Therapy Oncology Group. Cancer 1982; 50:893–899.

Vane JR. Inhibition of prostaglandin synthesis as a mechanism of action for aspirin-like drugs. Nature 1971; 234:231–238.

Correspondence to: Richard Payne, MD, Department of Neuro-Oncology, University of Texas M. D. Anderson Cancer Center, 1515 Holcombe Blvd., Box 8, Houston, TX 77030, USA. Tel: 713-794-4998; Fax: 713-794-4999; email: rp@utmdacc.mda.uth.tmc.edu.

Assessment and Treatment of Cancer Pain,
Progress in Pain Research and Management,
Vol. 12, edited by R. Payne, R.B. Patt, and
C.S. Hill, IASP Press, Seattle, © 1998.

18

Opioid Pharmacology: Tolerance, Receptor Modulation, and New Analgesics

Charles E. Inturrisi

*Department of Pharmacology, Cornell University Medical College,
New York, New York, USA*

CONCEPTS OF OPIOID TOLERANCE

Patients with pain who receive opioids repeatedly develop tolerance to the analgesic effects (Jacox et al. 1994). Opioid tolerance is manifest when a given dose of an opioid produces a decreased effect or when a larger dose is required to maintain the original effect. This tolerance is not due to pharmacokinetic changes in the disposition of the opioid but rather it is a pharmacodynamic type of tolerance that results from neuroadaptive processes (see below). In quantitative terms tolerance is demonstrated by a shift to the right of the dose-response curve and an increase in the opioid ED50 value (the dose required to produce an effect in 50% of the population) (Houde et al. 1966; Foley 1991).

In the clinical setting, dose escalation is used to assess the presence or absence of tolerance. Surveys using this criterion indicate that the rate and extent of tolerance differ dramatically among pain patients (Portenoy 1994; Foley et al. 1991). In pain patients it is usually difficult to separate a change in the pain stimulus (worsening pain) from the development of tolerance per se. Clearly, in those patients whose opioid dose must be rapidly escalated to maintain analgesia, a progression in the painful lesion must be sought (Portenoy et al. 1994). However, even the failure of some patients to escalate their analgesic dose over time does not rule out a change in pain or the development of some degree of tolerance. When patients are successfully maintained on a regular dosing schedule, as is appropriate, often the pain does not occur with a frequency that would allow an assessment of whether the level of pain has decreased over time. Thus, tolerance may be a primary "driving force" for analgesic dose escalation or it may develop following the escalation of the opioid dose to manage an increase in pain. In either case tolerance is a contributing factor to dose escalation. The loss of analgesic efficacy as a result of tolerance does not usually limit the clinical use of opioid drugs (Foley et al. 1991; Portenoy 1994). However, the development of tolerance to the respiratory depressant and other limiting effects allows the dose of opioid to be increased through dose titration. This can result in an increase in the intensity of some adverse effects (e.g., sedation or consti-pation) or the appearance at higher doses of other adverse effects (e.g., myoclonus) (Inturrisi 1990).

In contrast to the pain assessment methods used with patients, certain animal behavioral test paradigms such as the tail-flick and hot-plate tests are designed so as to maintain control of the nociceptive stimulus. While this is a desirable attribute, these animal tests do not mimic many of the important aspects of continuous or exacerbating pain seen in many pain patients. How-ever, these and other animal test paradigms have predicted both the clinical utility of many analgesics and their ability to produce morphine-like toler-ance and dependence and thus have an empirical validity. This chapter will provide a brief overview of two new approaches that seek to identify drugs that can prevent or reverse the development of morphine tolerance by modu-lating (i.e., blocking or down regulating) N-methyl-D-aspartate (NMDA) or delta-opioid receptors.

NMDA RECEPTOR ANTAGONISTS ATTENUATE
MORPHINE TOLERANCE

Recent studies (Marek et al. 1991; Trujillo and Akil 1991; Tiseo and Inturrisi 1993; Elliott et al. 1994a,b; 1995b; Tiseo et al. 1994; Mao et al. 1996; Shimoyama et al. 1996) have demonstrated that the excitatory amino acid (EAA) receptor system is involved in morphine tolerance and depen-dence. Since the 1980s, EAAs, including glutamate and aspartate, have been identified as neurotransmitters in the vertebrate central nervous system (CNS). An important aspect of the NMDA subtype of EAA receptor is that it opens a distinctive membrane channel, characterized by voltage-dependent Mg^{2+} blockade and high permeability to calcium ions (Mayer and Miller 1991). Physiological increases in intracellular calcium subsequent to receptor acti-vation can initiate several metabolic changes in the cell (Mayer and Miller 1991; Bading et al. 1993).

NMDA antagonists including MK801, LY274614, dextromethorphan, and ketamine can attenuate or reverse the development of tolerance to morphine's antinociceptive (analgesic) effects (Marek et al. 1991; Trujillo and Akil 1991; Tiseo and Inturrisi 1993; Elliott et al. 1994a,b; 1995b; Tiseo et al. 1994; Mao et al. 1996; Shimoyama et al. 1996). These NMDA antagonists do not affect the tail-flick or hot-plate measures of analgesia (Elliott et al. 1995b). Therefore, these behavioral measures can be used to assess the adaptations that result from chronic opioid exposure and the effects of NMDA antagonists on opioid tolerance. The characteristics of the effects of NMDA antagonists on morphine tolerance, as represented by LY274614, are of interest. The attenuation of morphine tolerance by LY274614 is dose dependent (Tiseo and Inturrisi 1993). Additionally, animals tested one week after the discontinuation of drug treatments (LY274614 plus morphine) retained their analgesic sensitivity to morphine whereas control animals (morphine only) remained relatively tolerant (Tiseo and Inturrisi 1993; Tiseo et al. 1994). LY274614 was administered to nontolerant animals for one week to determine whether such treatment modifies the subsequent development of tolerance. One week after LY274614 treatment was discontinued the animals were challenged with morphine and then implanted with morphine pellets. Comparison of LY274614 and saline-treated animals showed no differences in the expression of morphine analgesia or the development of morphine tolerance (Tiseo et al. 1994). Thus, the ability of LY274614 to affect the development of tolerance and the subsequent sensitivity of animals to morphine requires coadministration of LY274614 when morphine is present and therefore occupying opioid receptors. However, LY274614 administration does not alter the affinity or density of opioid receptors in the rat CNS nor does it alter opioid ligand binding in several standard equilibrium opioid-binding assays (Tiseo et al. 1994).

In contrast to MK801 or LY274614, ketamine is a clinically available drug with noncompetitive NMDA receptor antagonist activity. It is a phencyclidine (PCP) analog with many behavioral effects in common with other PCP-like drugs, including anesthetic, antinociceptive, psychotomimetic, anticonvulsant, neuroprotective, and amnesic effects (Church and Lodge 1990). Although it acts on many neurotransmitter systems, more recent studies suggest that the locus for many of these shared behavioral effects is its activity as a noncompetitive antagonist of the NMDA receptor (Martin and Lodge 1985; O'Shaughnessy and Lodge 1988). Fig. 1 shows that intrathecal (i.t.) ketamine can attenuate the tolerance produced by i.t. morphine. The intrathecal administration of morphine in escalating doses for three days (saline + morphine group) resulted in a large rightward shift of the dose-response curve for morphine on day 5 (Fig. 1), which indicates a significant degree of analgesic tolerance. The magnitude of this tolerance can be

C.E. INTURRISI

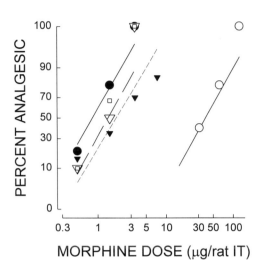

●   DAY 1 CONTROL
○   DAY 5 SALINE + MORPHINE
▼   DAY 5 KETAMINE + MORPHINE
▽   DAY 5 KETAMINE + SALINE
□   DAY 5 SALINE + SALINE

Fig. 1. Intrathecal (i.t.) ketamine prevents the rightward shift in the i.t. morphine (M dose-response curve on day 5). Tolerance was produced by t.i.d. administration of morphine at 10 µg on day 1, 20 µg on day 2, and 40 µg on day 3. Ketamine at 50 nmol or saline was administered 10 minutes prior to each morphine dose. On day 1 cumulative morphine dose-response assessment preceded each treatment. On day 5, the saline + morphine curve shifted 46-fold while the curves for day 5 ketamine + morphine, ketamine + saline, and saline + saline groups were not significantly different from the curve for day 1, which assessed the morphine dose-response relationship before t.i.d. treatment with morphine was initiated (Shimoyama et al. 1996).

expressed as a 46-fold increase in the ED50 value for i.t. morphine from 0.8 µg (0.5–1.3, 95% confidence interval; CI) in naive rats to 38.5 µg (26.9–54.9, 95% CI) in morphine-treated rats. In contrast, the rats that had been coadministered ketamine and morphine (ketamine + morphine group) showed only a slight rightward shift on day 5 (Fig. 1). The i.t. morphine ED50 for the ketamine + morphine group on day 5 was significantly different from that of the saline + morphine group on day 5, which indicated an attenuation in the development of tolerance to i.t. morphine (from a 46-fold increase in the ED50 value to a twofold increase in the ED50 value of i.t. morphine). Control groups (ketamine + saline; saline + saline) showed no difference in the ED50 value of i.t. morphine on either day 1 or day 5 as compared to that of day 1 saline + morphine group. No difference in baseline tail-flick latencies assessed prior to the morphine dose-response assessment were observed between day 1 and day 5 in any of the treatment groups (Shimoyama et al. 1996). Similar results were obtained in mice where systemically administered ketamine attenuated the tolerance seen after systemically induced morphine tolerance (Shimoyama et al. 1996). Ketamine at subanesthetic doses has analgesic effects in humans (Maurset et al. 1989) and may be of value in the management of neuropathic pain (Backonja et al. 1994; Eide et al. 1994; Max et al. 1995; Nikolajsen et al. 1996) and cancer pain (Oshima et al. 1990; Clark and Kalan 1995). The most likely side effects that may be encountered with the clinical usage of ketamine at subanesthetic doses are the dose-dependent psychotomimetic effects (Krystal 1994). The coadministration of a benzodiazepine is known to attenuate ketamine's postanesthetic emergence reactions (Cartwright and Pingel 1984) and may be useful in controlling this side effect. Thus, it will be of interest to learn whether ketamine may improve pain management in opioid-tolerant patients by virtue of its NMDA receptor-mediated effects on morphine tolerance and its direct analgesic effects.

In animal studies the reversal of established morphine tolerance by an NMDA receptor antagonist shows a pattern of gradual reversal over a period of at least two days (Tiseo and Inturrisi 1993; Tiseo et al. 1993; Elliott et al. 1994b). This time course differs from the immediate reversal of tolerance produced by drugs such as the cholecystokinin (CCK) antagonist proglumide (Watkins et al. 1984), which potentiates morphine analgesia. Table I shows the ability of dextromethorphan to reverse morphine tolerance. The morphine

Table I
Reversal of morphine tolerance by dextromethorphan

Treatment	Morphine Day	ED50 (95% CI)	Relative Potency
SAL	1	3.9 (2.8–5.4)	1.00
MOR-1	4	36.6* (25.2–52.9)	0.11
MOR-2	4	36.7* (25.3–53.1)	0.11
MOR-1 + DM	8	8.0*† (5.4–11.8)	0.49
MOR-2 + SAL	8	48.0 (33.5–69.3)	0.08

Source: Elliott et al. 1994b.

Note: ED50 values for morphine (MOR) with the 95% confidence interval (CI) were determined on days 1, 4 and 8. The MOR pretreatment was two 25-mg morphine pellets implanted on day 1 and removed on day 4. The dextromethorphan (DM) treatment was 30 mg/kg s.c. given once on day 4, following the removal of the pellets, and t.i.d. on days 5, 6, and 7. Controls received parallel saline (SAL) injections. The notation -1 and -2 identify separately treated MOR groups.

* Significantly different ($P < .05$) from day 1 SAL Group.
† Significantly different ($P < .05$) from day 4 MOR-1 and MOR-2 and day 8 MOR-2 + SAL Groups.

tolerance paradigm used involved the implantation of two 25-mg morphine pellets for three days followed by a morphine dose-response determination the morning of day 4.

A significant degree of analgesic tolerance developed, expressed as a nearly 10-fold increase in the morphine ED50 value (Table I). Following this cumulative dose-response assessment, the morphine pellets were removed and the treatment groups received either saline or dextromethorphan 30 mg/kg subcutaneously three times a day (s.c., t.i.d.) for the next three days. The ED50 value for morphine was determined on the morning of day 8. The tolerant animals that received saline for three days (MOR2+SAL) remained tolerant (Table I), while the administration of dextromethorphan (MOR-1+DM) nearly completely reversed morphine tolerance and resulted in an increase in the relative potency of morphine. As we have observed in the rat (Tiseo et al. 1994), morphine tolerance, once established, persists for several days following the removal of the morphine pellets. These results suggest that NMDA receptors are required for both the induction and the maintenance of morphine tolerance. Furthermore, they suggest that the induction and maintenance of tolerance involves time lags consistent with cellular biosynthetic processes.

Dextromethorphan also can suppress NMDA-provoked seizures (Ferkany et al. 1988), NMDA-induced neuronal firing of spinal cord neurons (Church et al. 1985), glutamate-induced neurotoxicity (Choi 1987), and the "wind-up" phenomenon (Dickenson et al. 1991). In other animal studies, dextromethorphan suppressed formalin-induced nociceptive behavior following systemic or intraspinal administration (Elliott et al. 1995a).

Central sensitization of the spinal cord projection neurons may be modulated by the release of EAAs, especially glutamate, and the subsequent activation of the NMDA receptor. These neuronal changes may be attenuated experimentally with NMDA receptor antagonists (Woolf and Thompson 1991). NMDA receptor antagonists can block this central hyperexcitability (Mao et al. 1992; Yamamoto and Yaksh 1992). A case report describes the analgesic activity of an experimental NMDA receptor antagonist, DL-CPP (3-[2-carboxypiperazin-4-yl]propyl-1-phosphonic acid), administered intrathecally to a patient with intractable neuropathic leg pain (Kristensen et al. 1992). Unfortunately, this trial was complicated by the development of drug-induced psychotomimetic side effects. Price et al. (1994) reported that the temporal summation of second pain, a psychophysical correlate of wind-up in humans, is attenuated by dextromethorphan. McQuay et al. (1994) used a double-blind crossover design and found no significant difference in analgesic effectiveness between dextromethorphan and placebo in patients with neuropathic pain. The relatively modest dosing schedule for dextromethorphan may have limited the efficacy of the drug in these patients. Because of the established safety of dextromethorphan, clinical evaluation of its analgesic efficacy alone or in combination with opioids will continue.

Studies both in vivo and in vitro are beginning to provide important new insights into the receptor and signal transduction events that appear to be involved in morphine tolerance. During morphine tolerance spinal cord levels of membrane-bound protein kinase C (PKC) increase, while GM1 ganglioside, a reported intracellular inhibitor of PKC translocation and activation, and H7 (a PKC inhibitor) both attenuate morphine tolerance in vivo (Mao et al. 1994, 1995; Mayer et al. 1995). H7 also blocks morphine-induced cyclic adenosine monophosphate (cAMP) superactivation in SH-SY5Y cells (Wang et al. 1994). Of interest are the observations that these same intracellular loci may also be involved in hyperalgesia associated with nerve injury and inflammation (Mao et al. 1995).

The development of tolerance to morphine's analgesic effects can also be attenuated by coadministration of nitric oxide synthase (NOS) inhibitors (Kolesnikov et al. 1993; Elliott et al. 1994a). Also, just as with the NMDA receptor antagonists, the NOS inhibitors can reverse morphine tolerance (Kolesnikov et al. 1993).

How are NMDA receptor-mediated events linked to those transduced at opioid receptors and how might these interactions be related to tolerance? Opioids have both presynaptic and postsynaptic actions (Yaksh 1986). The presynaptic inhibitory effects of opioids on the release of neurotransmitters or neuromodulators (e.g., glutamate and substance P) are unlikely to result in the activation of NMDA receptors that is required for the development of morphine tolerance (Mao et al. 1995). The postsynaptic actions could occur within the same neuron (Chen and Huang 1991) or involve additional neural circuits. While the latter possibility cannot be excluded, as Mao et al. (1995) point out, this circuit would require that the NMDA receptor be activated by EAAs released from interneurons that are excited by means of opioid-mediated disinhibition. A more direct explanation may be found in the observations by Chen and Huang (1991) that within a single neuron, expressing both NMDA and mu-opioid receptors, the magnitude of the NMDA receptor-mediated inward membrane current is enhanced by mu-opioid agonists. They also showed that mu receptor activation results in PKC translocation/activation (Chen and Huang 1992). The translocated PKC then phosphorylates the NMDA receptor and removes the Mg^{2+} blockade, which allows the NMDA receptor to be activated in the presence of an opioid. PKC may be involved in additional downstream events including the modulation of G-protein-coupled K^+ channels and the uncoupling of G proteins at the mu receptor (Mao et al. 1995). Thus, studies described above have linked mu receptor

occupancy by morphine to PKC activation of NMDA receptors, which results in a Ca^{2+} influx and the formation of NO. As shown in Fig. 2, these
events can result in longer lasting changes in gene expression that are the
basis of persistent tolerance and dependence (Elliott et al. 1995b).

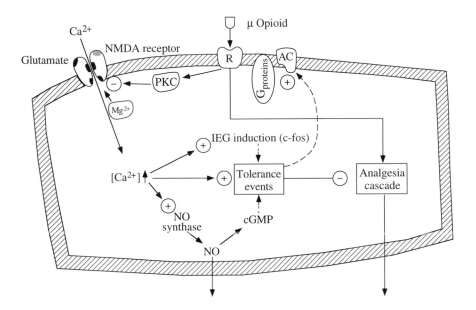

Fig. 2. A scheme that suggests some of the receptor-mediated signal transduction events
that may be involved in the attenuation of morphine (μ) opioid tolerance by NMDA
receptor antagonists or nitric oxide synthase (NOS) inhibitors. Morphine (μ-opioid agonist) occupation of the receptor results in an intracellular cascade mediated in part by a G-
protein-coupled inhibition of adenyl cyclase (AC). This cascade results in the cellular
changes, e.g., inhibition of neurotransmitter release, that are reflected at the behavioral
level (i.e., tail-flick or hot plate tests) as analgesia. Concurrently, μ-opioid receptor
occupancy results in the activation of protein kinase C (PKC), which then phosphorylates
the NMDA receptor and results in the removal of a Mg^{2+} block and the opening of Ca^{2+}
channel of the NMDA receptor. Ca^{2+} influx triggers the activation of several signal
transduction systems including nitric oxide synthase (NO synthase), which leads to NO
production and immediate early gene activation resulting in induction of c-fos, a transcription factor for several genes. Additional signaling events include the activation of Ca^{2+}-
mediated protein kinases. During persistent exposure to morphine these signal transduction
events result in neuronal plasticity changes labeled here as "tolerance events." These
tolerance events include the up-regulation of AC resulting in the accumulation of cAMP,
changes in ion channel currents, and other downstream events. The general result of these
tolerance events is antianalgesic effect on the analgesia cascade (e.g., a loss of the ability
of morphine to inhibit neurotransmitter release). NMDA receptor antagonists and NOS
inhibitors interfere with these tolerance events but have no direct effects on the analgesia
cascade. Note that not all tolerance events are the result of the entire scheme. For example,
activated PKC or activated Ca^{2+} mediated protein kinases may "directly" mediate AC or
ion channel changes. (Modified from Elliott et al. 1995 by permission of Elsevier Science
Inc. Copyright 1995 by The American College of Neuropsychopharmacology.)

ANTISENSE OLIGONUCLEOTIDES ATTENUATE
MORPHINE TOLERANCE

Studies from several laboratories indicate a modulatory role for the delta-opioid receptor (DOR) in morphine tolerance and dependence. The analgesic effects of morphine, which acts almost exclusively at the mu receptor to produce analgesia, can be modulated by delta-opioid receptor ligands. For example, nonantinociceptive doses of the delta-opioid receptor ligands leu-enkephalin, [D-Ala^2,Gluz^4]deltorphin, and [D-Pen^{2,5}]enkephalin (DPDPE) enhance, whereas met-enkephalin attenuates the analgesic effects of morphine (Vaught and Takemori 1979; Jiang et al. 1990; Porreca et al. 1992). A role for the delta receptor in these effects is strengthened by the observation that only the modulation of morphine potency by delta-receptor opioids, but not morphine analgesia per se, is blocked by the selective delta antagonists ICI17464 and naltrindole-5'-isothiocyanate (5'-NTII) (Cotton et al. 1984; Portoghese et al. 1990; Porreca et al. 1992). Furthermore, morphine tolerance produces changes in delta-opioid receptor binding capacity in mice and rats (Holaday et al. 1982; Rothman et al. 1986; Abdelhamid and Takemori 1991), while selective delta receptor blockade by naltrindole (Portoghese et al. 1988) or 5'-NTII prevents the development of morphine tolerance and dependence in mice (Abdelhamid et al. 1991; Miyamoto et al. 1993)]. Physiological and biochemical evidence indicating a close association of delta and mu binding sites, perhaps in an opioid receptor complex, has been reported (Traynor and Elliott 1993) and may account for the interaction between delta receptor ligands and morphine.

We evaluated the role of the DOR in morphine tolerance and acute dependence using an in vivo antisense knockdown strategy in mice (Kest et al. 1996). The antisense strategy involves the use of an oligonucleotide sequence that is complementary to a specific messenger RNA (mRNA) sequence and can attenuate or "knockdown" protein expression. Antisense can provide a highly selective receptor "antagonist" that can be used to identify receptor linked functions (Pasternak and Standifer 1995). Intracerebroventricular (i.c.v.) saline, antisense, or mismatch (a control that is different from antisense at four bases) oligodeoxynucleotide (ODN) that targeted nucleotides 7–26 of the coding region of the DOR-1 mRNA for three days did not affect tail-flick analgesia as measured by the s.c. morphine ED50 value (+ the 95% confidence interval, CI) on day 4 (Fig. 3). When s.c. morphine was coadministered with i.c.v. mismatch ODN or saline on days 4, 5, and 6, the morphine ED50 increased fourfold on day 7, which indicated the development of tolerance. However, in antisense treated mice, the morphine ED50 was increased less than twofold, which represented an attenuation of tolerance relative to saline and mismatch treated mice (Fig. 3). In a separate set of experiments the opioid antagonist naloxone when given s.c. three hours after a single s.c. dose of morphine produced vertical jumping that is indicative of morphine dependence in mice. Three days of i.c.v. antisense, but not mismatch, ODN reduced the incidence and magnitude of jumping (Fig. 4). Thus, antisense knockdown of the delta-opioid receptor can modulate morphine tolerance and dependence occurring at the mu-opioid receptor without affecting morphine analgesia (Kest et al. 1996).

These results demonstrate that compounds that act at NMDA or delta-opioid receptors may provide a new approach for improving pain management. This approach combines a drug that acts at a distinct receptor (NMDA or delta-opioid receptor) to modulate some of the limiting effects (e.g., tolerance or dependence) produced by morphine's activation of the mu-opioid receptor. Studies are evaluating the clinical utility of this strategy.

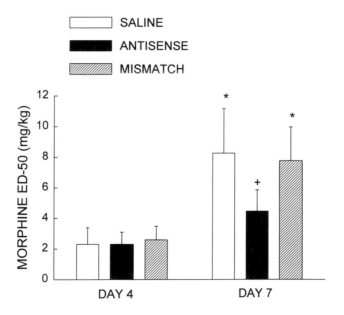

Fig. 3. Effect of delta-opioid receptor antisense and mismatch oligodeoxynucleotides (ODN) on morphine tolerance in mice. After three days of intracerebroventricular (i.c.v.) saline or ODN treatment the morphine ED50 values (and the 95% confidence limits) were determined on day 4 using cumulative dose-response analysis (see Fig. 1). Then morphine was administered subcutaneously t.i.d. for three days at 10, 20, and then 40 mg/kg while i.c.v. saline or ODN treatment was continued. Next, the morphine ED50 values were determined on day 7. *Significantly different ($P < 0.05$) from the corresponding day 4 morphine ED50 values. +Significantly different ($P < 0.05$) from saline or mismatch day 7 morphine ED50 values (modified from Kest et al. 1996).

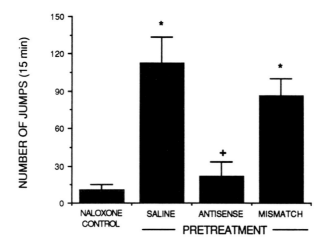

Fig. 4. Effect of delta-opioid receptor antisense and mismatch oligodeoxynucleotides (ODN) on acute morphine dependence in mice. After three days of intracerebroventricular saline or ODN treatment, a single dose of morphine (50 mg/kg, s.c.) was administered. This morphine dose was followed three hours later by naloxone (50 mg/kg, s.c.). The naloxone control group was not pretreated and received saline followed by naloxone. Bars represent mean number of jumps (a measure of acute morphine dependence) during the subsequent 15-minute period. *Significantly different ($P < 0.05$) from naloxone control group. +Significantly different ($P < 0.05$) from saline or mismatch groups (Kest et al. 1996).

ACKNOWLEDGMENTS

I thank Drs. R.W. Houde and K.J. Elliott for helpful discussions. This research was supported in part by NIDA Grants DA01457 and DA01530. Dr. Inturrisi is the recipient of a Research Scientist Award from NIDA (DA00198). The research described in this report was approved by the Cornell University Medical College Institutional Animal Care and Use Committee.

REFERENCES

Abdelhamid EE, Takemori AE. Characteristics of μ and δ opioid binding sites in striatal slices of morphine-tolerant and -dependent mice. Eur J Pharmacol 1991; 198:157–163.

Abdelhamid EE, Sultana M, Portoghese PS, Takemori AE. Selective blockage of delta opioid receptors prevents the development of morphine tolerance and dependence in mice. J Pharmacol Exp Ther 1991; 258:299–303.

Backonja M, Arndt G, Gombar KA, Check B, Zimmermann M. Response of chronic neuropathic pain syndromes to ketamine: a preliminary study. Pain 1994; 56:51–57.

Bading H, Ginty DD, Greenberg ME. Regulation of gene expression in hippocampal neurons by distinct calcium signaling pathways. Science 1993; 260:181–186.

Cartwright PD, Pingel SM. Midazolam and diazepam in ketamine anaesthesia. Anaesthesia 1984; 39:439–442.

Chen L, Huang L-YM. Sustained potentiation of NMDA receptor-mediated glutamate responses through activation of protein kinase C by a μ opioid. Neuron 1991; 7:319–326.

Chen L, Huang L-Y. Protein kinase C reduces Mg^{2+} block of NMDA-receptor channels as a mechanism of modulation. Nature 1992; 356:521–523.

Choi DW. Dextrorphan and dextromethorphan attenuate glutamate neurotoxicity. Brain Res 1987; 403:333–336.

Church J, Lodge D. N-methyl-D aspartate (NMDA) antagonism is central to the actions of ketamine and other phencyclidine receptor ligands. In: Domino EF (Ed). Status of Ketamine in Anesthesiology. Ann Arbor: NPP Books, 1990, pp 501–519.

Church J, Lodge D, Berry SC. Differential effects of dextrorphan and levorphanol on the excitation of rat spinal neurons by amino acids. Eur J Pharmacol 1985; 111:185–190.

Clark JL, Kalan GE. Effective treatment of severe cancer pain of the head using low-dose ketamine in an opioid-tolerant patient. J Pain Symptom Manage 1995; 10:310–314.

Cotton R, Giles MG, Miller L, Shaw JS, Timms D. ICI 174864: a highly selective antagonist for the opioid δ-receptor. Eur J Pharmacol 1984; 97:331–332.

Dickenson AH, Sullivan AF, Stanfa LC, McQuay HJ. Dextromethorphan and levorphanol on dorsal horn nociceptive neurones in the rat. Neuropharmacology 1991; 30:1303–1308.

Eide PK, Jørum E, Stubhaug A, Bremnes J, Breivik H: Relief of postherpetic neuralgia with the N-methyl-D-aspartic acid receptor antagonist ketamine: a double-blind, cross-over comparison with morphine and placebo. Pain 1994; 58:347–354.

Elliott K, Minami N, Kolesnikov YA, Pasternak GW, Inturrisi CE. The NMDA receptor antagonists, LY274614 and MK-801, and the nitric oxide synthase inhibitor, NG-nitro-L-arginine, attenuate analgesic tolerance to the mu-opioid morphine but not to kappa opioids. Pain 1994a; 56:69–75.

Elliott KJ, Hynansky A, Inturrisi CE. Dextromethorphan attenuates and reverses analgesic tolerance to morphine. Pain 1994b; 59:361–368.

Elliott KJ, Brodsky M, Hynansky A, Foley KM, Inturrisi CE. Dextromethorphan suppresses both formalin-induced nociceptive behavior and formalin-induced increase in spinal cord c-fos mRNA. Pain 1995a; 61:401–409.

Elliott K, Kest B, Man A, Kao B, Inturrisi CE. N-methyl-D- aspartate (NMDA) receptors, mu and kappa opioid tolerance, and perspectives on new analgesic drug development. Neuropsychopharmacology 1995b; 13:347–356.

Ferkany JW, Borosky SH, Clissold DB, Pontecorvo MJ. Dextromethorphan inhibits NMDA-induced convulsions. Eur J Pharmacol 1988; 151:151–154.

Foley KM. Clinical tolerance to opioids. In: Basbaum AI, Besson JM (Eds). Towards a New Pharmacotherapy of Pain. Chichester: John Wiley & Sons, 1991, pp 181–203.

Holaday JW, Hitzemann RJ, Curell J, Tortella FC, Belenky GL. Repeated electroconvulsive shock or chronic morphine treatment increases the number of ^3H-D-Ala^2,D-Leu^5-enkephalin binding sites in rat brain membranes. Life Sci 1982; 31:2359–2362.

Houde RW, Wallenstein SL, Beaver WT. Evaluation of analgesics in patients with cancer pain. In: Lasagna L (Ed). Clinical Pharmacology. Vol. 1 of International Encyclopedia of Pharmacology and Therapeutics. Oxford: Pergamon, 1966, pp 59–98.

Inturrisi CE. Opioid analgesic therapy in cancer pain. In: Foley KM, Bonica JJ, Ventafridda V (Eds). Advances in Pain Research and Therapy, Vol. 16. New York: Raven Press, 1990, pp 133–154

Jacox A, Carr DB, Payne R, et al. Management of Cancer Pain. Clinical Practice Guideline no. 9. AHCPR Publication no. 94-0592. Rockville, MD: U.S. Department of Health and Human Services, Public Health Service, Agency for Health Care Policy and Research, 1994.

Jiang Q, Mosberg HI, Porreca F. Modulation of the potency and efficacy of mu-mediated antinociception by delta agonists in the mouse. J Pharmacol Exp Ther 1990; 254:683–689.

Kest B, Lee CE, McLemore, GL Inturrisi, CE. An antisense oligodeoxynucleotide to the delta opioid receptor (DOR-1) inhibits morphine tolerance and acute dependence in mice. Brain Res Bull 1996; 39:185–188.

Kolesnikov YA, Pick CG, Ciszewska G, Pasternak GW. Blockade of tolerance to morphine but not to κ opioids by a nitric oxide synthase inhibitor. Proc Natl Acad Sci USA 1993b; 90:5162–5166.

Kristensen JD, Svensson B, Gordh T. The NMDA-receptor antagonist CPP abolishes neurogenic "wind-up pain" after intrathecal administration in humans. Pain 1992; 51:249–253

Krystal JH, Karper LP, Seibyl JP, et al. Subanesthetic effects of noncompetitive NMDA antagonist, ketamine, in humans. Arch Gen Psychiatry 1994; 51:199–214.

Mao J, Price DD, Mayer DJ, Lu J, Hayes RL. Intrathecal MK-801 and local nerve anesthesia synergistically reduce nociceptive behaviors in rats with experimental peripheral mononeuropathy. Brain Res 1992; 576:254–262.

Mao J, Price DD, Mayer DJ. Thermal hyperalgesia in association with the development of morphine tolerance in rats: roles of excitatory amino acid receptors and protein kinase C. J Neurosci 1994; 14:2301–2312.

Mao J, Price DD, Mayer DJ. Mechanisms of hyperalgesia and morphine tolerance: a current view of their possible interactions. Pain 1995; 62:259–274.

Mao J, Price DD, Caruso FS, Mayer DJ. Oral administration of dextromethorphan prevents the development of morphine tolerance and dependence in rats. Pain 1996; 67:361–368.

Marek P, Ben-Eliyahu S, Gold M, Liebeskind JC. Excitatory amino acid antagonists (kynurenic acid and MK-801) attenuate the development of morphine tolerance in the rat. Brain Res 1991; 547:77–81.

Martin D, Lodge D. Ketamine acts as a non-competitive N-methyl-D-aspartate antagonist on frog spinal cord in vitro. Neuropharmacology 1985; 24:999–1003.

Maurset A, Skoglund LA, Hustveit O, Øye I. Comparison of ketamine and pethidine in experimental and postoperative pain. Pain 1989; 36:37–41.

Max MB, Byas-Smith MG, Gracely RH, Bennett GJ. Intravenous infusion of the NMDA antagonist, ketamine, in chronic posttraumatic pain with allodynia: a double-blind comparison to alfentanil and placebo. Clin Neuropharmacol 1995; 18:360–368.

Mayer ML, Miller RJ. Excitatory amino acid receptors, second messengers and regulation of intracellular Ca^{2+} in mammalian neurons. Trends Pharmacol Sci 1991; Special Report:36–42.

Mayer DJ, Mao J, Price DD. The development of morphine tolerance and dependence is associated with translocation of protein kinase C. Pain 1995; 61:365–374.

McQuay HJ, Carroll D, Jadad AR, et al. Dextromethorphan for the treatment of neuropathic pain: a double-blind randomized controlled cross-over trial with integral n-of-1 design. Pain 1994; 59:127–133.

Miyamoto Y, Portoghese PS, Takemori AE. Involvement of delta² opioid receptors in the development of morphine dependence in mice. J Pharmacol Exp Ther 1993; 264:1141–1145.

Nikolajsen L, Hansen CL, Nielsen J, et al. The effect of ketamine on phantom pain: a central neuropathic disorder maintained by peripheral input. Pain 1996; 67:69–77.

O'Shaughnessy CT, Lodge D. N-methyl-D-aspartate receptor-mediated increase in intracellular calcium is reduced by ketamine and phencyclidine. Eur J Pharmacol 1988; 153:201–209.

Oshima E, Tei K, Kayazawa H, Urabe N. Continuous subcutaneous injection of ketamine for cancer pain. Can J Anaesth 1990; 37:385–386.

Pasternak G, Standifer KM. Mapping of opioid receptors using antisense oligodeoxynucleotides: correlating their molecular biology and pharmacology. Trends Pharmacol Sci 1995; 16:344–350.

Porreca F, Takemori AE, Sultana M, et al. Modulation of mu-mediated antinociception in the mouse involves opioid delta-2 receptors. J Pharmacol Exp Ther 1992; 2.63:147–152.

Portenoy RK. Tolerance to opioid analgesics: clinical aspects. Cancer Surv (US) 1994; 21:49–65.

Portoghese PS, Sultana M, Takemori AE. Naltrindole, a highly selective and potent non-peptide δ opioid receptor antagonist. Eur J Pharmacol 1988; 146:185–186.

Portoghese PS, Sultana M, Takemori AE. Naltrindole 5'-isothiocyanate: a nonequilibrium, highly selective δ opioid receptor antagonist. J Med Chem 1990; 33:1547–1548.

Price DD, Mao J, Frenk H, Mayer DJ. The N-methyl-D-aspartate receptor antagonist dextromethorphan selectively reduces temporal summation of second pain in man. Pain 1994; 59:165–174.

Rothman RB, Danks JA, Jacobson AE, et al. Morphine tolerance increases μ-noncompetitive δ binding sites. Eur J Pharmacol 1986; 124:113–119.

Shimoyama N, Shimoyama M, Inturrisi CE, Elliott KJ. Ketamine attenuates and reverses morphine tolerance in rodents. Anesthesiology 1996; 85:01–10.

Tiseo PJ, Inturrisi CE. Attenuation and reversal of morphine tolerance by the competitive N-methyl-D-aspartate receptor antagonist, LY274614. J Pharmacol Exp Ther 1993; 264:1090–1096.

Tiseo PJ, Cheng J, Pasternak GW, Inturrisi CE. Modulation of morphine tolerance by the competitive N-methyl-D-aspartate receptor antagonist LY274614: Assessment of opioid receptor changes. J Pharmacol Exp Ther 1994; 268:195–201.

Traynor JR, Elliott J. δ-Opioid receptor subtypes and cross-talk with μ-receptors. Trends Pharmacol Sci 1993; 14:84–86.

Trujillo KA, Akil H. Inhibition of morphine tolerance and dependence by the NMDA receptor antagonist MK-801. Science 1991; 251:85–87.

Vaught JL, Takemori AE. Differential effects of leucine and methionine enkephalin on morphine-induced analgesia, acute tolerance and dependence. J Pharmacol Exp Ther 1979; 208:86–90.

Wang Z, Bilsky EJ, Porreca F, Sadee W. Constitutive μ opioid receptor activation as a regulatory mechanism underlying narcotic tolerance and dependence. Life Sci 1994; 54: PL339–350.

Watkins LR, Kinscheck IB, Mayer DJ. Potentiation of opiate analgesia and apparent reversal of morphine tolerance by proglumide. Science 1984; 224:395–396.

Woolf CJ, Thompson SWN. The induction and maintenance of central sensitization is dependent on N-methyl-D-aspartic acid receptor activation: Implications for the treatment of post-injury pain hypersensitivity states. Pain 1991; 44:293–299.

Yaksh TL. The effects of intrathecally administered opioid and adrenergic agents on spinal function. In: Yaksh TL (Ed). Spinal Afferent Processing. New York: Plenum Press, 1986, pp 505–539.

Yamamoto T, Yaksh TL. Studies on the spinal interaction of morphine and the NMDA antagonist MK-801 on the hyperesthesia observed in a rat model of sciatic mononeuropathy. Neurosci Lett 1992; 135:67–70.

Correspondence to: Charles E. Inturrisi, PhD, Pharmacology LC524, Cornell University Medical College, 1300 York Ave., New York, NY 10021, USA. Tel: 212-746-6235; Fax: 212-746-8835; email: ceintur@med.cornell.edu.

Assessment and Treatment of Cancer Pain,
Progress in Pain Research and Management,
Vol. 12, edited by R. Payne, R.B. Patt, and
C.S. Hill, IASP Press, Seattle, © 1998.

19

Nonopioid Analgesics for Cancer Pain: Update on Clinical Pharmacology

Richard Payne

*Pain and Symptom Management Section, Department of Neuro-Oncology,
The University of Texas M. D. Anderson Cancer Center, Houston, Texas, USA*

Two major groups of nonopioid pharmacological agents are commonly used to manage cancer-related pain: nonsteroidal anti-inflammatory drugs (NSAIDs) and adjuvant analgesic drugs. Adjuvant analgesics are a heterogeneous group of compounds that provide analgesia in specific pain syndromes (e.g., tricyclic antidepressants or anticonvulsant drugs for relief of neuropathic pain) or that counteract a side effect of opioids so as to allow continued dosing of the drug (e.g., methylphenidate to counteract opioid-induced sedation). Adjuvant drugs may also be called "coanalgesics," especially when used to provide additive analgesia in combination with opioids.

The basic principles of pain assessment and management apply when using these agents (Table I). A comprehensive assessment of the patient should include a complete history and physical examination and a focused neurological examination. The latter is particularly important because adjuvant analgesic drugs are often used to treat neuropathic pain, and appropriate definition of sensory, motor, and reflex changes on examination often confirms the sites of dysfunction in the central and peripheral nervous system responsible for pain. Adjuvant drugs and NSAIDs are seldom the sole agents used to treat pain, and are more often a part of a multimodal approach to management, which could include the use of physical, psychological, and even anesthetic treatments. The clinician should address a specific pain and consider use of several agents in the same drug class, because sequential drug trials are often necessary to select the best drug for an individual patient. Adjuvant analgesic drugs usually require a several-week trial to determine their utility, and seldom offer complete analgesia; patients should be educated to increase the likelihood of compliance.

Table I
Basic principles in use of nonopioid drugs

---

1. Perform a comprehensive assessment of the patient.
   • Thorough history and physical examination
   • Focused neurological examination
   • Assessment of psychosocial complications of the pain and the underlying disorder

2. Use the drugs as part of a multimodal approach to pain treatment.
   • Physical treatments (e.g., physical therapy, massage, ultrasound for musculoskeletal pain)
   • Psychological/behavioral treatments
   • Anesthetic treatments
   • Neurosurgical treatments

3. Target a specific pain.

4. Use sequential drug trials.
   • Prepare patient for several drugs and to accept partial analgesia as outcome.
   • Perform adequate trial (may need several weeks).
   • Consider drug combinations (e.g., NSAIDs + opioids).
   • Limit side effects (if possible).

ACETAMINOPHEN AND NSAIDS

NSAIDs constitute a large class of compounds with analgesic, anti-inflammatory, and antipyretic effects. Of course, aspirin is the prototype drug in this class. Acetaminophen (APAP) is also considered to be in this class, even though it has only weak anti-inflammatory potency (Hanel and Lands 1982) (Table II). Acetaminophen and the NSAIDs constitute the first line of management in the pharmacotherapy of acute and cancer pain, as recommended by the World Health Organization guidelines (WHO 1996) and the acute pain and cancer pain clinical practice guidelines of the Agency for Health Care Policy and Research (AHCPR) (Jacox et al. 1992, 1994a,b).

NSAIDs and acetaminophen have a ceiling effect to their analgesic efficacy in that increasing the dose beyond this level will produce no increase in therapeutic effect, though it may produce more side effects (Inturrisi 1989). Thus, their use as sole agents should be restricted to the management of mild to moderate pain because severe pain above the ceiling dose of analgesic efficacy usually cannot be relieved. Opioids (alone or in combination with NSAIDs and APAP) are used for severe pain because they do not have an intrinsic ceiling for analgesic efficacy. The opioid analgesics are discussed in several references (Portenoy and Kanner 1996; Foley 1996, Levy 1996; Payne et al. 1996) and in the chapter by Inturrisi. Also, in contrast to the opioid analgesics, these drugs do not produce physical dependence or tolerance.

Table II
Partial list of acetaminophen and nonsteroidal
anti-inflammatory drugs used for cancer pain

Drug	Proprietary Name	Typical Starting Dose
Acetaminophen	Tylenol and others	650 mg q4h p.o.
Aspirin	multiple	650 mg q4h p.o.
Ibuprofen	Motrin and others	200–800 mg q6h p.o.
Choline-magnesium trisalicylate	Trilisate	1000–1500 mg t.i.d. p.o.
Diclofenac sodium	Voltaren	50–75 mg q8–12h p.o.
Diflunisal	Dolobid	500 mg q12h p.o.
Etodolac	Lodine	200–400 mg q8–12h p.o.
Flurbiprofen	Ansaid	200–300 mg q4–8h p.o.
Naproxen	Naprosyn	250–750 mg q12h p.o.
Naproxen sodium	Anaprox	275 mg q12h p.o.
Oxprozin	Daypro	600–1200 mg daily p.o.
Sulindac	Clinoril	150–200 mg q12h p.o.
Piroxicam	Feldene	10–20 mg daily p.o.
Nabumetone	Relafen	1000–2000 mg daily p.o.
Ketoprofen	Orudis	50 mg q6h p.o.
Ketorolac	Toradal	10 mg q4–6h p.o. (not to exceed 10 days??)
Ketorolac	Toradal	60 mg (initial), then 30 mg q6h i.v. or i.m. (not to exceed 5 days)

The minimum effective dose and the ceiling dose of a specific NSAID may vary among patients, however, so that some dose titration may be necessary within a narrow range of doses (Portenoy and Kanner 1996). Patients also vary in their responses to the different NSAIDs, both in respect to analgesic effects and side effects. If a satisfactory balance between analgesia and side effects cannot be achieved with one NSAID, a trial of an alternative drug in the same class may be justified (Portenoy and Kanner 1996).

The NSAIDs inhibit cyclooxygenase, thereby inhibiting prostaglandin synthesis. The cyclooxygenase enzyme converts arachidonic acid into prostaglandin (Vane 1971). Prostaglandins are important mediators of the inflammatory process and may sensitize nociceptors; the ability of the NSAIDs to inhibit prostaglandin synthesis in the periphery may underlie their analgesic properties (Portenoy and Kanner 1996). Recent data indicate that NSAIDs may exert a central action in the brain or spinal cord that may be important for their analgesic effects (Malmberg and Yaksh 1992).

Two isoforms of the enzyme cyclooxygenase (COX-1 and COX-2) are selectively inhibited by NSAIDs (Mitchell et al. 1993). The COX-1 isoenzyme

normally is found in blood vessels, the stomach, and the kidney, while
COX-2 is induced in peripheral tissues by inflammation. Inhibition of
COX-1 is associated with the well-known gastric and renal side effects
associated with NSAID use, while COX-2 inhibition produces therapeutic
effects (Fig. 1). Most NSAIDs inhibit both forms of the COX isoenzyme,
thereby producing toxic and therapeutic effects. Relatively selective COX-2
inhibitors, such as meloxicam and nabumetone, have fewer gastrointestinal
(GI) and renal side effects (Laneuville et al. 1994).

As recommended by the WHO three-step analgesic ladder approach,
NSAIDs or acetaminophen may be used as single agents for patients with
mild pain in step 1 of the ladder, or in combination with opioids and adjuvant analgesic drugs (defined below) in steps 2 or 3 of the ladder. These
agents thus are essential in the pharmacotherapy of acute and cancer pain
and are widely used by the public for general aches and pains. A 1995
survey estimated the annual U.S. sales of acetaminophen and NSAIDs to be
more than $3 billion, with Tylenol brand of acetaminophen accounting for
almost $800 million in sales (Wall Street Journal, 1996).

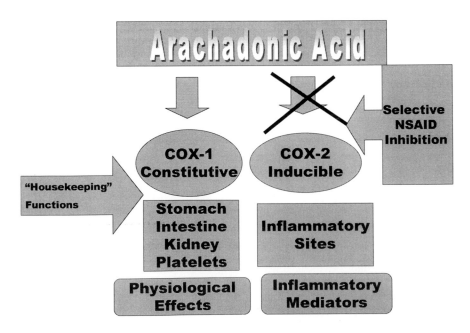

Fig. 1. Pharmacological actions of NSAIDs are thought to be dependent on the inhibition of
the cyclooxygenase (COX) enzyme, which exists in at least two isoforms, COX-1 and
COX-2. NSAIDs that selectively inhibit the COX-2 isoform may still produce analgesia,
but may have fewer serious adverse effects than do nonselective COX inhibitors because the
mucosal integrity of the stomach and intestinal tract is dependent on the function of the
COX-1 isoenzyme.

Acetaminophen is equipotent to aspirin in analgesic efficacy, and is generally well tolerated and not associated with the risks of GI hemorrhage. Acetaminophen is a weak inhibitor of COX, which presumably explains its poor anti-inflammatory potency. This analgesic is the principal metabolite of phenacetin, which was removed from use because of nephrotoxicity; renal failure has been described with long-term use of acetaminophen (Perneger et al. 1994). Acute hepatotoxicity such as occurs during overdosage is correlated with acetaminophen plasma concentrations above 200 mg/ml at four hours after ingestion, and is also probable if plasma concentrations persist above 10 mg/ml at 24 hours (Rumack et al. 1981). Although not as well correlated with plasma concentrations, that chronic ingestion of acetaminophen ranging from 2.5 to 4 g/day is well known to increase the risk for hepatotoxicity. More recently it has been observed that the odds of chronic renal failure doubled for patients who had a cumulative lifetime intake of more than 1000 pills of acetaminophen (Perneger et al. 1994). These data combined with the well-known risks of GI bleeding and platelet dysfunction that occur with acute and chronic NSAID use indicate that these drugs should not be used with impunity.

Many NSAIDs are now available; they differ in dosing interval and cost, and to some extent in analgesic ceiling and safety. The choice of NSAID must be individualized to the patient's needs (Table II). Certain adverse effects are common to most of the drugs in this group. All may be associated with gastrointestinal toxicity, with ulceration and bleeding the most serious complications. A recent meta-analysis of NSAID use compared 12 studies in which comparative data regarding risk of GI toxicity could be determined. In this study, ibuprofen in doses less than 1600 mg/day was associated with the least risk for serious GI hemorrhage. Aspirin, indomethacin, naproxen, and sulindac were associated with intermediate risk, and ketoprofen and peroxicam with the highest risk (Henry et al. 1996).

NSAIDs also inhibit platelet function to a variable degree; aspirin is the strongest platelet inhibitor, while the nonacetylated salicylates, such as choline magnesium trisalicylate, have minimal effects on platelets (Ehrlich 1983). All NSAIDs must be used with caution in patients with coagulopathies, including chemotherapy-induced thrombocytopenic. It is prudent to avoid the simultaneous administration of NSAIDs and corticosteroids because of the significant risk of GI toxicity. Another relative contraindication to the use of NSAIDs relates to their antipyretic effects, which may mask fever as an early sign of infection in immunocompromised patients.

Ketorolac is available in an oral formulation and is the only NSAID now available in parental formulation. Ketorolac may be given by intravenous or intramuscular administration and is often used in hospitalized patients to manage postoperative pain and other acute pains, including exacerbations of chronic pain problems that occur in cancer and sickle cell patients. In patients experiencing side effects such as opioid-induced ileus or delirium, the addition of oral NSAIDs or Ketorolac may have important "opioid-sparing" effects to allow dose reduction and the lessening of side effects without compromising analgesia.

Several studies have confirmed the effectiveness of the NSAIDs in the treatment of cancer pain (Levick et al. 1988; Eisenberg et al. 1994). Of interest, the additive analgesic effects of NSAIDs when combined with opioids as documented in single-dose postoperative pain studies (Houde et al. 1965) have not been confirmed in a more recent meta-analysis of repeated dose studies (Eisenberg et al. 1994). This finding is puzzling because it is intuitively plausible that NSAIDs and opioids given together should have additive effects given their different mechanisms of action. Furthermore, much anecdotal clinical data suggest that additive analgesic effects do occur when NSAIDs and opioids are coadministered (WHO 1996). It is common clinical practice to use NSAIDs and opioids in combination despite the findings of this recent meta-analysis.

ADJUVANT ANALGESICS IN CANCER PAIN MANAGEMENT

As noted above, the adjuvant analgesics are a heterogeneous group of drugs that were marketed and approved for indications other than pain, but that may be analgesic in certain clinical conditions, or that may counteract adverse effects of conventional opioid and nonopioid analgesics. (Portenoy 1993). Three broad categories of adjuvant analgesics are: (1) general purpose drugs (e.g., tricyclic antidepressants); (2) drugs used in specific pain syndromes such as neuropathic, bone, or visceral pain (e.g., anticonvulsants for neuropathic pain; radiopharmaceutical for bone pain; octreotide for visceral pain); and (3) drugs used to counteract opioid analgesic side effects (e.g., caffeine, methylphenidate, phenothiazine antiemetics) (Table III).

GENERAL-PURPOSE ADJUVANT ANALGESICS

These drugs are used for a variety of pains, including those of musculoskeletal, neuropathic, and visceral origin, and also for chronic headache. The tricyclic antidepressants are commonly employed effectively as adjuvant analgesics. It is hypothesized that these drugs act by increasing levels of norepinephrine or serotonin, and thus may enhance the activity of endogenous pain-modulating pathways (Hammond 1985). Amitriptyline, imipramine, nortriptyline, and desipramine all have some analgesic efficacy

(Kvinesdal et al. 1984; Gomez-Perez et al. 1985; Max et al. 1987; Kishore-Kumore et al. 1990) in chronic pain, especially pain of neuropathic origin. The doses required to produce analgesia are generally lower than those required to treat depression, and the analgesic effect can occur within one week, which is much quicker than the onset of antidepressant effects. These drugs are most useful in the management of neuropathic pain states; examples in the cancer population include postmastectomy pain, postherpetic neuralgia, and painful peripheral neuropathy complicating administration of cancer chemotherapies such as vinca alkaloids, plaxitaxel, and cisplatin.

The new selective serotonin reuptake inhibitors (SSRIs), although accompanied by fewer side effects than the tricyclic antidepressants, have a mixed picture as analgesics. For example, one randomized controlled trial using fluoxetine in diabetic neuropathy could not demonstrate an analgesic effect in nondepressed patients (Max et al. 1992), although paroxetine has at least some analgesic effect in the management of painful diabetic neuropathy (Sindrup et al. 1990).

In general, treatment should begin with relatively low doses of tricyclic antidepressants (especially in elderly patients), with a dose increase every three days. For example, a typical regimen for amitriptyline begins with a 10-mg dose at bedtime that increases to 25 mg in three days, and then increases by 25 mg every three to seven days until a dose of 75–150 mg is reached. Sequential trials of different tricyclics should be considered, especially selection of drugs in the secondary amine family (e.g., desipramine or nortriptyline) if the tertiary amine drugs such as amitriptyline are not tolerated because of adverse effects. The SSRIs are generally used as second- or third-line agents because the data supporting their efficacy in neuropathic pain is not as strong as that for the tricyclic antidepressant family.

Adrenergic receptor activation in the spinal cord may produce analgesia through systems that interact with opioid systems (Payne and Gonzales 1998). Clonidine, an α_2 adrenergic receptor agonist can be classified as a "general purpose" adjuvant analgesic because it has been used in neuropathic pain, postoperative pain, and headache. However, as described below, it may have a specific application in neuropathic pain. Clonidine can be administered by the oral and transdermal routes, and recently has been approved by the Food and Drug Administration for spinal administration. Clonidine is also an α_1 antagonist at peripheral adrenergic receptors and can block the effect of sympathetic nervous system activity. It is thus useful as an antihypertensive medication and has also been used to block the sympathetically mediated effects related to opioid withdrawal (Jasinski et al. 1985). Effects of clonidine include dry mouth, somnolence, and orthostatic hypotension when given by oral, transdermal, or spinal routes.

Table III
Adjuvant analgesic drugs used to treat cancer-related pain

Drug Class and Category	Usual Dose	Indications
GENERAL PURPOSE, NONSPECIFIC		
Tricyclic antidepressants	Amitriptyline 10–25 mg p.o. every hour of sleep up to 150 mg/day Nortriptyline 25 mg every hour of sleep up to 100–150 mg/day	Neuropathic and musculoskeletal pain
Corticosteroids	Dexamethasone 4–16 mg/day p.o. (2–4 divided doses) Prednisone 60–80 mg/day p.o. (2–4 divided doses)	Essential for spinal cord compression and brain herniation; also useful in malignant bone and nerve pain
Phenothiazine	Methotrimeprazine 10–15 mg i.m. q6h	Useful for opioid sparing in very tolerant patients and opioid-induced ileus
Marijuana and cannabinoids	Drabinoil 2.5–5.0 mg b.i.d. p.o.	No firm evidence for analgesic effects at usual doses; effects of smoked marijuana as analgesic in anecdotal reports only; possibly useful as appetite stimulant, anti-emetic, and anti-glaucoma agent
USED IN SPECIFIC PAIN SYNDROMES		
Neuropathic Pain		
Anticonvulsants	Carbamazepine 200–800 mg/day p.o. (divided doses) Valproic acid 15–60 mg/kg/day p.o. (divided doses) Gabepentin 300–400 mg t.i.d. p.o. Clonazapam 0.5–1.0 mg t.i.d. p.o.	Useful for dysesthetic and paroxysmal lancinating pain
Antieurhythmics and local anesthetics	Lidocaine 5 mg/kg i.v. continuous infusion in 30 minutes Mixelitine 450–600 mg/day in divided doses p.o.	Usually reserved for neuropathic pain refractory to anticonvulsants and opioids
Topical creams and ointments	Capsaicin 0.075% cream; apply to site of pain at least 4 times a day Eutectic mixture of local anesthetics (EMLA) cream; apply to site 60–90 minutes site prior to procedure	Capsaicin most often used for postherpetic neuralgia; EMLA used often in children

(continued)

Table III—Continued

Drug Class and Category	Usual Dose	Indications
Baclofin	5 mg b.i.d. p.o.—150 mg/day (divided doses)	Useful as second-line agent in neuropathic pain in combination with anticonvulsants; also used in spinal spasticity.
Dissociative "anesthetics"	Ketamine 0.1–0.5 mg/kg per hour i.v. or s.c.	Effects on NMDA receptors occur at lower doses than anesthetic effects; psychotomimetic effects may still occur.
Dextrorphan	Delsym 15 mg b.i.d. day p.o.— 1000 mg/day	Delsym is a single-entity slow-release preparation. Dextromethorphan also is contained in common cough syrups such as Robitussin-DM.
Bone Pain		
Radiopharmaceutical	Strontium-89 4 μCurie/dose i.v.	Dose may be repeated if positive analgesic response and adequate marrow reserve.
Bisphosphonates	Pamidronate 90 mg i.v. over 2 hours, monthly	Inhibits bone resporation and improves bone pain.
Other osteoclast inhibitors	Calcitonin 25 IU i.v. b.i.d.— 150 IU b.i.d.	Also used in Paget's disease, phantom pain, and complex regional pain syndromes such as reflex sympathetic dystrophy (RSD).
Visceral Pain		
Octreotide	Octreotide 100–600 μg/day via s.c. bolus or infusion	Useful for secretory diarrhea and malignant bowel obstruction
Calcium channel blockers	Diltiazam —180–240 mg/day	
Scopolamine	Scopolamine—0.5 mg every 72 hours, transdermal	
USED TO COUNTERACT OPIOID-INDUCED SIDE EFFECTS		
Over-the-counter preparations	Caffeine 100–200 mg/day p.o.	One cup of coffee or 12 oz caffeinated beverage contains 65 mg caffeine.
Controlled substances	Methylphenidate 5–20 mg/day p.o. Dextroamphetamine sulfate 5–15 mg/day p.o.	Act additively with opioids for analgesia and improve alertness.

Epidural clonidine may be effective in selected patients with cancer pain, particularly for neuropathic pain. In a recent study, 85 cancer patients were titrated to pain relief on epidural morphine and then randomized to receive epidural clonidine (30 μg/hr) or placebo, with either group receiving epidural morphine rescue doses as needed. Analgesia was reestablished in 45% of the epidural clonidine group but only 21% of the placebo group, and was more likely to occur when a neuropathic pain mechanism was the predominant pain (Eisenach et al. 1995). Hypotension occurred as a serious complication in only two patients on epidural clonidine.

Methotrimeprazine is a phenothiazine compound with analgesic activity (Bronwell et al. 1996). Analgesic studies have confirmed that 15 mg of i.m. methotrimeprazine is equipotent to 10 mg of i.m. morphine. This drug produces analgesia through a nonopioid mechanism, however. It is most useful in for hospitalized patients with opioid-induced ileus because it can provide an opioid-sparing analgesic effect (Table III). The side-effect profile is the same as for other phenothiazines, and orthostatic hypotension and sedation can be dose-limiting effects. Other limitations to its use are its relative expense and lack of availability in an oral formulation in the United States. The parenteral formulation has been used orally by mixing it in juice.

Corticosteroids may enhance analgesia in a variety of situations, including metastatic bone pain, pain related to nerve compression, and pain from epidural spinal cord compression (Bruera et al. 1985; Ettinger and Portenoy 1988). The response to corticosteroids may be rapid and dramatic, but they are best reserved for patients with advanced disease or for short-term use because of the potential for serious adverse effects with prolonged use.

ADJUVANT ANALGESICS USED IN SPECIFIC PAIN SYNDROMES

Neuropathic pain

Many types of pharmacological agents have been used to manage neuropathic pain. Although tricyclic antidepressant drugs are considered the agents of first choice, in fact, anticonvulsants, systemic local anesthetic agents, topical anesthetic creams and capsaicin, baclofen, and clonidine have been used, either in anecdotal reports or clinical trials. In addition, two old drugs, ketamine and dextromethorphan, are being reevaluated in neuropathic pain because of their ability to inhibit N-methyl-D-aspartate (NMDA) receptors, which are now considered important in neuropathic pain states (Fig. 2) (Felsby et al. 1996). The tricyclic antidepressants were discussed above as general purpose adjuvant analgesic drugs, but they find their most widespread use in neuropathic pain. Finally, cannabinoids have received recent renewed attention as potential analgesics in terminally ill patients such as

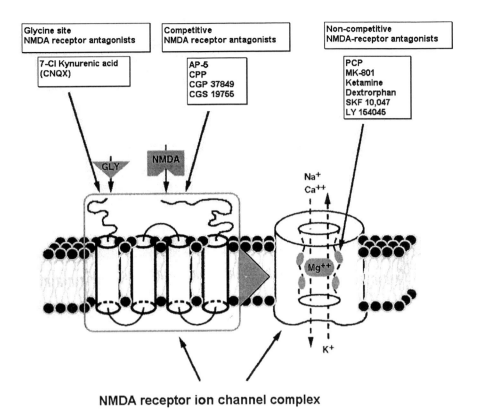

NMDA receptor ion channel complex

Fig. 2. NMDA receptor complex (by Ke Ren; reprinted from Pain (57)1994, cover illustration, with kind permission of Elsevier Science-NL, Sara Burgerhartstraat 225, 1055 KV Amsterdam, The Netherlands).

those with cancer and AIDS; this chapter will review the sparse extant data regarding the analgesic use of marijuana (Noyes and Baram 1947; Noyes et al. 1975).

Anticonvulsant drugs are generally used to manage pain refractory to conventional analgesic drugs and as first-line agents to treat lancinating pain of neuropathic origin (Swerdow 1984). Current estimates indicate that about 5% of anticonvulsant drug prescriptions are written for neuropathic pain (Anonymous 1996). Generally these drugs are given in the dose ranges usually administered to treat epilepsy (Table III). These drugs may produce analgesia through a variety of mechanisms. Carbamazepine and phenytoin act as membrane stabilizers, blocking sodium channels and suppressing neuronal firing. Valproic acid and clonazepam, which enhance γ-aminobutyric acid (GABA)-mediated neuronal inhibition, may also be useful in these situations. The risk of leukopenia associated with carbamazepine may complicate the use of this drug in cancer patients receiving concurrent chemotherapy or radiotherapy. Examples of cancer pain syndromes potentially responsive to the anticonvulsants include cranial neuralgias, postherpetic neuralgia, and neoplastic brachial or lumbosacral plexopathy, especially when lancinating and paroxysmal pain is prominent.

Gabapentin, a GABA analog, is a relatively new anticonvulsant that has received recent attention for its use in pain treatment, particularly for neuropathic or sympathetically maintained pain, or for other complex regional pain syndromes (Mellick et al. 1995) This drug is relatively free of side effects, although drowsiness, dizziness, and ataxia have been associated as dose-related effects, and weight gain and hair loss (Watling et al. 1996) as idiosyncratic effects. Unlike other anticonvulsant drugs, gabapentin has no established therapeutic blood concentrations.

Systemically administered local anesthetics may have a role in the management of neuropathic pain. Intravenous lidocaine is usually given as a 2–5 mg/kg dose over 20–30 minutes. Most clinicians do the infusion while continuously monitoring blood pressure and heart rate. Intravenous lidocaine often provides dramatic relief of neuropathic pain (Kastrup et al. 1987; Rowbotham et al. 1991; Marchettini et al. 1992), but the analgesic effect is usually short lived, although it may persist well beyond the duration of the infusion (Kastrup et al. 1987). Lidocaine blocks sodium channels, but its mechanism of analgesia is uncertain; both peripheral and central mechanisms have been proposed. The efficacy of intravenous lidocaine in the management of cancer-related neuropathic pain has not been established definitively, because a placebo-controlled trial could not demonstrate a difference between lidocaine and the inactive treatment (Bruera et al. 1992).

Mexiletine is an oral analogue of lidocaine that is effective in treating certain neuropathic pain states (Dejgard et al. 1988). Its oral formulation makes it a practical alternative to lidocaine for patients requiring chronic treatment, and it is typically given in divided doses of 150–600 mg/day (Table II). Although it has not yet been shown that a response to intravenous lidocaine fully predicts a response to oral mexiletine, an empiric trial of a local anesthetic is indicated for patients with refractory neuropathic pain; these drugs should be considered second-line agents (Glazer and Portenoy 1991).

Peripheral neuropathic pain syndromes may sometimes be responsive to topical agents. Capsaicin cream, 0.075%, is of some benefit in diabetic neuropathy, postherpetic neuralgia, and postmastectomy pain when applied regularly to painful areas (Watson et al. 1988, 1989; Capsaicin Study Group 1991). Capsaicin often produces a burning discomfort, which may limit its use in some patients. A eutectic mixture of local anesthetics (EMLA cream) may also be helpful in some patients, particularly children undergoing venipuncture or other painful procedures (Stow et al. 1989). This compound contains the local anesthetics pilocaine and lidocaine Topical lidocaine cream was effective in a clinical trial as treatment for postherpetic neuralgia pain (Rowbotham et al. 1996). As they are relatively free of systemic side effects, topical agents represent low-risk interventions worthy of trials in patients with neuropathic pain, and are attractive because they can avoid or minimize the risk of side effects mediated side by the central nervous system.

Baclofen is a GABA agonist that has been used for many neuropathic pain syndromes, most notably in combination with carbamazepine for trigeminal neuralgia that is refractory to carbamazepine alone (Fromm 1994). The drug inhibits firing in spinal trigeminal neurons, similar to the action of carbamazepine (Fromm et al. 1980). Baclofen is also used to manage pain and spasticity from spinal cord injury. A wide range of effective oral doses range from 5 mg twice a day (b.i.d.) up to 150 mg a day. This drug is used in combination with carbamazepine for the treatment of postherpetic neuralgia.

As mentioned above, activation of the NMDA receptor by endogenous ligands such as the excitatory amino acids glutamate and aspartate promotes pain and hyperalgesia following experimental peripheral nerve injury, and blockade of this receptor by drugs such as dextromethorphan relieves pain (Tal and Bennett 1993). As depicted in the cartoon shown in Fig. 2, the NMDA receptor is a complex molecule that can be inactivated by competitive and noncompetitive antagonists acting at different sites of the molecule. Two old drugs, ketamine and dextromethorphan, are competitive NMDA receptor antagonists and produce analgesia in neuropathic pain (Mercandante 1996). Ketamine blocks NMDA receptors and produces analgesia in doses much lower than those needed to produce anesthesia and is typically given by continuous infusion at 0.1–1.5 mg/kg per hour. The infusion can be repeated as needed. Dextromethorphan is an antitussive included in many cough-syrup formulations. It also can be given as a single entity in a slow-release preparation know as Delsym, in doses ranging from 15 mg to 500 mg b.i.d. Better controlled trials of these agents are required to determine the ultimate usefulness of ketamine and dextromethorphan as NMDA receptor blockers in neuropathic pain. Side effects common to these agents include sedation for ketamine and dextromethorphan and delirium for ketamine.

Marijuana has attracted renewed attention as an analgesic given recent passage of voter referendums in California and Arizona that approved use in medical conditions such as pain, cachexia, glaucoma, and nausea. When smoked, the marijuana plant delivers more than 60 cannabinoid compounds with known or potential pharmacological activity, although the δ-9 tetrahydrocannabinoid (Δ-9 THC) metabolite is the most pharmacologically active (Adams and Martin 1996). This compound, Δ-9 THC, is also available as a medicinal dronabinol in doses of 2.5 mg per capsule. A recent placebo-controlled trial demonstrated effectiveness of dronabinol in doses of 2.5 mg b.i.d. in increasing appetite, improving mood, and decreasing nausea in patients with AIDS-related anorexia and weight loss (Beal et al. 1995).

The data regarding the efficacy of Δ-9 THC as an analgesic are less clear. A controlled trial comparing 10- and 20-mg oral doses to placebo and to oral doses of codeine at 30 and 60 mg demonstrated that only the 20-mg dose could be distinguished from placebo in patients with cancer pain (Noyes et al. 1975). Although the 20-mg dose was equipotent to 60 mg codeine, patients did not tolerate this dose because of the associated dysphoria, and the authors did not deem it a useful analgesic dose for that reason (Noyes et al. 1975). There are no studies of the analgesic effect of smoked marijuana, although there are anecdotal reports (Noyes and Baram 1947). Future studies of the analgesic effects of smoked marijuana and Δ-9 THC must account for the difficulties in blinding of treatment and nontreatment groups, and stratification of patient populations for those with prior experience with marijuana, which is a large percentage of the population In summary, the data are unclear as to whether inhaled marijuana or Δ-9 THC have any advantage over existing analgesics in analgesic efficacy or side-effect profile.

Of interest to neuropathic pain is the recent finding of NMDA-receptor blocking activity by the cannabinoid derivative, WIN 55.212-2 mesylate. This compound is a cannabinoid agonist, and in the chronic constriction nerve injury model in the rat, it reversed thermal and mechanical hyperalgesia and modified pain behaviors in doses ranging from 0.43 to 4.3 mg/kg, given by intraperitoneal injection (Herzberg et al. 1997). It is thus attractive to speculate that this drug, or other cannabinoid derivatives, may have efficacy in neuropathic pain states in humans.

Bone pain

NSAIDs used with or without opioids are the drugs of choice for metastatic bone pain of mild to moderate intensity (Levick et al. 1988; Payne et al. 1996). However, radiotherapy is highly effective in relieving metastatic bone pain. For localized bone pain, external beam treatment will reduce pain in up to 80% of patients (Hoskin 1988). Single-fraction treatment appears to be as effective as more prolonged regimens (Price et al. 1986; Cole 1989). For widespread bony metastases causing more generalized pain, wide-field or hemibody irradiation may be highly effective (Salazar et al. 1986). The administration of systemic radioisotopes such as strontium-89 also is effective in treating diffuse pain from bone metastases (Porter et al. 1993). Unlike external beam treatment, where the analgesic response may be seen within days of treatment, pain relief with strontium-89 may not occur until the third or fourth week after treatment. The response to external beam and radio-pharmaceutical may be sustained for several months (Hoskin 1988). Bisphosphonate compounds inhibit the reabsorption of bone and reduce bone pain in lytic bone metastasis, such as is typical of breast cancer (Hortobagyi et al. 1996). A recent randomized controlled trial of pamidronate for stage IV breast cancer showed that this drug reduced further skeletal complications and significantly reduced bone pain, when compared to placebo controls.

Calcitonin has been used in Paget's disease, reflex sympathetic dystrophy, phantom pain, and metastatic bone pain (Roth and Kolari'c 1986). The well-known effects of calcitonin on osteoclasts and its use in the treatment for metastatic bone disease and the hypercalcemia associated with malignancy make it an attractive agent for consideration in treatment malignant bone pain. Calcitonin has been used by the intravenous and intranasal routes, although the optimal dose and route of administration are unknown. Similar to most agents used as adjuvant analgesics, the dose range varies widely. Typically, intravenous calcitonin is given as a 25 international unit (IU) test dose, then in doses ranging from 25 IU b.i.d. to 100–150 IU b.i.d./q.i.d.

Visceral pain

Pain of visceral origin occurs in response to tumor infiltration of thoracic, abdominal, or pelvic internal organs. Perhaps the most common types of visceral pain are related to bladder and rectal spasm and bowel obstruction. Many types of adjuvant drugs have been used to treat the intermittent colicky pain that often results from visceral pathology. NSAIDs, diltiazem, and clonidine have been used for bladder and rectal spasm. Scopolamine and, especially, octreotide, have received much attention for bowel obstruction. A recent review has described the use of these drugs as adjuvant analgesics (Portenoy 1993).

Octreotide, a synthetic analogue of somatostatin, has been given by intrathecal and intraventricular administration to relieve pain in patients (Candrina and Galli 1992; Paice et al. 1996). This drug also has been used to manage nausea, vomiting, and diarrhea associated with bowel obstruction in a variety of clinical circumstances, such as malignant bowel obstruction associated with gastrointestinal and gynecological cancers, radiation and chemotherapy-induced diarrhea, AIDS, short bowel syndromes, and dumping syndrome, among many others (Ippoliti et al. 1997) The drug is given as a subcutaneous bolus or infusion in doses ranging from 100–600 mg/day.

ADJUVANT ANALGESIC DRUGS USED TO COUNTERACT OPIOID-INDUCED SIDE EFFECTS

Psychostimulants such as caffeine (Laska et al. 1994), methylphenidate, pemoline, and dextroamphetamine also have a place in cancer pain treatment (Table III). Methylphenidate enhances the analgesic effect of opioid drugs and decreases the sedation associated with opioid use (Bruera et al. 1987). These stimulant medications are most useful in patients who are receiving adequate analgesia from opioids but whose quality of life is compromised by excessive sedation (Foley 1996).

SUMMARY

Nonsteroidal anti-inflammatory analgesics, and the heterogenous class of drugs collectively known as adjuvant analgesic drugs, are essential medications in the management of cancer pain. They can be used alone to achieve analgesia in specific pain syndromes (e.g., anticonvulsants used to manage lancinating neuropathic pain), but are most often used in combination with opioids to produce additive analgesia, or to counteract a side effect. They can be used at any stage in the WHO analgesic ladder, and the judicious use of these agents often allows successful pharmacotherapy of cancer pain.

REFERENCES

Adams IB, Martin BR. Cannabis: pharmacology and toxicology in animal and humans. Addiction 1996; 91:1585–1614.
Anonymous. Emerging Applications for Anticonvulsant Therapy: Use of Antiepileptic Drugs in the Treatment of Chronic Pain Syndromes. Secaucus, NJ: Physicians World Communications Group, 1996, p 17.
Bauman J. Treatment of acute herpes zoster neuralgia by epidural injection or stellate ganglion block. Anesthesiology 1979; 31:S223.
Beal JE, Olson R, Laubenstein L, et al. Dronabinol as a treatment for anorexia associated with weight loss in patients with AIDS. J Pain Symptom Manage 1995; 10:89–97.
Bronwell AW, Rutledge R, Dalton ML. Analgesic effect of methotrimeprazine and meperidine in postoperative patients: double-blind study in 24 cases. Am Surg 1996; 32:641–644.
Bruera E, Roca E, Cedaro L, et al. Action of oral methylprednisolone in terminal cancer patients: a prospective randomized double-blind study. Cancer Treat Rep 1985; 69:751–754.
Bruera E, Chadwick S, Brenneis C, et al. Methylphenidate associated with narcotics for the treatment of cancer pain. Cancer Treat Rep 1987; 71:67–70.
Bruera E, Ripamonti C, Brenneis C, et al. A randomized double-blind crossover trial of intravenous lidocaine in the treatment of neuropathic cancer pain. J Pain Symptom Manage 1992; 7:138–140.
Candrina R, Galli G. Intraventricular octreotide for cancer pain. J Neurosurg 1992; 76:336–337.
Capsaicin Study Group. Treatment of painful diabetic neuropathy with topical capsaicin: a multicenter, double-blind, vehicle-controlled study. Arch Int Med 1991; 151:2225–2229.

Cole DJ. A randomized trial of a single treatment versus conventional fractionation in the palliative radiotherapy of painful bone metastases. Clin Oncol 1989; 1:59–62.

Dejgard A, Petersen P, Kastrup J. Mexiletine for treatment of chronic painful diabetic neuropathy. Lancet 1988; 1:9–11.

Ehrlich GE (Ed). The Resurgence of Salicylates in Arthritis Therapy. Norwalk, CT: Scientific Media Communications, Inc, 1983, pp 75–90.

Eisele JH, Grigsby EJ, Dea G. Clonazepam treatment of myoclonic contractions associated with high-dose opioids: case report. Pain 1992; 49:231–232.

Eisenach JC, DuPen SL, Dubois M, et al. Epidural clonidine analgesia for intractable cancer pain. Pain 1995; 61:391–399.

Eisenberg E, Berkey CS, Carr DB, et al. Efficacy and safety of nonsteroidal anti-inflammatory drugs for cancer pain: a meta-analysis. J Clin Oncol 1994; 12:2756–2765.

Elliott KJ. Taxonomy and mechanisms of neuropathic pain. Semin Neurol 1994; 14(3):195–205.

Ettinger AB, Portenoy RK. The use of corticosteroids in the treatment of symptoms associated with cancer. J Pain Symptom Manage 1988; 3:99–103.

Felsby S, Nielsen J, Arendt-Nielsen L, Jensen TS. NMDA receptor blockade in chronic neuropathic pain: a comparison of ketamine and magnesium chloride. Pain 1996; 64:283–291.

Foley KM. Pain syndromes in patients with cancer. In: Portenoy RK and Kanner RM (Eds): Pain Management: Theory and Practice. Philadelphia: F.A. Davis, 1996, pp 191–215.

Foley KM. Supportive care and the quality of life of the cancer patient. In: DeVita VT, Hellman S, Rosenberg SA (Eds). Cancer: Principles and Practice of Oncology, 5th ed. Philadelphia: J.B. Lippincott, 1997, pp 2807–2841.

Fromm GH. Baclofen as an adjuvant analgesic. J Pain Symptom Manage 1994; 9:500–509.

Fromm GH, Terrence CF. Chattha AS, Glass JD. Baclofen in trigeminal neuralgia: its effect on the spinal trigeminal nucleus: a pilot study. Arch Neurol 1980; 37:768–771.

Galer BS, Coyle N, Pasternak GW, et al. Individual variability in the response to different opioids: report of five cases. Pain 1992; 49:87–91.

Glazer S, Portenoy RK. Systemic local anesthetics in pain control. J Pain Symptom Manage 1991; 6(1):30–39.

Gomez-Perez FJ, Rull JA, Dies H, et al. Nortriptyline and fluphenazine in the symptomatic treatment of diabetic neuropathy: a double-blind cross-over study. Pain 1985; 23:395–400.

Hammond DL. Pharmacology of central pain-modulating networks (biogenic amines and non-opioid analgesics). In: Fields HL, Dubner R, Cervero F (Eds). Advances in Pain Research and Therapy, Vol. 9. New York: Raven Press, 1985, pp 499–513.

Hanel AM, Lands WEM. Modification of anti-inflammatory drug effectiveness by ambient lipid peroxides. Biochem Pharmacol 1982; 31:3307–3311.

Henry D, Lim LL-Y, Rodriguez LAG, et al. Variability in risk of gastrointestinal complications with individual non-steroid anti-inflammatory drugs: results of a collaborative meta-analysis. BMJ 1996; 312:1563–1566.

Herzberg U, Eliav E, Bennett GJ, Kopin IJ. The analgesic effects of R (+)-WIN 55,212-2 mesylate, a high affinity cannabinoid agonist, in a rat model of neuropathic pain. Neurosci Lett 1997; 221:157–160.

Hortobagyi GN, Theriault RL, Porter L, et al. Efficacy of pamidronate in reducing skeletal complications in patients with breast cancer and lytic bone metastasis. New Engl J Med 1996; 335:1785–1791.

Hoskin PJ. Scientific and clinical aspects of radiotherapy in the relief of bone pain. Cancer Surv 1988; 7:69–86.

Houde R, and Wallenstein SL, Beaver WT. Clinical measurement of pain. In: deStevens G (Ed). Analgesics. New York: Academic Press, 1965, pp 75–122.

Inturrisi CE. Management of cancer pain: pharmacology and principles of management. Cancer 1989; 63:2308–2320.

Ippoliti C, Champlin R, Bugazia N, et al. Use of octreotide in the symptomatic management of diarrhea induced by graft-versus-host disease in patients with hematologic malignancies. J Clin Oncol 1997; 15:3350–3354.

Jacox A, Carr DB, et al. Acute pain management: operative or medical procedures and trauma. Clinical Practice Guideline no.1. AHCPR Publication no. 92-0021. Rockville, MD: U.S. Department of Health and Human Services, Public Health Service, Agency for Health Care Policy and Research, 1992.

Jacox A, Carr DB, Payne R. Special report: new clinical practice guidelines for the management of pain in patients with cancer. N Engl J Med 1994a; 330:651–655.

Jacox A, Carr DB, Payne R, et al. Management of cancer pain. Clinical Practice Guideline no. 9. AHCPR Publication no. 94-0592. Rockville, MD: U.S. Department of Health and Human Services, Public Health Service, Agency for Health Care Policy and Research, 1994b.

Jasinski DR, Johnson RE, Kocher TR. Clonidine in morphine withdrawal. Arch Gen Psychiatry 1985; 42:1063–1066.

Kastrup J, Petersen P, Dejgard A, et al. Intravenous lidocaine infusion: a new treatment of chronic painful diabetic neuropathy? Pain 1987; 28:69–75.

Kishore-Kumar R, Max MB, Schafer SC, et al. Desipramine relieves post-herpetic neuralgia. Clin Pharmacol Ther 1990; 47:305–312.

Kvinesdal B, Molin J, Froland A, et al. Imipramine treatment of painful diabetic neuropathy. JAMA 1984; 251(13):1727–1730.

Laneuville O, Breuer DK, DeWitt DL, et al. Differential inhibition of human prostaglandin endoperoxide H synthetase-1 and -2 by nonsteroidal anti-inflammatory drugs. J Pharmacol Exp Ther 1994; 271:927–934.

Laska EM, Sunshine A, Mueller F, et al. Caffeine as an analgesic adjuvant: review of the evidence. Headache 1994; 34:10–12.

Levick S, Jacobs C, Loukas DF, et al. Naproxen sodium in the treatment of bone pain due to metastatic cancer. Pain 1988; 35:253–258.

Levin AB, Katz J, Benson RC. Treatment of pain of diffuse metastatic cancer by stereotactic chemical hypophysectomy: long term results and observations on mechanism of action. Neurosurgery 1980; 6:258–262.

Levin DN, Cleeland CS, Dar R. Public attitudes toward cancer pain. Cancer 1985; 56:2337–2339.

Levy MH. Pharmacologic treatment of cancer pain. New Engl J Med 1996; 335:1124–1132.

Malmberg AB, Yaksh TL. Hyperalgesia mediated by spinal glutamate or substance P receptor blocked by spinal cyclooxygenase inhibition. Science 1992; 257:1276–1279.

Marchettini P, Lacerenza M, Marangoni C, et al. Lidocaine test in neuralgia. Pain 1992; 48:377–382.

Max MB, Culnane M, Schafer SC, et al. Amitriptyline relieves diabetic neuropathy pain in patients with normal or depressed mood. Neurology 1987; 37:589–596.

Max MB, Lunch SA, Muir J, et al. Effects of desipramine, amitriptyline, and fluoxetine on pain in diabetic neuropathy. New Engl J Med 1992; 326:1287–1288.

Mellecik LB, Mellick GA, Mellicy LB. Gabapentin in the management of reflex sympathetic dystrophy. J Pain Symptom Manage 1995; 10:265–266.

Mercadante S. Ketamine in cancer pain: an update. Palliat Med 1996; 10:225–230.

Mitchell JA, Akarasereenomt P, Thiemermann C, Flower RJ, Vane JR. Selectivity of nonsteroidal anti-inflammatory drugs as inhibitors of constitutive and inducible cyclooxygenase. Proc Natl Acad Sci USA 1993; 90:11693–11697.

Noyes R, Baram DA. Cannabis analgesia. Compr Psychiatry 1947; 15:531–535.

Noyes R, Brunk SF, Avery DAH, Canceter AC. The analgesic properties of delta-9-tetrahydrocannabinol and codeine. Clin Pharmacol Ther 1975; 18:84–89.

Paice JA, Penn RD, Kroin JS. Intrathecal octreotide for relief of intractable nonmalignant pain: 5-year experience with two cases. Neurosurgery 1996; 38:203–207.

Payne R, Weinstein SM, Hill CS. Assessment and management of pain. In: Levin VL (Ed). Cancer in the Nervous System. New York: Churchill-Livingstone, 1996, pp 411–448.

Payne R, Gonzales GR. Pathophysiology of cancer pain. In: Doyle D, Hanks GW, MacDonald N (Eds). Oxford Textbook of Palliative Medicine. Oxford: Oxford University Press, 1998.

Perneger TV, Whelton PK, Klag MJ. Risk of kidney failure associated with the use of acetaminophen and nonsteroidal anti-inflammatory drugs. N Engl J Med 1994; 331:1675–1679.

Portenoy RK. Adjuvant analgesics in pain management. In: Doyle D, Hanks GW, MacDonald N (Eds). Oxford Textbook of Palliative Medicine. Oxford: Oxford University Press, 1993, pp 187–203.

Portenoy RK, Kanner RM. Non-opioid and adjuvant analgesics. In: Portenoy RK, Kanner RM (Eds). Pain Management: Theory and Practice. Philadelphia: F.A. Davis, 1996, pp. 219–276.

Porter AT, McEwan AJB, Powe JE, et al. Results of a randomized phase-III trial to evaluate the efficacy of strontium-89 adjuvant to local field external beam irradiation in the management of endocrine resistant metastatic prostate cancer. Int J Radiation Oncol Biol Phys 1993; 25:805–813.

Price P, Hoskin PJ, Easton D, et al. Prospective randomized trial of single and multi fraction radiotherapy schedules in the treatment of painful bony metastases. Radiother Oncol 1986; 6:247–255.

Roth A, Kolari'c K. Analgesic activity of calcitonin in patients with painful osteolytic metastases of breast cancer: results of a controlled randomized study. Oncology 1986; 43:283–287.

Rowbotham MC, Reisner-Keller LA, Fields HL. Both intravenous lidocaine and morphine reduce the pain of post-herpetic neuralgia. Neurology 1991; 41:1024–1028.

Rowbotham MC, Davies PS, Verkempinck C, Galer BS. Lidocaine patch: double-blind controlled study of a new treatment method for post-herpetic neuralgia. Pain 1996; 65:39–44.

Rumack BH, Peterson RC, Koch GG, Amara IA. Acetaminophen overdose: 662 cases with evaluation of oral acetylcysteine treatment. Arch Intern Med 1981; 141:380–385.

Salazar OM, Rubin P, Hendrickson FR, et al. Single-dose half-body irradiation for palliation of multiple bone metastases from solid tumors. Cancer 1986; 58:29–36.

Sindrup SH, Gram LF, Brosen K, et al. The selective serotonin re-uptake inhibitor paroxetine is effective in the treatment of diabetic neuropathy symptoms. Pain 1990; 42:135–144.

Stow PJ, Glynn CJ, Minor B. EMLA cream in the treatment of post-herpetic neuralgia: efficacy and pharmacokinetic profile. Pain 1989; 39:301–305.

Swerdlow M. Anticonvulsant drugs and chronic pain. Clin Neuropharmacol 1984; 7:51–82.

Tal M, Bennett GJ. Dextorphan relieves neuropathic heat-evoked hyperalgesia in the rat. Neurosci Lett 1993; 151:107–110.

Vane JR. Inhibition of prostaglandin synthesis as a mechanism of action for aspirin-like drugs. Nature 1971; 234:231–238.

Ventafridda V, Tamburini M, Caraceni A, et al. A validation study of the WHO method for cancer pain relief. Cancer 1987; 59:850–856.

Waitling CJ, Allen RR, Hassenbusch S, Payne R. Case reports from M. D. Anderson Cancer Center: Commissural myelotomy for intractable cancer pain: report of two cases. Clin J Pain 1996; 12.

Watson CPN, Evans RJ, Watt VR. Post-herpetic neuralgia and topical capsaicin. Pain 1988; 33:333–340.

Watson CPN, Evans RJ, Watt VR. The post-mastectomy pain syndrome and the effect of topical capsaicin. Pain 1989; 38:177–186.

World Health Organization. Cancer Pain Relief. Geneva: World Health Organization, 1996.

Correspondence to: Richard Payne, MD, Department of Neuro-Oncology, University of Texas M. D. Anderson Cancer Center, 1515 Holcombe Blvd., Box 8, Houston, TX 77030, USA. Tel: 713-794-4998; Fax: 713-794-4999; email: rp@utmdacc.mda.uth.tmc.edu.

Assessment and Treatment of Cancer Pain,
Progress in Pain Research and Management,
Vol. 12, edited by R. Payne, R.B. Patt, and
C.S. Hill, IASP Press, Seattle, © 1998.

20

Alternative Routes for Administering Analgesics at Home

Porter Storey

The Hospice at the Texas Medical Center, Houston, Texas, USA

Controlling pain in the home has become increasingly important as more patients with cancer or human immunodeficiency virus (HIV) are being discharged from the hospital after shorter stays and are dying at home. The routine methods for administering analgesics in the hospital, such as intravenous infusions, injections, and patient-controlled analgesia (PCA) pumps, are costly and their maintenance requires skilled nursing care. Therefore, alternative means are needed to ensure that pain is managed safely and cost effectively at home. Techniques such as radiation therapy and nerve blocks, which are discussed elsewhere in this book, can be effective but have limited indications. This chapter focuses on the assessment and management of pain in the home, particularly in patients with advanced cancer and HIV. The chapter will examine the reasons that oral agents sometimes do not work at home and how to correct this problem. It will evaluate the limiting factors and useful preparations that can be given by the sublingual route, the rectal route, and the subcutaneous route. The chapter concludes with brief mention of some novel routes of administration such as nebulized and topically applied agents.

ASSESSMENT

Improper assessment and poor prescribing are common reasons for failure of oral analgesics at home. These problems can be avoided by developing expertise in the essentials of symptom management (Storey and Knight 1996), making a home visit, performing a careful history and physical examination, and collaborating with an interdisciplinary team (Storey and

Table I
Components of total pain

Physical problems, often multiple
Anxiety, anger, and depression
Interpersonal, social, financial, and family distress
Non-acceptance, existential or spiritual distress

Source: Adapted from Storey 1996.

Knight, in press) to address the physical, psychological, social, and spiritual aspects of the patient's problems (Table I). Pain is multifactorial. Dr. Cicely Saunders (1976) emphasized the concept of "total pain" in which discrete components of pain need to be identified and addressed by different members of the interdisciplinary team. The physician can often identify multiple causes of physical pain with a good history and a careful physical examination. With this approach, problems such as oral candidiasis, constipation, and bladder spasms can be treated specifically rather than with opioid analgesics. Psychological problems such as anxiety, anger, and depression also exacerbate pain for patients treated in the home. It is important to provide appropriate information about the disease and treatment plan, to listen in a kind and caring way, and to use counseling skills to help patients overcome these problems. In addition, medications for anxiety and depression can be quite useful.

Interpersonal problems at home are common. Tension between the patient and the family or between different family members can result in failure to purchase, give, or take analgesics on schedule. Tension and anger can multiply the distress caused by the disease. Although the role of the primary physician and visiting nurse remains pivotal, the contributions of social workers and psychologists can be extremely useful in addressing these difficulties (Rusnack et al. 1990). "Nonacceptance" and "spiritual pain" are terms that refer to the search for meaning, hope, and wholeness in the context of advancing cancer or HIV disease (Kearney 1996). Patients with religious backgrounds may seek answers within their religious tradition (Storey and Knight 1997). Belief systems may emphasize sin as a cause of illness or state emphatically that healing is available to those with sufficient faith. Chaplains and clergy can be enormously helpful in this situation. Although teamwork is often adequate for resolving these problems at home (Storey and Knight 1997), a short stay in an inpatient environment can sometimes be useful for assessing these multifaceted problems.

MAINTENANCE OF ORAL ANALGESIA AT HOME

Oral analgesics are the least expensive, simplest, and most effective way to manage pain in most ambulatory patients treated at home. To ensure their success, it is important that practitioners have a good knowledge of available drug formulations. For example, patients with advanced cancer and HIV may find it difficult to swallow some tablets, such as those containing large amounts of acetaminophen. Many liquid preparations are extremely dilute and require that large volumes be consumed, or they have a *very* disagreeable taste. Some tablets can be readily crushed or dissolved, but breaking, crushing, or chewing slow-release or enteric coated tablets is contraindicated. Consultation with an expert pharmacist can be extremely helpful. Scheduling considerations are also important. If some medicines are prescribed every four hours and other medicines every six hours, the family will be giving medicines roughly every two hours, around the clock, and no one sleeps soundly. Often the result is poor medication compliance, stress, and inadequate pain control. Usually, immediate-release opioids can be prescribed every four hours on a regular schedule until bedtime, when a double dose to last eight hours can be given. Often medicines that are usually prescribed every six hours can be administered every eight or 12 hours to simplify the schedule. The clinician should foresee and aggressively treat complications such as constipation, nausea, or oversedation that would otherwise interfere with the intake of oral medicines. The provision of adequate laxatives, the timely use of antiemetics, and close monitoring of the patient's mental status are essential to maintaining oral therapies.

SUBLINGUAL OR BUCCAL ROUTE

The sublingual or buccal route often constitutes the route of second choice when the volume and taste of oral preparations are acceptable. There is argument in the literature about whether opioids such as morphine are absorbed sublingually. Bardgett et al. (1984) measured plasma concentrations and the bioavailability of buccal morphine tablets (7.4 mg or 13.3 mg) and reported that plasma concentrations and the area under the curve were *greater* for the buccal preparations than the same dose given intramuscularly. These results conflict with those reported by Weinberg et al. (1988), who placed 1-ml aliquots of opioids in acidic solutions under the tongue for a 10 minutes and then aspirated the remainder. Weinberg and coworkers estimated the absorption of morphine as only 18% compared to buprenorphine

(55%), fentanyl (51%), and methadone (34%). Part of this discrepancy may have been due to the acidic solutions used, because the team documented a doubling (to 75%) of methadone absorption when the oral cavity was buffered to pH 8.5. The short study interval and strict efforts to prevent swallowing may also have contributed to outcome. Apparent efficacy in the home may be due to a proportion of concentrated agents simply trickling down the throat rather than passing through the mucous membranes directly into the bloodstream. Pitorak and Kraus (1987), two hospice nurses, reported their impression that patients required lower doses of sublingual versus oral morphine. The water-soluble tablets were well tolerated and less expensive than slow-release or rectal preparations of morphine.

In any case, agents such as morphine, oxycodone, and hydromorphone often appear to be effective when given in a small volume inside the buccal mucosa or under the tongue. Teaching families to give opioids in this way often postpones the need for parenteral infusions, or may serve as a supplement to transdermal or slow-release rectal opioids for breakthrough pain. Fentanyl, an opioid previously available only for parenteral use in anesthesia and in a transdermal patch, has recently been marketed as a raspberry-colored lozenge on a plastic handle so as to resemble a lollipop. The new formulation has been approved by the U.S. Food and Drug Administration for pre-anesthesia use in adults and for use in anesthesia or "monitored anesthesia care" in adults and children. The lozenges are supplied in 200-, 300-, and 400-µg sizes, and the recommended dose is 5 µg/kg in adults and 5–15 µg/kg in children. One study has found they are effective for breakthrough cancer pain (Ashburn et al. 1989).

TRANSDERMAL ROUTE

The transdermal route is an effective and convenient method for maintaining consistent blood levels of nitroglycerin, scopolamine, clonidine, and now fentanyl. The delivery system consists of a drug reservoir interposed between an impermeable backing membrane and a microporous membrane that controls the rate of drug delivery across the layer of contact adhesive to the skin. The absorption of fentanyl into the bloodstream is also affected by variations in the lipid layer, moisture content, thickness, intactness, and temperature of the skin. These factors account for its wide range of absorption rates and the slow but highly variable time to steady-state levels (Portenoy et al. 1993). This transdermal system is useful in cancer patients who cannot (or will not) swallow slow-release morphine tablets and who do not need close monitoring of their opioid intake to avoid side effects. Several authors have noted that the manufacturer's recommendations overestimate the potency of these patches (Zech et al. 1991; Donner et al. 1996; Korte et al. 1996). Clinicians who prescribe the transdermal fentanyl system should also prescribe an immediate-release oral or sublingual opioid for breakthrough pain and should be prepared to escalate the dose, as at least 50% of patients will not achieve adequate analgesia with the manufacturers' dosing recommendations (Ahmedyai et al. 1994). Usual opioid side effects (constipation, nausea, sedation) should be anticipated.

RECTAL ROUTE

The rectal route of drug administration has several advantages for patients who cannot take oral analgesics: no equipment and little patient and family education are required, it is inexpensive, and several adjuvant analgesics can be given rectally that are not available in transdermal or injectable formulations. The surface area of the rectum available for drug absorption is 200–400 cm^2 compared to 2,000,000 cm^2 available in the small intestine. The blood supply of the middle and lower parts of the rectum, however (unlike colostomies), avoids first-pass hepatic metabolism by draining directly into the inferior vena cava. The decreased surface area and increased access to the systemic circulation account for the wide variations in rectal absorption observed.

Morphine is as reliably absorbed from the rectum as it is when taken orally (Ellison and Lewis 1984; DeConno et al. 1995). Morphine is commercially available in suppositories doses ranging from 5 to 30 mg. Hydromorphone 3-mg suppositories are available in the United States, and oxycodone 30-mg suppositories are available in Australia (Leo et al. 1992). The need for frequent insertion and the limited variety of available dosage forms limit the applicability of these preparations. High-dose, custom-made suppositories of methadone are useful in opioid-tolerant cancer patients (Bruera et al. 1992). Although it is an off-label use, the most practical method for opioid administration via the rectum is the twice daily insertion of slow-release morphine tablets, which are inexpensive and are widely available in dosage strengths ranging from 15 to 200 mg. Multiple tablets can be placed in gelatin capsules to ease administration. Both brands of commercially available 12-hour morphine preparations are effective rectally (Kaiko et al. 1989; Grauer et al. 1992). Serum concentration-time profiles following oral or rectal administration of slow-release morphine tablets showed no significant differences in the areas under the curve, although the maximal concentration achieved was lower and the time to maximal concentration was longer following rectal administration, so some dose adjustment may be needed (Wilkinson et al. 1992).

Adjuvant analgesics are often prescribed to manage neuropathic and other types of pain. When crushed tablets, opened capsules, or concentrated liquid preparations cannot be tolerated orally or put through an existing gastrostomy or nasogastric tube, rectal administration may become the route of choice at home. Indomethacin and ibuprofen suppositories are available commercially and rectal naproxen is well absorbed (bioavailability 80%) (Calvo et al. 1987). Valproic acid (in a 500-mg suppository) is absorbed rectally at least as well as by mouth (Yoshiyama et al. 1989). Carbamazepine also is well absorbed rectally from a suspension or crushed tablets in gelatin capsules, but often causes a strong urge to defecate (Graves et al. 1985). Phenytoin 250-mg suppositories were *not* absorbed (undetectable serum levels) when given to volunteers (Meijer and Kalff 1975). Amitriptyline suppositories were clinically effective in one case (Adams 1982), and 50-mg doxepin capsules given rectally twice daily have produced therapeutic serum levels and pain relief (Storey and Trumble 1992).

The following recommendations should be considered to maximize drug absorption from the rectum, especially if commercial or custom-made suppositories are not readily available.

1. The rectum should be relatively empty and moist. Treat constipation first to avoid premature expulsion of the medication.
2. If tablets or capsules are used, instill 10 ml of warm water to ensure that the dosage form dissolves. Use a gelatin capsule if multiple tablets are to be given in a single dose. Avoid enteric-coated tables as they are unlikely to dissolve in the alkaline environment of the rectum.
3. Oral suspensions can be administered with an enema tip fitted to a standard syringe, a small enema bulb, or by putting a 6–8 cm length of tubing (as is used for oxygen administration) on the end of a syringe and guiding it into the rectum with the index finger. Limit volume to less than 60–80 ml to reduce the likelihood of spontaneous expulsion. Avoid repeated instillations of drugs in vehicles that contain alcohol or that use glycols as solubilizing agents (e.g., parenteral forms of lorazepam, diazepam, chlordiazepoxide, or phenytoin) to reduce rectal irritation (Warren 1996).
4. Make sure rectal administration is understood by and acceptable to the patient and family. If the medication is not given, it will not be effective.
5. Absorption is highly variable, so consider monitoring serum levels if desired effects are not forthcoming.

6. Remember that the side effects of most analgesics (e.g., peptic ulcers from NSAIDs or constipation from opioids) occur independent of route of administration.

SUBCUTANEOUS ADMINISTRATION

When patients cannot be treated effectively with oral medications due to nausea, xerostomia, or delirium, they also often resist taking bitter-tasting opioids sublingually or by the rectal route, which may be regarded as intrusive. If a central venous catheter is already in place, it can be used effectively at home with a portable pump. If a central venous line is not available, subcutaneous infusion is usually the most effective and least invasive route in such settings.

This method was first described by Russell (1979) in the United Kingdom for adults and Miser et al. (1983) in the United States for children. A small-gauge butterfly needle is gently inserted under the skin of the upper arm, abdomen, or thigh and connected to a portable low-volume pump or syringe for bolus doses. The volume of infusion is usually limited to less than 2 ml per hour (unless hyaluronidase is added for clysis). Large studies have shown that this method is safe and effective for morphine or hydromorphone (Bruera et al. 1988). Other agents such as metoclopramide, haloperidol, and methotrimeprazine can be added to the infusion to control nausea, agitation, and refractory pain (Storey et al. 1990). Serum concentrations of morphine (Waldmann et al. 1984) and hydromorphone (Moulin et al. 1991) achieved by subcutaneous administration are comparable to those obtained from the same intravenous doses. Cultures of pumps and cost analysis indicate that this method is safe and efficacious in the home setting (Ohlsson et al. 1995). Reported complications include rare occurrences of pneumothorax from needles in the upper chest (Ingham and Cooney 1992) (other sites are preferable) and local irritation at the infusion site, which is relatively common. Usually the needle is simply moved to a new site, but when problems persist, the addition of 25 mg of hydrocortisone (Shvartzman and Bonneh 1994) or 1 mg of dexamethasone can reduce the frequency of site changes. Teflon (MacMillan et al. 1994) or Vialon (Currow and Cooney 1994) cannulas may last longer than butterfly needles but are more expensive and can cause sterile abscess if deep irritation goes unrecognized. Higher infusion volumes appear to be associated with the need for more frequent site changes. Highly concentrated hydromorphone (30 ± 15 mg/ml) did not increase the need for site changes (Bruera et al. 1993). Biopsies of irritated subcutaneous sites have revealed lobular inflammation in the subcutaneous tissue with necrosis of the subdermal panniculus (Adams et al. 1989). In this study skin sensitivity testing for hydromorphone reactivity was negative in patients' biopsies and a dummy needle left in place for five days did not produce the reaction, so the authors hypothesized that a hydraulic irritation effect was responsible for plaque formation.

NEBULIZED OR INHALED ANALGESICS

A few agents such as morphine and hydromorphone are safe and effective for dyspnea when administered in a nebulized form (Stegman and Stoukides 1995). One opioid, butorphanol, is marketed in a commercial nasal spray for relief of migraine headaches. Calcitonin nasal spray can relieve pain from osteolytic metastases (Back and Finlay 1995), and patient-controlled nitrous oxide can be safe and effective for breakthrough cancer pain (Farncombe et al. 1994).

TOPICAL ROUTE

Small studies have shown that a few agents are effective when administered topically. Local anesthetics such as lidocaine/prilocaine (EMLA cream) are effective on intact skin and have been quite helpful in pediatric palliative care. One 69-year-old patient with advanced colorectal carcinoma and perirectal pain that was resistant to morphine achieved complete pain relief from the perirectal application of lidocaine/prilocaine cream (Szanto et al. 1992). For broken skin, as in decubitus ulcers, local anesthetics can be combined with saline to provide comfort during dressing changes. Lidocaine jelly has been particularly useful as a lubricant and anesthetic during Foley catheter insertion. Opioids also are helpful when applied topically (Keating and Kundrat 1996). A dose of 10–30 mg of morphine can be mixed with 30 ml of saline and applied to a dressing or mixed with a hydrogel for application to a wound. We have found this method even more effective than the topical use of local anesthetics.

SUMMARY

In summary, pain can often be managed at home if alternative routes of administration are used in combination with careful assessment and interdisciplinary teamwork. When discrete pains are treated specifically and physician, nurse, social worker, chaplain, volunteer, and physical therapist work as a team, optimal pain management can be achieved for most patients in their homes. A knowledge of the available routes of administration provides the interdisciplinary team with increased options to help these very ill patients, which makes the medical care for the patient and the experience of palliative care for the professional much more satisfying.

REFERENCES

Adams F. Amitriptyline suppositories. N Engl J Med 1982; 306:996.

Adams F, Cruz L, Deachman MJ, Zamora E. Focal subdermal toxicity with subcutaneous opioid infusion in patients with cancer pain. J Pain Symptom Manage 1989; 4:31–33.

Ahmedyai S, Allan E, Fallon M, et al. Transdermal fentanyl in cancer pain. J Drug Dev 1994; 6(3):93–97.

Ashburn MA, Fine PG, Stanley TH. Oral transmucosal fentanyl citrate for the treatment of breakthrough cancer pain: a case report. Anesthesiology 1989; 71:615–617.

Back IN, Finlay I. Analgesic effect of topical opioids on painful skin ulcers. J Pain Symptom Manage 1995; 10:493.

Bardgett D, Howard C, Murray GR, Calvey TN, Williams NE. Plasma concentration and bioavailability of a buccal preparation of morphine sulfate. Br J Clin Pharm 1984; 17:198–199.

Bruera E, Brenneis C, Michaud M, et al. Use of subcutaneous route for administration of narcotics in patients with cancer pain. Cancer 1988; 62:407–411.

Bruera E, Schoeller T, Fainsinger RL, Kastelan C. Custom-made suppositories of methadone for severe cancer pain. J Pain Symptom Manage 1992; 7(6):372–374.

Bruera E, MacEachern T, Macmillan K, Miller MJ, Hanson J. Local tolerance to subcutaneous infusions of high concentrations of hydromorphone: a prospective study. J Pain Symptom Manage 1993; 8:201–204.

Calvo MV, Lanao JM, Cominguez-Gil A. Bioavailability of rectally administered naproxen. Int J Pharmaceutics 1987; 38:117–122.

Currow D, Cooney N. Comparison of metal versus Vialon subcutaneous catheters in a palliative care setting. Palliative Med 1994; 8:33–336.

DeConno F, Ripamonti C, Saita L, et al. Role of rectal route in treating cancer pain: a randomized crossover clinical trial of oral versus rectal morphine administration in opioid-naive cancer patients with pain. J Clin Oncol 1995; 13:1004–1008.

Donner B, Zeny M, Tryba M, Strumph M. Direct conversion from oral morphine to transdermal fentanyl: a multicenter study in patients with cancer pain. Pain 1996; 64:527–534.

Ellison NM, Lewis GO. Plasma concentrations following single doses of morphine sulfate in oral solution and rectal suppository. Clin Pharm 1984; 3:614–617.

Farncombe M, Chater S, Gillin A. The use of nebulized opioids for breathlessness: a chart review. Palliat Med 1994; 8:306–312.

Grauer PA, Bass J, Wenzel E, Wheeler W, Shepard KV. An evaluation of the analgesic effect of Oramorph SR tablets when administered rectally or vaginally in patients with terminal cancer [meeting abstract]. Proc Annu Meet Am Soc Clin Oncol 1992; 11, A1392.

Graves NM, Riel RL, Sones-Saete C, Cloyd JC. Relative bioavailability of rectally administered carbamazepine suspension in humans. Epilepsia 1985; 26:429–433.

Ingham JM, Cooney NJ. Pneumothorax following insertion of subcutaneous needle. Palliat Med 1992; 6:343–344.

Kaiko RF, Healy N, Pav J, Thomas GB, Goldenheim PD. The comparative bioavailability of MS Contin tablets (controlled-release oral morphine) following rectal and oral administration. In: Turncross RG (Ed). The Edinburgh Symposium on Pain Control and Medical

Education. Royal Society of Medicine Services International Congress Symposium Series 1989, 149:235–241.

Kearney M. Mortally Wounded: Stories of Soul Pain, Death, and Healing. New York: Scribner, 1996.

Keating HJ, Kundrat M. Patient-controlled analgesia with nitrous oxide in cancer pain. J Pain Symptom Manage 1996; 11:126–130.

Korte W, Stouty N, Morant R. Day-to-day titration to initiate transdermal fentanyl in patients with cancer pain: short- and long-term experiences in a prospective study of 39 patients. J Pain Symptom Manage 1996; 11:139–146.

Leo KP, Smith MT, Watt JA, Williams BE, Cramond T. Comparative oxycodone pharmacokinetics in humans after intravenous, oral, and rectal administration. Ther Drug Monit 1992; 14:479–484.

MacMillan K, Bruera E, Kuehn IV, Selmser P, MacMillan A. A prospective comparison study between a butterfly needle and a Teflon cannula for subcutaneous narcotic administration. J Pain Symptom Manage 1994; 9:82–84.

Meijer JWA, Kalff R. Less usual ways of administering antiepileptic drugs. In: Schmeider H, Jany D, Gardner-Thorpe C, Meinordi H, Sherwin AL (Eds). Clinical pharmacology of antiepileptic drugs. Berlin: Springer-Verlag, 1975, pp 223–228.

Miser AW, Davis DM, Hughes CS, Muline AF, Miser JS. Continuous subcutaneous infusion of morphine in children with cancer. Am J Dis Child 1983; 137:383–385.

Moulin DE, Kreeft JH, Murray-Parsons N, Bouquillon AI. Comparison of continuous subcutaneous and intravenous hydromorphone infusions for management of cancer pain. Lancet 1991; 337:465–468.

Ohlsson LJ, Rydberg TS, Eden T, Grimhall BAK, Thulin LA. Microbiologic and economic evaluation of multi-day infusion pumps for control of cancer pain. Ann Pharmacother 1995; 29:972–976.

Pitorak EF, Kraus JC. Pain control with sublingual morphine: the advantages for hospice care. Am J Hospice Care 1987; 4:39–41.

Portenoy RK, Southam MA, Gupta SK, et al. Transdermal fentanyl for cancer pain: repeated dose pharmacokinetics. Anesthesiology 1993; 78:36–43.

Rusnack B, Schaefer SM, Moxley D. Hospice: social work's response to a new form of social caring. Soc Work Health Care 1990; 15(2):95–119.

Russell PSB. Analgesia in terminal malignant disease. Br Med J 1979; 1:1561.

Saunders CM. The challenge of terminal care. In: Symington T, Carter RL (Eds). Scientific Foundations of Oncology. London: Heinemann, 1976, pp 673–679.

Shvartzman P, Bonneh D. Local skin irritation in the course of subcutaneous morphine infusion: a challenge (case report). J Palliat Care 1994; 10:44–45.

Stegman MB, Stoukides CA. Resolution of tumor pain with EMLA cream: a case report. Am J Hospice and Palliative Care 1995; 1:19–21.

Storey P. Primer of Palliative Care. Gainesville, FL: American Acacemy of Hospice and Palliative Medicine, 1996.

Storey P, Knight C. UNIPAC 3: Assessment and Treatment of Pain in the Terminally Ill. Gainesville, FL: American Academy of Hospice and Palliative Medicine, 1996.

Storey P, Knight C. UNIPAC 2: Alleviating Psychological and Spiritual Pain in the Terminally Ill. Gainesville, FL: American Academy of Hospice and Palliative Medicine, 1997.

Storey P, Knight C. UNIPAC 5: Caring for the Terminally Ill: Communication and the Physician's Role on the Interdisciplinary Team. Reston, VA: American Academy of Hospice and Palliative Medicine, in press.

Storey P, Trumble M. Rectal doxepin and carbamazepine therapy in patients with cancer [letter]. N Engl J Med 1992; 327:1318–1319.

Storey P, Hill Jr. HH, St. Louis RH, Tarver EE. Subcutaneous infusions for control of cancer symptoms. J Pain Symptom Manage 1990; 5:33–41.

Szanto J, Ady N, Jozsef S. Pain killing with calcitonin nasal spray in patients with malignant tumors. Oncology 1992; 49:180–182.

Waldmann CS, Bason JR, Rambohul E, et al. Serum morphine levels: a comparison between continuous subcutaneous infusion and continuous intravenous infusion in postoperative patients. Anesthesia 1984; 39:768–771.

Warren DE. Practical use of rectal medications in palliative care. J Pain Symptom Manage 1996; 11:378–387.

Weinberg DS, Inturrisi CE, Reidenberg B, et al. Sublingual absorption of selected opioid analgesics. Clin Pharmacol Ther 1988; 44:335–342.

Wilkinson TJ, Robinson BA, Begg EJ, et al. Pharmacokinetics and efficacy of rectal versus oral sustained-release morphine in cancer patients. Cancer Chemother Pharmacol 1992; 31:251–254.

Yoshiyama Y, Nakano S, Ogawa N. Chronopharmacokinetic study of valproic acid in man: comparison of oral and rectal administration. J Clin Pharmacol 1989; 29:1048–1052.

Zech D, Gornd S, Lynch J. Clinical experience. In: Lehmann KA, Zech D (Eds). Transdermal Fentanyl. Berlin: Springer-Verlag, 1991, pp 171–187.

Correspondence to: Porter Storey, MD, Vice President, Medical and Academic Affairs, The Hospice at the Texas Medical Center, 1905 Holcombe Blvd., Houston, TX 77030 USA, Tel: 713-467-7423; Fax: 713-677-7177.

Index

Locators in *italic* refer to figures.
Locators followed by t refer to tables.

A

Abdominopelvic pain
  drug therapy, 209t
  neural blockade, 209t
  neurosurgery, 214
Acculturation, 38
Acetaminophen
  for cancer pain, 290–294
  efficacy, 293
  in elderly, 5
  hepatotoxicity, 293
Acid phosphatase, 262
Acute pain services, 179–180
Adaptation, and emotion, 113–114
Adjuvants
  analgesic. *See* Analgesics, adjuvant
  unfavorable attributes, 204t
Afferents, nociceptive, 223
A-fibers
  in anesthesiology, 176
  in nociception, 175–176, 223
Aged. *See* Elderly
Agency for Health Care Policy and
    Research (AHCPR), cancer care
    guidelines, 17–21
Aging. *See also* Elderly
  body composition, 56
  pathophysiology, 54–57
AIDS (Acquired Immunodeficiency
    Syndrome)
  acute pain management, 179–180
  incidence, 11
  marijuana for, 301–302
  pain and mortality, 149
Alendronate, 266
Allergy, 233
Allodynia, 168
Amino acids, excitatory
  in central sensitization, 280
  in morphine tolerance, 276, 280
  in neuropathic pain, 165

Amitriptyline, 295
Amygdala, 117
Analgesic ladder, 292
Analgesics
  adjuvant
    for cancer pain, 296t–297t
    categories, 294
    defined, 289
    in elderly, 59
    general purpose, 294–298
    for neuropathic pain, 298–302
    for opioid side effects, 297t, 304
    tricyclic antidepressants, 294–295
  home administration, 309–317
    buccal, 311–312
    inhaled, 316
    interpersonal issues, 310
    nebulized, 316
    oral, 311
    rectal, 313–315
    subcutaneous, 315–316
    sublingual, 311–312
    topical, 316
    transdermal, 312–313
  non-opioid, 289–304, 290t
  oral, 58–59
  patient controlled, 60, 180
  spinal, 186, 206t
  topical, 300–301
Ancestry
  defined, 37
  in Hispanics, 39
Anesthesia
  approaches to, 195–210
  techniques, 175–186
Anesthetics, local
  for cancer pain, 198–200
  diagnostic nerve blocks, 182–183
  in elderly, 59
  indications, 199t
  for neuropathic pain, 300
Angina
  analgesia, 148–149
  pain interactions, *147*

Angina *(cont.)*
  as pain model, 146–149
Animal models, 135–142
Anticonvulsants, 299
Antidepressants
  in elderly, 59
  tricyclic
    as adjuvant analgesics, 294–295
    for central pain lesions, 162, 165
    dosage, 295
    for neuropathic pain, 298–299
    pharmacodynamics, 294–295
Antisense oligonucleotides, 282–284
Argentina, 6–9
Arginine-glycine-aspartate sequence,
      263–264
Aspirin, 290
Assimilation, 38
Autonomic nervous system, 124

B
Back pain
  brachial plexus in, 80, 82–86
  in degenerative spinal disease, 68
  leptomeningeal disease in, 80, *81–82*
  lumbosacral plexus in, 86–88
  from neoplasm metastasis, 73, 75
  osteomyelitis in, *79, 80*
  radiation-induced, 68–72
  radiologic imaging, 67–89
  vertebral fractures in, 72–77
  vertebral inflammation in, 78–79
Baclofen, 301
Batimastat, 260–261
Behavior
  and emotions, 114
  exploratory, 139–140
  hypothalamo-pituitary-adrenocortical
      axis in, 124
Bisphosphonates, 265–266, 271
Blood-brain barrier, *230*
Body composition, 56
Bone abnormalities, radiation-induced,
      68–72
Bone marrow, 261
Bone matrix, *262*
Bone metastasis
  bone pain management, 269–272
  bone scans, 261
  bony reaction, 262
  cell surface receptors, 263–164
  experimental therapeutics, 264–266
  incidence, 257, 269
  lytic lesions, 263
  marrow displacement, 261

  mechanisms, 257–267
  pain management, *270*
  pathophysiology, 261–264
  resorption in, 261, 263
Bone morphogenetic proteins, 262
Bone pain
  adjuvant analgesics, 271–272, 297t
  corticosteroids for, 272
  management, 302–303
    in bone metastasis, 269–272
    flowchart, *270*
    with radiopharmaceuticals, 270
  in metastasis, 261
  in metastatic carcinoma, 257
  radiotherapy, 269, 302
Bone resorption
  bisphosphonates for, 265–266
  calcitonin for, 265
  cytokine mediation, 263
  etidronate for, 265
  in Ewing's sarcoma, 263
  in lymphoma, 263
  in metastasis, 261
  osteoclastic, 265–266
Bone scans
  in metastasis, 261
  spinal, 67
Brachial plexus
  anatomy, *83*
  in back pain, 80, 82–86
  fibrosis, radiation-induced, *84*
  neurofibroma in, 86
  radiation injuries, 83
Breast neoplasms, *82*
Brief Pain Inventory, 91
Brudzinski's sign, 249
Butamben, 176

C
Caffeine, 304
Calcitonin
  for bone pain, 272, 303
  for bone resorption, 265
Calcitonin gene-related peptide, 262
Calcium channel blockers, 254
Cancer. *See also* Specific types
  incidence, 11
  metabolism, 153–154
  metastasis. *See* Metastasis
  radiation-induced, 68
Cancer pain
  acute care, 179–180
  analgesia and anesthesia
    approaches to, 195–210
    management role, 196–197

study design, 186
techniques, 175–186
analgesics
adjuvant, 294–304, 296t–297t
non-opioid, 289–304
nonsteroidal anti-inflammatory
drugs, 290–294
anesthetics, local, 198–200
assessment, *23*
celiac plexus block, 184
clinical model, 175–176
electrical stimulation for, 200
incidence, 6, 17, 213
interventional therapies, 196–197
management
guidelines, 17–30, 42
integrated, 180–181
services for, 177–180
marijuana for, 301–302
neural blockade, 182t
diagnostic, 182–183
drug therapy integration, 197–198
neuroablation for, 200–208
neuropathic. *See* Neuropathic pain
neurosurgery for, 213–219
outcome measures, 195–196
palliative care, 3–16
in Argentina, 6–9
in Columbia, 11–15
patient education, 25–29
psychological interventions, 109–132
and survival, 150–151
undertreatment, 42
Cannabinoids, 301–302
Capsaicin, 300–301
Carbamazepine
adverse effects, 300
for neuropathic pain, 162, 299
Caregivers
characteristics, 61
for elderly, 60–63
Catheters
percutaneous, 236–237
Totally implanted, 237
CD44, 263
Celiac plexus block. *See also* Nerve
block
effectiveness, 184
evidence ratings, 185t
outcome, 208
in pancreatic cancer, 153
techniques, 184–185
Cell lines, 264–265
Cell surface receptors, 263–164
Central nervous system

aging and, 54–55
pain mechanisms, 165–166
Centro de Cuidados Paliativos, 8, 9t
Cervix neoplasms, *88*
Chest pain, 146–149
Chest syndrome, 150
Chlorobutanol, 242
Cholecystokinin, 165
Chronic pain, 295
Clinical practice guidelines, 17–30
content, 21–22
criteria, 18t
development rationale, 17–22
evidence-based, 19, 20t
implementation barriers, 22, 24–25
peer review process, 21
Clinical trials
design, 189–193
efficacy vs. safety in, 190
ethics, 192–193
placebo
controls, 189–190
properties, 190–192
Clodronate, 266
Clonazepam, 299
Clonidine
administration and dosage, 295, 298
epidural, 298
intrathecal administration, 254
Coagulopathy, 233
Cognition
in elderly pain assessment, 57–58
and emotion, 118
Colonic neoplasms, 260–261
Columbia
AIDS incidence, 11
cancer incidence, 11
drug legislation, 13–14
illegal drug trade, 13–15
opioid availability, 12–13
palliative care, 11–15
Conditioning
classical, 116
emotional response, 117
pain phobia, 116–118
Constipation, 252
Coping skills, 127
Cordotomy, 216–217
Corticosteroids, 272, 298
Cost-effectiveness analysis, 100–102
COX inhibitors, 291–292, 293
Cross-cultural comparisons, 37–38
Cryoanalgesia, 206–207
Culture
assessment tools, 44–45

Culture *(cont.)*
  and assimilation, 38
  in pain assessment, 35, 43–48, 103
  terminology, 37–38
  as world view, 36–38
Cyclooxygenase inhibitors, 291–292
Cytokines, 263

D
Decision making, medical, 91–104
  clinical outcome evaluation, 93–94
  clinical perspective, 92
  cost-effectiveness analysis, 100–102
  decision analysis tools, 92–93
  pain health state evaluation, 94–95
  prescriptive aspects, 92
  principles, 106
  in terminal illness, 106–107
  utility assessment, 93–94
    process, 95–100
    quality-adjusted life year in, 94, 100
    standard gamble, 96–97
    visual analog rating scale in, 99, *100*
Deep brain stimulation, 200
Depression, 153
Desipramine, 295
Dextroamphetamine, 304
Dextromethorphan
  in morphine tolerance, 279–281
  for neuropathic pain, 301
Dextrorphan, 254
DL-CPP, 279–281
Dorsal horn
  anatomy, 226–228
  input modulation, *226*
  marginal zone, 226, *227*
  sensory processing, 223
  substantia gelatinosa, 227
Dose-response, 275
Drug delivery systems, implanted
  complications, 247–250
  constant infusion system, *239*
  infusate selection, 241–242
  intracerebroventricular, 239
  intraoperative bleeding, 247–248
  mechanical pump, 238
  mental confusion and, 241
  percutaneous catheters, 236–237
  placement techniques, 243–247
  postoperative bleeding, 248
  programmable infusion system, *239,*
    240
  selection of, 234–241
  types of, 234, 236t

Drug therapy
  for abdominopelvic pain, 209t
  adjuvant. *See also* Analgesics,
    adjuvant
    unfavorable attributes, 204t
  failure measures, 207t
  favorable attributes, 203t
  integration with neural blockade, 197–
    198
  patient attitude in, 204
  rectal administration, 12–13, 313–315
  unfavorable attributes, 204t
Drug tolerance
  in drug delivery system implantation,
    250–251
  to morphine, 276–285
  to opioids, 275–276
Drugs
  availability of, 4
  illegal
    in Columbia, 13–15
    drug control agencies, 12
    and palliative care, 11–15
    Single Convention on Narcotic
      Drugs, 11–12
    legislation, 13–14
    national policy, 4
Dural puncture, 249
Dysesthetic pain, delayed-onset, 217
Dysphoria, 252

E
Education, and palliative care, 4, 5
Elderly. *See also* Aging
  adjuvant analgesics in, 59
  alternative care facilities, 60–63
  caregivers for, 60–63
  defined, 53
  demographics, 53
  functionally impaired, 60–61
  nonsteroidal anti-inflammatory drugs
    in, 58–59
  opioids in, 59
  oral analgesics for, 58–59
  pain assessment, 57–58
  pain epidemiology, 54
  pain management, 53–63
    nonpharmacologic, 59–60
  transdermal fentanyl in, 59
  underreporting of pain, 57
Emotions
  adaptive functions, 113–114
  basic types, 112t
  and behavior, 114

cognition and, 118
definitions, 111–113
in learning, 116–118
memory and, 116–118
neuroanatomy, 114–116
and pain, 126, 153
Ethics, professional, 192–193
Ethnicity
in Hispanics, 39
vs. culture, 37
Etidronate, 266
EuroQol instrument, 94
Ewing's sarcoma, 263
Excitatory amino acids
in central sensitization, 280
in morphine tolerance, 276, 280
in neuropathic pain, 165
Exercise, 50
Exploratory behavior, 140

F
FACT (Functional Assessment of Cancer
Therapy), 91
Failure, defined, 204
Family relations
in Hispanics, 40–41
and pain management, 45–47
FEMEBA, 6–9
Fentanyl
intraspinal, 241
transdermal, 59, 313
Fibroblast growth factor, 262
Fluoxetine, 295
Functional Assessment of Cancer
Therapy (FACT), 91
Functional evaluation, 57

G
Gabapentin, 300
Gastrointestinal disorders, 252
Gastrointestinal system, 56
Gate control theory, 109–110
Geriatric patients. *See* Elderly
GM1 ganglioside, 281
Guidelines, clinical practice. *See* Clinical
practice guidelines

H
H-7, 281
Headache, 249
Health care interventions, 102t
Health economics, 100–102
Health Utilities Index, 95
Hematoma, 248
Hemorrhage, operative, 247–248

Hepatotoxicity, of acetaminophen, 293
Hispanics
acculturation, 38
demographics, 38–41
ethnicity, 39
family relations, 40–41
pain assessment, 35–49
barriers, 43–48
cultural factors, 45–48
family role, 45–47
steps in, 48t
support systems, 47t
values, 40–41
Home care
analgesia administration, 309–317
buccal, 311–312
inhaled, 316
nebulized, 316
oral, 311
rectal, 313–315
subcutaneous, 315–316
sublingual, 311–312
topical, 316
transdermal, 312–313
assessment, 309–310
of cancer pain, 7–9
interpersonal issues, 310
and patient compliance, 311
Hydroxamates, 260
Hygroma, 248
Hypercalcemia, systemic, 261
Hyperesthesia, 253
Hypnosis, 126–127
Hypothalamo-pituitary-adrenocortical
(HPA) axis, *123*
and behavior, 124
feedback activation, *123*
paraventricular nucleus, 122–123
and stress, 124
and ventral noradrenergic bundle,
122–124
Hypothalamus, 124

I
Ibandronate, 266
Imipramine, 295
Immunosuppression, 140–141
Implanted devices. *See* Drug delivery
systems, implanted
INCB (International Narcotics Control
Board), 12
Infusion pumps
constant infusion system, 238
programmable, 239, *240*
totally implanted, 238–239

Institute of Medicine, clinical practice guidelines, 17–18
Insufficiency fractures, radiation-induced, 68, 70–72
Integrins, 263–264
Interleukins
    in bone resorption, 263
    in hyperalgesia, 135–136
International Narcotics Control Board (INCB), 12
Intrathecal opioids. *See* Opioids, intrathecal
Islet cells, 227

K
Kernig's sign, 249
Ketamine
    for cancer pain, 182
    in morphine tolerance, 277–279, *278*
    for neuropathic pain, 165, 301
Ketorolac, 293–294
Kidney function, 55–56
Killer cells, natural. *See* Natural killer cells

L
Laminae, Rexed's, 226–227
Latin America, palliative care, 3–16
League table, of health care interventions, 102t
Learning
    by association, 116
    and emotions, 116–118
    operant, 116
    reinforcement in, 116
Leptomeningeal disease, 80, *81–82*
Lidocaine
    for cancer pain, 162–163
    for neuropathic pain, 162, 300
    topical administration, 301
Life expectancy
    and intrathecal opioids, 233
    and neuroablation, 201
    and pain management, 151–152
Lignocaine, 182
Limbic brain, 114–116
Liver
    acetaminophen toxicity, 293
    function in elderly, 56–57
Liver enzymes, 56–57
Lobotomy, 115
Locus coeruleus
    and dorsal noradrenergic bundle, 120–122
    neuroanatomy, 120–121

in nociception, 120
Lumbar radiculopathy, *82*
Lumbosacral plexus
    anatomy, 86, *87*
    in back pain, 86–88
    in cervix carcinoma, *88*
    neurofibromas in, 88, *89*
    in pelvic neoplasms, 88
Lung neoplasms
    back pain in, 73
    cell line 1, 264–265
    experimental therapeutics, 264–266
    invading brachial plexus, *85*
    metastasis, *78*
        to bone, 258
        from osteosarcoma, 258
LY274614, 277
Lymphoma, of bone, 263

M
MADB106 tumor cells
    culture, 137–138
    lung retention, 139–140
    neoplasm metastasis, 136
Magnetic resonance imaging (MRI)
    in metastasis diagnosis, 68
    of spine, *73–76*
Marijuana, 301–302
Memory, and emotions, 116–118
Meningitis, 249
Mental status, in opioid therapy, 233, 252–253
Meperidine, 56, 59
Metalloproteinases
    matrix, 259t
        binding domains, 260
        drug effects, 260–261
        in neoplasm metastasis, 259–261
    tissue inhibitors, 260
Metastasis
    to bone. *See* Bone metastasis
    cellular properties, 258
    killer cells for, 136
    from lung carcinoma, *78*
    MADB106 model, 136
    magnetic resonance imaging diagnosis, 68
    matrix metalloproteinases in, 259–261
    organ specificity, 258
    "seed and soil" hypothesis, 257–258
    surgically induced, 138–140
        morphine effects on, 138–139
        pain effects on, 141–142
    vertebral fractures in, 72–77
Methotrimeprazine, 298

Methylphenidate, 304
Mexiletine, 162, 163, 300
Mitoxanthrone, 272
Models
    pain neuroimmunology, 135–142
    pain survival, 146–149
Mood, and pain, 153–154
Morphine
    challenge, 234
    consumption, in Latin America, 5t
    intraspinal, 241
    pre- vs. postoperative, 139–140
    rectal administration, 313–314
    and surgically induced metastasis,
        138–139
    tolerance
        antisense oligonucleotides in, 282–
            284
        delta opioid receptors in, 282–284,
            285
        excitatory amino acids in, 280
        NMDA antagonists and, 276–282
        protein kinase C inhibitors in, 281–
            282
        signal transduction, 281, 283
Mortality, and pain, 135–156
    in AIDS, 149
    in cancer, 150–151
    emotions in, 153–154
    models, 146–149
    in sickle cell disease, 150
Myelotomy, midline C1-C2, 217
Myocardial ischemia
    analgesia, 148–149
    stress response, 147

N
Natural killer cells
    immunosuppression, 154
    metastasis control, 136–137
    pain management and, 154
    surgery effects on, 138–140
    surgical suppression, 140–142
Nausea, 252
Neoplasm metastasis. *See* Metastasis
Neoplasms. *See* Cancer; specific
    neoplasm types.
Nerve block. *See also* Celiac plexus block
    in cancer pain, 182t, 182–183
    diagnostic, 182–183
    early implementation, 209t
    indications for, 200–201
    integration with drug therapy, 197–
        198
Nervi nervorum, 164

Nervous system, aging and, 54–55
Neural activity, ectopic, 162
Neural blockade. *See* Nerve block
Neural compression, 164
Neuroablation
    attributes, 205t
    for cancer pain, 200–208
    controlled studies, 209–210
    early consideration of, 208t
    limitations, 205t
Neuroanatomy, 114–116
Neurofibroma
    in brachial plexus, 86
    in lumbosacral plexus, 88, 89
Neuroimmunology, of pain, 135–142
Neuroleptics, 59
Neurolysis
    adverse effects, 202–203
    indications, 202t
    opioid therapy with, 195–196
    outcomes, 195–196, 206–208
    subarachnoid, 184–185
Neuronal-specific calcium channel
        blockers, 254
Neurons, in aging, 54–55
Neuropathic pain, 159–170
    in cancer patients, 159–161
        clinical syndromes, 160t
        dimensions of, 167
        M.D. Anderson Cancer Center
            Neuropathic Pain Questionnaire,
            167, 168
        multidimensional assessment, 167
        numbness, 167
        paroxysms, 166–167
        patient history, 166–167
        physical examination, 167–169
        prophylactic therapy, 166
        vs. noncancer population, 159–161
    clinical assessment, 166–169
    clinical features, 161t
    drug therapy
        adjuvant analgesics, 296t–297t,
            298–302
        anticonvulsants, 299
        lidocaine, 162
        local anesthetics, 300
        marijuana, 301–302
        topical agents, 300–301
        tricyclic antidepressants, 162, 165,
            295, 298–299
    excitatory amino acids in, 165
    mechanisms, 161t, 162–166
        central, 165–166
        nervi nervorum, 164

Neuropathic pain *(cont.)*
　neurogenic inflammation, 163–164
　neuromodulator up-regulation, 165
　neuropathy symptom score, 169
　neurosurgery for, 215
　physical examination, 167–169
　plasticity in, 165–166
　positive vs. negative symptoms, 167–168
　quantitative sensory testing, 169
　refractive nature of, 165–166
　sodium channel abnormalities in, 162–163
　static vs. dynamic allodynia, 168
　sympathetic dysfunction in, 163
Neurosurgery
　for abdominopelvic pain, 214
　for cancer pain, 213–219
　guidelines
　　generic, 214
　　procedure-specific, 214–216
　intervention sites, 214
　for neuropathic pain, 215
　patient criteria, 215
　procedures, 216–219
　for visceral pain, 215
Nitric oxide synthase inhibitors, 281
Nm23 (nonmetastatic 23), 261
N-methyl-D-aspartate (NMDA) antagonists
　intrathecal administration, 254
　in morphine tolerance, 276–282
　for neuropathic pain, 301
　in opioid tolerance, 165
Nociception
　A-fibers in, 175–176
　age-associated changes, 55
　anatomy, 223–226
　central noradrenergic processing, 119
　locus coeruleus in, 120–121
Nociceptive pathways, 119–120
　anatomy, 224–225
　ascending, 224–225
　central mechanisms, 119
　descending, 226
Nonmetastatic 23 (Nm23), 261
Nonsteroidal anti-inflammatory drugs
　　(NSAIDs)
　adverse effects, 293
　for cancer pain, 290–294, 291t
　clinical trials, 59
　cyclooxygenase inhibition by, 291
　efficacy, 294
　in elderly, 58–59
　gastrointestinal effects, 293
　usage of, 289

Noradrenergic pathways
　dorsal bundle, 120–122
　locus coeruleus, 119, 120–122
　ventral bundle, 122–124
Nortriptyline, 295
NSAIDs. *See* Nonsteroidal anti-
　　inflammatory drugs (NSAIDs)
Nursing homes
　elderly population, 61–62
　pain management in, 62–63

O

Ocreotide, 303
Oligonucleotides, antisense, 282–284
Opioid receptors
　anatomy, 228
　of dorsal horn, 228, 230
Opioids
　administration, 228
　availability of, 4, 5, 12–13
　delta receptors, 282–284, *285*
　distribution of, 11–12
　epidural, 235, 236
　intraspinal, 199–200
　　administration and dosage, 241
　　advantages, 231–232
　　adverse effects, 251–253
　　continuous infusion vs. bolus, 242–243
　　device placement, 243–247, *245*
　　drug tolerance, 250–251
　　epidural vs. intrathecal, 235
　　favorable response to, 232
　　hydrophilicity, 241
　　nonopioid additives, 241–242
　　properties, 231t
　　respiratory depression in, 251–252
　　surgical complications, 247–250
　　test doses, 232, 234
　intrathecal
　　administration, *229*
　　advantages, 235–236
　　clinical applications, 233–253
　　complications, 251–253
　　contraindications, 233–234
　　future research needs, 253–254
　　implanted devices, 234–241
　　indications, 232–233
　　life expectancy and, 233
　　neurotoxicity, 231
　　patient selection, 232–234, 254
　　troubleshooting, 253
　intraventricular infusion, 219
　with neural blockade, 197–198
　neuroaxial, 235t

pharmacokinetics, 228–231
pharmacology, 275–285
spinal infusion, 217–218
systemic infusion, *229*
tolerance, 165, 275–276
unfavorable attributes, 204t
Osteitis, vertebral, radiation-induced, 68, *71*
Osteoblasts, 262
Osteoclasts, 262
Osteolysis, 261
Osteomyelitis, *79, 80*
Osteosarcoma, metastasis to lung, 258
Ovarian neoplasms, 260–261

P
Pain. *See also specific organ or area* pain
and AIDS survival, 149
biomedical vs. biocultural models, 40–41
Cartesian model, 175
clinical, 175–176, *176*
components, 310t
conditioning and, 116
and depression, 153
and disease survival, models, *146*
in elderly, 54
emotion in, 119–26
fear of, 116–118
immunology, 154
interaction with angina, *147*
and metastasis resistance, 141
modulation, *225*
physiological, *176*
in sickle cell disease, 150
and stress, 124–126
and surgically induced immunosuppression, 141
and survival, 135–156
Pain assessment, *23*
clinical decision analysis, 92–93
cultural factors, 35, 43–48, *49,* 103
in elderly, 57–58
cognitive impairment, 57–58
functional evaluation, 57
preexisting conditions, 57
underreporting of symptoms, 57
with EuroQol instrument, 94
health state evaluation, 94–95
in Hispanics, 35–49, 43–48
instruments, 43–48, 91
M.D. Anderson Cancer Center
Neuropathic Pain Questionnaire,
167, *168*
neuropathy symptom score, 169
of neuropathic pain, 166–169
pain health state evaluation, 94–95

patient preferences in, 91–92, 103
utility assessment, 103
Pain centers
acute pain services, 177–180
in cancer pain management, 177–180
organization, 177
patient controlled analgesia in, 180
Royal North Shore Hospital, University of Sydney, 177–180
Pain management
clinical practice guidelines, 17–30, 42
content of, 21–22
evidence-based criteria, 19, 20t
implementation barriers, 22, 24–25
rationale for, 17–22
coping skills, 127
culture in, 45–46, 48–49
in elderly, 53–63
invasive methods, 60
nonpharmacologic, 59–60
with opioid analgesics, 59
with oral analgesics, 58–59
patient-controlled analgesia, 60
strategies for, 58–60
gate control theory, 110
hypnosis in, 126–127
integration of techniques, 180–181
and life expectancy, 151–152
in nursing homes, 62–63
outcome measures, 195–196
in pancreatic cancer, 152
patient education, 25–29
psychological, 109–132
relaxation in, 126
strategies, *24*
in terminal illness, 145–155
undertreatment, 145
Pain perception. *See* Nociception
Palliative care
in Argentina, 6–9
barriers, 6–7
in Latin America, 3–16
volunteer services, 7–9
Pamidronate
for bone metastasis, 266, 271
for bone pain, 303
Pancreatic neoplasms
celiac plexus block, 153
pain management, 152
Parathyroid hormone-related peptide, 164
Paraventricular nucleus, hypothalamic,
122–123
Paroxetine, 295
Patient attitudes, 204
Patient care team, 8

Patient-controlled analgesia
in elderly, 60
in pain centers, 180
Patient education
materials for, 26t
development of, 26–27
dissemination of, 27–29
in pain management, 25–29
Patient noncompliance, 234
Pelvic neoplasms
lumbosacral plexus involvement, 88
radiation injury in, 68, 70
Pemoline, 304
Pentazocine, 59
Peripheral infections, 248–249
Peripheral nervous system, central pain in,
165–166
Pharmacotherapy. *See* Drug therapy
Phenytoin, 162, 299
Phosphodiesterase, 261
Placebos
in clinical trials, 189–190
drug mimicking by, 191
object end points in, 192
persistence of effects, 191–192
properties, 190–192
variable response, 191
Plasticity, neuronal, 165–166
Platelet inhibitors, 293
Postoperative complications, 247–248
Potassium conductance, 228
Preexisting conditions, in pain assessment, 57
Propoxyphene, 59
Prostaglandin E, 135–136
Prostaglandin inhibitors, 261
Prostatic neoplasms, 262
Protein kinase C inhibitors, 281–282
Pruritus, in opioid therapy, 252
Psychological interventions, 109–132
Psychotherapy, 153
Public policy, and palliative care, 4, 5
PuF tumor marker, 261

Q
Quality-adjusted life year (QALY)
cost-effectiveness analysis, 100, 102t
as outcome measure, 94
in terminal illness, 107

R
Radionuclide imaging, 68
Randomized clinical trials. *See* Clinical
trials
Rapid eye movement (REM) sleep, 121–122
Rectal drug administration, 313–315

Reinforcement, 116
Relaxation, 126
REM sleep, 121–122
Research methods, 189–193
Reservoir refilling, 249–250
Respiratory depression, 251–252
Retinoids, 261
Rexed's laminae, 226–227
Risk-benefit ratio, 204–205

S
Sacral fractures, radiation-induced, 68, 70
Samarium, 271
Sarcoma, radiation-induced, 72
Seroma, 248
Serotonin, 148
Serotonin reuptake inhibitors, selective
(SSRI), 295
Sickle cell pain, 150
Signal transduction, 281, *283*
Single Convention on Narcotic Drugs,
11–12
Sodium bisulfate, 231
Sodium channels
abnormalities, 162–163
blocking agents, 162
Spanish language, 40
Spinal cord compression, 236
Spinal cord stimulation, 200
Spinal diseases, degenerative, 68
Spinal nerve, mixed, 224t
Spinomesencephalic tract, 224–225
Spinoreticular tract, 224–225
Spinothalmic tract, 224–225
Spondylosis
bone scans, 68
degenerative, *69*
SSRI (Selective serotonin reuptake
inhibitors), 295
Stalk cell, 227
Standard gamble, in utility assessment,
96–97
Stress
and hypothalamo-pituitary-adrenocor-
tical axis, 124
in ischemia, 147
and pain, 124–126
physical vs. psychological, 125–126
Strontium 89, 271, 302–303
Substance P, 223
Substantia gelatinosa
anatomy, 227
opioid receptors in, 228
Sufentanil, intraspinal, 241–242
Suppositories, 313–314

Surgery
  drug delivery system implantation
    complications, 247–250
    hematoma in, 248
    hygroma in, 248
    intraoperative bleeding, 247–248
    meningitis in, 249
    peripheral infection in, 248–249
    postoperative bleeding, 248
    seroma in, 248
    techniques, 243–247
  and natural killer cell cytotoxicity,
    138–140
  neuroimmunology, 135–136
Survival. *See* Mortality
Sympathetic nervous system, 163

T
Team care, 8
Terminal illness
  medical decision making, 106–107
  pain management in, 145–155
Tetracyclines, 260
Tetrahydrocannabinoid, 302
Thermal lesions, 207
Time trade-off, 98–99
Tolerance
  to morphine, 276–285
  to opioids, 275–276
Transcription factors, 261
Transcutaneous electrical nerve stimula-
    tion (TENS), 200
Tricyclic antidepressants. *See* Antidepres-
    sants, tricyclic
Tumor cells
  MADB106, 136
  murine lung carcinoma, 264–265
Tumor markers, 261
Tumor necrosis factor-a, 263

U
Underreporting of pain, 57
Undertreatment
  in minority groups, 42
  in pain management, 145
Urinary retention, 252
Utility assessment
  in clinical decision analysis, 93–94
  defined, 93
  methods, 95
  process, 95–100
  quality-adjusted life year in, 94, 100
  standard gamble, 96–97
  time tradeoff, 98–99
  visual analog rating scale, 99, *100*

V
Valproic acid, 299
Vertebral fractures, *73–75*
  bone scans, 72–77
  malignant vs. nonmalignant, 72–77
  metastatic, 75, *76–78*
  non-metastatic, 72, *73*
Visceral pain
  adjuvant analgesics for, 297t
  drug therapy, 303
  neurosurgery for, 215
Visual analog rating scale, 99, *100*
Vitronectin, 263–164
Volunteers
  in Argentine, 7–9
  duties, 8–9, 9t
  for palliative care, 7–9
  training, 8t
Vomiting, 252

W
WIN 55.212-2 mesylate, 302
World Health Organization
  congresses, 4–5, 5t
    Palliative Care Program for Latin
      America, 3